A History of Western Pharmacy in China

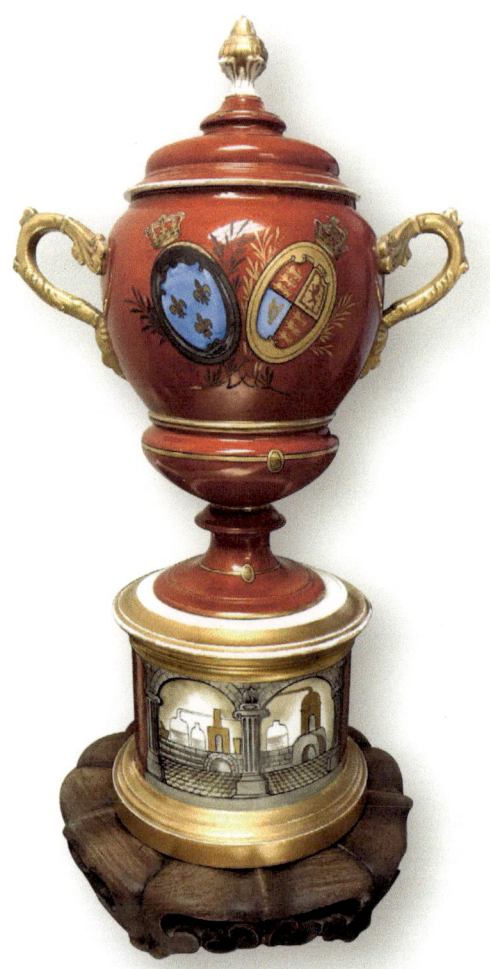

Porcelain *Vase de montre* (Watch Vase) with two handles on wooden vase stand, St. Paul's Hospital Pharmacy. @ 1920. *Courtesy* St. Paul's Hospital, Hong Kong. The front face of the pharmacy vase features two oval-shaped crests of arms, each adorned with a crown on top. The left crest of arms displays three lily flowers, known as *fleur-de-lis* in French, was a national symbol of France in the early 20th century. On the right crest of arms, the royal coat of arms of Edward, Prince of Wales (1984–1972) is displayed, consisting of four quadrants. The top left and bottom right quadrants showcase three lions each, representing England, while the top right quadrant depicts a lion, symbolizing Scotland. The bottom left quadrant features a harp, which is the emblem of Wales. The base of the vase shows two images related to modern pharmaceutical production. St. Paul's Hospital's *Vase de montre* was specially designed and ordered from France and was displayed centrally on the wall shelves of its pharmacy as a symbol of healing.

Patrick Chiu

A History of Western
Pharmacy in China

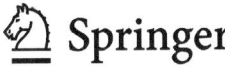 Springer

Patrick Chiu
Hong Kong Society for the History
of Pharmacy
Hong Kong, Hong Kong SAR

ISBN 978-981-99-8634-7   ISBN 978-981-99-8635-4 (eBook)
https://doi.org/10.1007/978-981-99-8635-4

This Springer imprint is published by the registered company Springer Nature Singapore Pte Ltd.
The registered company address is: 152 Beach Road, #21-01/04 Gateway East, Singapore 189721,
Singapore

Paper in this product is recyclable.

To My Loving Wife, Helen

Foreword by Dr. Stuart Anderson

Pharmacy history in its international context—relations between east and west, between imperial powers and colonies, and between neighbouring countries—has been a neglected field for too long. Only now is it receiving the attention it deserves. My own interest in the subject began in the 1990s as a result of informal discussions that took place at International Congresses for the History of Pharmacy and other conferences. Pharmaceutical historians came together from many countries, including several former British colonies and Dominions. Those conversations revealed—amongst other things—that British pharmaceutical colonialism had left a lasting legacy, and that experiences in former colonies were very different as a result of local contexts, climates, and cultures.

It soon became clear that little had been written about many of these issues, and efforts were made to explore the subject further. Detailed histories of pharmacy for some countries had been written, such as Reg Coombes's history of New Zealand pharmacy, Greg Haines's history of pharmacy in Australia, and Mike Ryan's history of pharmacy in South Africa. But these were essentially national accounts which only referred to other countries including Great Britain in passing, although some of Harkishan Singh's work prompted wider discussions with his account of the 'imperialization' of the British Pharmacopoeia in the late nineteenth century.

Some pharmaceutical histories of former British non-Dominion colonies have been published. These include Andrew Egboh's volume on pharmacy in Nigeria, John Joseph Borg's studies on the history of pharmacy in Malta, Thomas Paraidathathu's book on the history of pharmacy in Malaysia, and Ellen Grizzle's work in Jamaica. Together these provided a basis for an analysis of pharmacy professionalization across the British Empire and of the relationship between metropole and periphery. Fortunately, I was able to begin work on such a project alongside my duties as Associate Dean of Studies at the London School of Hygiene and Tropical Medicine.

By this time, I had already published a number of articles on the subject of pharmacy and Empire, and it was through one of these that the work of Patrick Chiu first came to my attention. Patrick had read one of my articles, 'Outposts of Empire: the Dawn of Pharmacy in the Straits Settlements, 1786–1867,' which had been published in the *Pharmaceutical Historian* in 2012. He contacted me to say that he had been researching the history of pharmacy in Hong Kong, and wondered if I might be willing to read through a draft of his findings and advise about how to present them. I was delighted to do so, and we have been in regular contact ever since.

Patrick's scholarship, thoroughness and attention to detail were clear from the beginning. We have since shared a stage on a number of occasions, at meetings including annual conferences of the British Society for the History of Pharmacy and International Congresses on the History of Pharmacy. We both gave presentations at a Workshop organised by the Shanghai Pharmaceutical Association when I was leading a pharmacy tour group to China in 2016. It was clear even then that Patrick had an impressive knowledge of the impact of western medicine on Traditional Chinese Medicine (TCM) and the impact of TCM on western medicine.

Over the last few years Patrick has been a prolific researcher and writer on the history of pharmacy in Hong Kong and China. His first article, on the 'First 100 years of Western pharmacy in colonial Hong Kong,' was published in the *Pharmaceutical Historian* in 2016. As its editor, I have been delighted to publish his subsequent work on this subject in a series of eight articles. Patrick has since brought the story up to date with an account of the development of pharmacy in Hong Kong in the post-colonial period, 1997–2022. I was delighted to hear that a book on the subject has since been published in Chinese.

Patrick has also been instrumental in persuading some of his Chinese colleagues to research and write about aspects of western pharmacy and medicine in English, and I have been very pleased to publish one or two of these in *Pharmaceutical Historian*. Patrick's own interests led to researching the history of the global retailer, A.S. Watson's, and to publication of his book *Transformation from Colonial Chemist to Global Health and Beauty Retailer* in 2022. Amongst his many commitments he is also the founder and president of the Hong Kong Society for the History of Pharmacy.

In this his latest book Patrick has taken on his largest project to date, the history of western pharmacy in China. He set himself some ambitious goals: to stimulate further debate about the movement of people, materia medica, and ideas between China and its neighbours in Central and South Asia in the period between 200 BCE and 1500 CE; and to explore China's interactions with the wider western world, starting with Europe around 1500, including Britain from the late 1600s, and the United States from the early 1800s. In addition, he aimed to explore China's relationship with her eastern neighbours, particularly with Japan in the late nineteenth century.

At the heart of this book, then, is the exchange of medical and pharmaceutical practices between Chinese, Western, and Japanese cultures, which reached its peak during the relatively brief Republican era between 1912 and 1949. Those with little knowledge of the subject often suppose that TCM and western medicine developed independently of each other, with little overlap and few external influences. In meeting his goals, Patrick unmasks the complex relationship between the two systems, exploring how each was influenced by the other, and how the relationship changed over time.

The story is told against a background of Chinese imperial and political history and within its wider social, economic, and religious frameworks. The opening of the Silk Roads between the Western Han and its northern neighbours followed the Emperor's expeditions to Central Asia between 135 and 115 BCE. The beginnings of western influences on Chinese medicine go back to at least 200 BCE, with knowledge and practices reaching China through Buddhist monks, Muslim imams, and later Jesuit missionaries. The arrival of Ayurvedic medicine and Buddhism enriched Chinese medicine and prompted Chinese medical philosophers to experiment with non-Chinese materia medica; Ayurvedic medicines from India underwent a process of sinification.

Traders originating from Arabia, India, Java and Europe introduced 'exotic' items from overseas markets, with many being incorporated into Chinese medical practice. Separate systems were initially recognised for Islamic medicine and TCM but attempts to introduce Islamic medicine into China in the late fourteenth century failed. After 1500 western influences became stronger as the Columbian exchange extended to China. The arrival of Portuguese traders in Macau in 1557 opened a new phase in relations between China and western nations. Macau became the main gateway for trade with Canton, attracting British, European, and later American traders. The first western hospital was opened in Macau in 1569. Dutch gifts to the Emperor in 1656 to help open trade links included cloves, cinnamon, and sandalwood; Christianity was approved by the authorities in 1692.

The Opium Wars, the First Sino-Japanese War, and the Boxer Movement in the late nineteenth and early twentieth centuries played decisive roles in China's adoption of western medicine and pharmacy. The first half of the twentieth century witnessed increased tensions between supporters of TCM and western medicine, with some advocating a complete move from one to the other. A conference on TCM in 1930 and the subsequent publication of a Chinese Pharmacopoeia were clearly defining moments prior to the Revolution in 1949 and the eventual implementation of the 'one country, two pharmacy systems' that exists today.

This book thus brings together a wide range of information covering a vast range of themes drawn from a wide variety of sources. It includes several biographies of important individuals, companies, and organisations, and is lavishly illustrated with a large number of figures, tables, and charts. Other themes include trade wars, establishment of the Peking Union Medical College, the rise of western chemists in China, and pharmaceutical manufacturing, along with opium cures, proprietary medicines, and soda water preparations. But discussion also extends to pharmaceutical education and manpower development, pharmacy laws, and the development of the Chinese Pharmacopoeia. Patrick is probably the only pharmaceutical historian able to do so.

The book represents an important contribution to the field as it is the first to provide a detailed account of the interaction between Chinese and western medicine from a pharmacy perspective. None of the existing historiography on the relationship between TCM and western medicine has so far explored pharmaceutical aspects in detail. This book therefore fills an important gap in the literature and is likely to become a key resource for further study. It will be of interest to a wide audience, including pharmaceutical, imperial, and business historians, and should be essential reading for pharmacy students. But it will also be of interest to a general readership curious about the history of pharmacy in China and of western influences on Chinese medicine.

Dr. Stuart Anderson, B.Sc., MA, Ph.D.,
FRPharmS
Editor-in-Chef
Pharmaceutical Historian
Emeritus Professor of Pharmacy
History
London School of Hygiene
and Tropical Medicine
Author, of Pharmacy
and Professionalization in the British
Empire, 1780–1970 (2021)
Pharmacopoeias, Drug Regulation,
and Empires: Making Medicines
Official in Britain's Imperial World,
1618–1968 (2024)
London, UK

Foreword by Dr. Lucas Richert

I first encountered Patrick Chiu in Washington, D.C. during the International Society for the History of Pharmacy (ISHP) biennial meeting in 2019. Intrigued by his paper title, *"The Beginnings of Western Pharmacy Practice in Modern China, 1910–1941: A Case Study of the Peking Union Medical College Hospital Pharmacy Department,"* I attended his talk and was immediately struck by how he exemplified the modern hybrid pharmacist-historian. His podium presentation combined technical knowledge of plants and medicines, insider knowledge of the healthcare and pharmaceutical industries, and a focus on significant historical characters. I was also struck by the originality of his presentation, which represented robust analysis of Western-Chinese pharmacy practices, institutions, and actors—but was recounted from the Chinese perspective, using Western and non-Western sources.

Now, years later, I am privileged to help introduce and contextualize A History of Western Pharmacy in China, a book that was more than a decade in the making and which broadens that 2019 paper both temporally and thematically. At the American Institute of the History of Pharmacy, where I serve as the Executive Director, and as one of the editors-in-chief of History of Pharmacy and Pharmaceuticals as well as The Social History of Alcohol and Drugs, I am lucky to have a birds-eye view of new scholarship; and I have tracked closely how the history of pharmacy and pharmaceuticals subfield has engaged with East-West interactions. To put it bluntly, the subfield has—for several reasons—lagged behind the larger history of science, medicine, and technology community when it comes to the topic of China-Western pharmacy. Chiu's book addresses that problem head on.

Since leaving the pharmacy and pharmaceutical space, Chiu has positioned himself as an authority in pharmacy history. Throughout his career as a pharmacist-historian, he has sought to explore the exchange of medicinal and pharmacy practices and substances within China during ancient times as well as assess the influence of Europe and the United States on those internal practices from the 19th century onwards. His intellectual and academic influences have ranged widely, but in Jimin Wong's and Lien-teh Wu's Chinese History of Medicine, we see an early model and shades of Chiu's work. First published in 1932, Chinese History of Medicine marked an early historical intervention into the nature of syncretical Chinese-Western medicine and, moreover, it was presented by two Chinese physicians in the English language. A History of Western Pharmacy in China ably builds on that foundation.

Readers of this book, to Chiu's credit, will be exposed to the nuanced cultural, medico-scientific, and business interactions that shaped Western pharmacy in China. Chiu puts a spotlight on the various materials, techniques, and processes of drug formulation and mass manufacture—and he rightly illustrates how pharmacy was substantiated as big business and mass manufacture. In analyses that incorporate materia medica and so-called dangerous drugs, such as opium, Chiu also articulates the complicated entangled histories of the movement, circulation, and translation of both pharmacy knowledge and goods. Yet, he appropriately acknowledges and evaluates non-Western epistemologies and practices that intermingled with Western ideas to create a novel type of pharmacy and pharmaceutical industry in China.

By his own admission, Chiu has been driven to write and share A History of Western Pharmacy in China for many years. Over a decade ago, while at Cambridge University taking a summer course, his desire to write this book was amplified. I am thankful he did write it. We now have a deeper understanding of how pharmacy theory and practice, knowledge, and technique was mediated and reshaped over time. We can, with greater certainty, identify how pharmacy has operated as a "science" and part of a bounded medical structure, but simultaneously as an art and craft tradition in early human communities.

Dr. Lucas Richert, Ph.D.
Professor and George Urdang Chair
in Pharmacy History, UW-Madison
Executive Director, American Institute
of the History of Pharmacy
Transdisciplinary Center for Research
on Psychoactive Substances
Editor at Social History of Alcohol
and Drugs/History of Pharmacy
and Pharmaceuticals
Madison, WIS

Preface

The shifting relationship between Chinese medicine to modern biomedicine is a complex story. My research of the transition of Chinese materia medica (本草, "bencao") to modern biologicals and chemical drugs is a long journey. In following the footsteps of Zhang Qian (张骞, 164–113 BCE), an official and diplomat of the Western Han period, to Kashgar, a border town near Krygystan of the Silk Road in 2000, I was fascinated by the display of decorated bottle gourds (葫芦 "hulu", Lagenaria siceraria) in several bazaar stalls managed by Chinese Muslim Uyghur traders. The gourd, reportedly originated from Africa, has been used as a container for water or alcohol in East Asia for a couple of millennia. The gourd is also a symbol of Chinese medicine carried by apothecaries when visiting households with sick patients in ancient China. As a pharmacy practitioner who has transcended the multiple sectors of community, hospital and industry in the past four decades, I began researching why are animal and plant products imported for medicinal purposes? What are the origins of these exotic materia medica or non-Chinese materia medica from faraway lands (海药, "haiyao") after my first trip to Kashgar.

My particular interest is the transition period from 1800 to 1949 when European and North American missionaries and traders brought the gospel, opium and "opium cures" to China, and Japanese educators who began teaching pharmacy courses in the two military academies of medicine in Guangzhou and Tianjin in the early-1900s. Many scholars have published excellent papers on western medicine in China. However, few books or publications have addressed the interactions between the stakeholders, such as opium traders, ship surgeons, chemists and druggists, medical missionaries, pharmacy educators, philanthropists, politicians, and public health policy makers. These pioneers have left undeletable marks in their contributions to modern China's pharmacy practice and the development of its pharmaceutical industry in the first hundred years of Shanghai's opening up to the outside world, soon after the first Sino-British War (1839–1842) had ended.

The main objective of this book is to stimulate discussions surrounding the movement of people, materia medica, and ideas between China and its neighbours in Central and South Asia from 200 BCE to 1500 CE. The book's scope will then expand to include interactions with Europe starting in 1500, Britian in the late

1600s, the United States in the early 1800s, and Japan in the late 19th century. Western traders and medical missionaries introduced various items as tributary gifts to the imperial courts. These gifts included tobacco, opium, American ginseng, and other exotic elements of materia medica, as well as consumer and industrial products such as clocks, watches, scientific instruments, and textiles. Furthermore, the expansion of western medicine in the coastal ports of Macau, Canton, Hong Kong, Shanghai, Ningbo, Tianjin, and beyond is extensively discussed. One focal point of the book will be the significant exchange of medical and pharmaceutical practices between Chinese, Western, and Japanese cultures, which reached its pinnacle during the relatively brief Republican era from 1912 to 1949.

When I started to write this book, three questions came across to me, as were often asked but without an answer. First, what events led diplomats, religious men and traders to export exotic materia medica to China from faraway lands over the past two millennia, particularly in the 19th and 20th centuries? Second, what sparks occurred when western chemists clashed with Chinese medicine apothecaries in the nineteenth century? Third and finally, what drove the shifting relationship between Chinese materia medica and biologicals, alkaloidal extracts, and chemical drugs during the late Manchu Qing dynasty to the early Republican period in China.

The book offers a comprehensive exploration of the history of western pharmacy in China, utilizing diverse sources such as original research works, biographies, corporate records, and oral histories. Chapter 1 takes a chronological approach, tracing influential arrivals from Buddhists monks who transmitted Ayurvedic Medicine to Jesuits who brought cinchona bark to China, spanning 200 BCE to 1800 CE. Subsequent chapters adopt a thematic approach, examining various topics from 1800 to 1949. Multiple chapters address the interplay of the retail, wholesale, and manufacturing sectors, providing an in-depth study of individuals, companies, and medical institutions. Their collective efforts profoundly shaped the adoption of western medicine in modern China, leaving a lasting impact on today's healthcare system. The book also traces the evolution of China's pharmaceutical industry, from local Chinese medicine dispensaries to an industrial exporter, during the period of European and Japanese colonialism from 1850 to 1949.

This book caters to a diverse audience, encompassing pharmaceutical, social, political, imperial, and business historians and general readers interested in the history of Western and Far Eastern influences on Chinese medicine, specifically focusing on the history of pharmacy. It is a valuable resource for researchers exploring Chinese medicine and pharmacy in contemporary China and the introduction of western medicine in China since 200 BCE. Additionally, the author aims to inspire graduate students to pursue doctoral theses by examining various sectors or periods within the history of pharmacy in modern China.

During my career as a pharmacist, I had the opportunity to work in various sectors of the pharmacy profession, including hospitals, retail chemists, and industrial pharmaceutical and consumer health companies, in the UK, Canada, and Asia. This diverse experience allowed me to gain a deep understanding of the actions of John Cameron at the Peking Union Medical College Hospital between 1921 and 1940, as described in Chap. 3. Furthermore, I could relate to the challenges faced by Henry

Humphreys, the pharmacist and managing director of A.S. Watson, who operated as the leading wholesaler and retailer of "opium cures", proprietary medicines and soda water in China and Southeast Asia, as discussed in Chaps. 4 and 5. Moreover, the accounts of entrepreneurs promoting their proprietary medicines and generics in 1930s and 1940s Asia offer valuable insights into the astute navigation of the intricate and frequently nebulous realm of intellectual property laws, as detailed in Chaps. 7 and 8. In the concluding Chap. 9, a comprehensive review is conducted, highlighting the interconnected nature of trade conflicts, wars, and political decision-making. The analysis reveals a cyclical pattern in which trade conflicts frequently escalate into armed conflicts, leading to further trade disputes, and ultimately placing the power of decision-making in the hands of politicians.

From the 1870s onwards, both local entrepreneurs and expatriates began importing and marketing "opium cures" as a substitute for opium smoking, which had exacerbated narcotic addiction. By the 1910s, the production of new dosage forms such as tablets, pills, and injections of "opium cures" became widespread, catering to the needs of drug users and replacing traditional forms like laudanum liquid, powder, and tincture. Consequently, millions of drug addicts turned to equally addictive options such as morphine injections, "red pills," and "white powders" at the turn of the twentieth century. Ironically, this development played a significant role in shaping the modern retail pharmacy and pharmaceutical industry in China.

With rapidly increasing trade and transshipments of bonded labourers and cargoes along the China coast in the late nineteenth century, import drug houses such as the British Dispensary, Koeffer Dispensary, Laou Teh Kee, A. S. Watson and others served as the drivers in the rapid transmission of western pharmacy. This book addresses the motivational factors for enterprising Chinese medicine owners to enter the western retail and wholesale drug market. Firstly, they learned business practices in marketing "opium cures" from western retail chemists in the 1880s. Secondly, retailing became wholesaling and local production of lucrative "opium cures" in the 1890s. Lastly, launching branded proprietary medicines in the 1900s eventually led to the modern pharmaceutical industry from the 1910s to the 1940s during the Nationalist Era.

When the China Medical Board (CMB) of the Rockefeller Foundation acquired the Union Medical College (UMC, Xiehe Yi Xuetang) and Hospital from the London Missionary Society in 1914, western medicine and pharmacy soon began to take root during the infancy of the Nationalist government. In 1921, the opening of the new Peking Union Medical College Hospital (Beijing Xiehe Yi Yuan) buildings turned a new chapter in the development of biomedicine in the young Nationalist government's private hospital. Best practice management in clinical pharmacy, zero tolerance for dispensing mistakes, publication of hospital formularies, and control of poisons and dangerous drugs were a few of many measures implemented at the PUMC Hospital pharmacy department from the 1920s to 1940s.

Modern pharmaceutical education was initiated by Japanese pharmacy lecturers in the early-1900s and training of industrial pharmacists by Dr. E. N. Meuser, a Canadian pharmaceutical missionary, began at the West China School of Pharmacy in Chengdu (Chengtu) in 1918. The latter was a classic example of developing local talents for China's modern pharmaceutical industry. Another classic example of this transition is the foundation of modern China's Central Epidemic Prevention Bureau to produce vaccines in 1919. The dissemination of vaccine production technology over the next century in mainland China and its mass immunization programme of children after 1949 led to the development of attenuated or inactivated SARS-CoV-2 vaccines in 2010 and COVID-19 vaccines, respectively, in 2020.

Today, China's bi-centennial journey to the modernity of pharmacy practice could date back to Dr. Alexander Pearson's variolation of smallpox in the British East India Company compounds in Canton and Macau in 1805. However, a story the global press has failed to cover is that the learnings in vaccine and pharmaceutical production technologies since the time of Dr. Pearson have enabled China's two largest vaccine manufacturers, Sinopharm and SinoVax, to produce five billion or 50% of the 11 billion vaccine doses to its home market and the Global South countries during the COVID-19 pandemic in 2021!

With the initiation of China's "New Journey for the New Era" in early 2023, the contemporary history of pharmacy in China, spanning from 1950 to the present, becomes a subject worthy of focused exploration. This period of pharmacy history will be extensively scrutinized in an upcoming open-access publication project titled *"Chinese History of Pharmacy: From Shennong to Tu Youyou"* jointly undertaken by Dr. Michael Shiyong Liu of Pittsburg University/Shanghai Jiaotong University and me. It aims to shed light on the crucial milestones that have shaped China's journey over the course of two millennia, as it navigates the transition from traditional medicine to modern pharmacy. Notably, a significant portion of this transformation has taken place in the past 70 years of the People's Republic of China.

Lastly, this book commemorates the remarkable centennial anniversary of Moody Meng's membership with the Pharmaceutical Society of Great Britain in 1924. Meng, a true pioneer in the realm of pharmaceutical education, also played a pivotal role in the creation of the first five editions of the Chinese Pharmacopoeia since 1930. His enduring contributions have withstood the test of time, spanning both the Republican and the People's Republic eras, and have left an indelible mark on the field of pharmacy. His remarkable legacy continues to shape and influence the discipline to this very day in China.

Hong Kong   Patrick Chiu

Acknowledgements

In my pursuit of researching the social history of pharmacy and the pharmaceutical market in Colonial Hong Kong and China's treaty ports, I have been fortunate to receive generous advice from Dr. Stuart Anderson, an esteemed authority on imperial pharmacy history. Dr. Anderson, the Editor-in-Chief of the *Pharmaceutical Historian*, has kindly agreed to write a foreword for this book and allowed me to incorporate materials from my previous publications in the *Pharmaceutical Historian*. I would also like to express my gratitude to Dr. Lucas Richert, a distinguished historian specializing in narcotic drugs and modern medicine, is the George Urdang Chair in the History of Pharmacy at the University of Wisconsin- Madison, for his gracious contribution of a foreword. Furthermore, I extend my thanks to Dr. Kazushige Morimoto, the president of the Japanese Society for the History of Pharmacy, for providing a kind book review.

As Britain, Japan, and the United States were the three most influential countries shaping China's modern pharmacy profession and pharmaceutical industry in the first half of the twentieth century, receiving personal forewords and reviews from these esteemed pharmacy historians on "*A History of Western Pharmacy in China*" is a great honour for me as a writer and pharmaceutical historian.

I am grateful to Dr. Fan Ka Wai, an authority in the history of Chinese Medicine, of The City University of Hong Kong who kindly reviewed my first manuscript draft and offered further insights, including the rationale for omitting the incorporation of Islamic Pharmacy in the "*Great Yuan Bencao Gangmu*" during the Mongolian rule of China from 1217–1368. Additionally, I would like to thank Dr. Arnab Chakraborty, an assistant professor at the Shanghai University Department of History, for his insightful feedback on my book. Three academics who have made significant contributions to the history of the transmission of Buddhist, Christian, and Islamic faiths and medical knowledge from India, West Asia and Europe to China via the ancient Silk Roads have kindly provided their book reviews: Dr. Vijaya Deshpande, a renowned Sanskrit scholar and historian of Ayurvedic medicine, Dr. Halil Tekiner, an authority on Islamic pharmacy, and the President of the International Society for the History of Pharmacy, and Rector Stephen Morgan, a theologian and philosopher and Rector of the University of St. Joseph of Macau, which traces its history back to St. Paul's College since the Portuguese traders settled there in the mid-16th century. Additionally, three internationally acclaimed historians specializing in Western medicine, narcotic drugs, and Chinese Medicine in modern China, namely Dr. Zhang Daqing of Peking University, Dr. Zhang Yongan of Shanghai University, and Dr. Pi Kuo-li of National Central University in Taiwan, have shared their respective his views on the transformation of medical culture from the late Manchu Qing to the Republican era.

Apart from conducting visits to archives and libraries in Beijing, Hong Kong, Shanghai, and Taipei, the essence of this book also stems from my oral history sessions with individuals or their immediate family members who lived during the pre-Communist era. These individuals include the late Dr. Thomas Cochrane, Chen Lifu, Moody Meng, and Dr. Minglu King. Their contributions have indelibly shaped China's healthcare system on both the mainland and Taiwan. I would also like to express my gratitude to Roy Delbyck, and Kate Petrusa for granting me permission to use images of original antique pieces, publications, and posters from the 19th and early 20th centuries, which are preserved in their respective museums in Hong Kong, Shanghai, and Vancouver. Lastly, but certainly not least, I want to extend my appreciation to Ms. Floor Oosting, the editorial director, and Mrs. Alex Campbell, the senior editor of social sciences and humanities at Springer Nature, for granting me the opportunity to publish this book.

Book Reviews

In his seminal work, *A History of Western Pharmacy in China*, Patrick Chiu furnishes an unparalleled investigation into the intricate relationship between China and the Western world through the lens of pharmaceutical history. This book traces China's transmogrification from the opening of the ancient Silk Road by Zhang Qian in Han Dynasty in 138 BCE with the pinnacle of her interactions with the West during the late Qing Dynasty, leading up to the intercourse of Eastern and Western medicine and pharmacy. Rapid transformation of modern China's pharmacy systems evolved during the short Republican period which gave rise to the birth of the People's Republic of China in 1949.

Emphasizing an array of subjects from the transmission of Ayurvedic medicine from India, Islamic pharmacy from West Asia, medical missionaries from Europe and North America, trade wars and institutional transformations to the foray into modern medicinal practices, Chiu's narrative offers an incisive understanding of the labyrinthine developments in Chinese pharmacy during the past two millennia.

The manifold roles enacted by medical missionaries, naval medical officers, and local apothecaries from Ningbo in the 19th century are examined scrupulously. Chiu inspects the multifaceted challenges and prospects that unfurled as Western medical methodologies—such as variolation and opiate-based therapies—found their place alongside indigenous practices. These Western interventions were not limited to therapeutics but extended to revolutionary pharmaceuticals like arsphenamine, insulin, and penicillin, forever altering China's pharmaceutical landscape.

One of the most enlightening aspects of Chiu's work is its multidimensionality. The book isn't confined to purely medical perspectives but encompasses broader socio-economic and industrial implications. It delves into the entrepreneurial ambitions of Chinese businesspersons in the Western pharmaceutical sphere, the shift from retail to wholesale pharmaceutical trade, and the nascent stages of China's contemporary pharmaceutical industry. Moreover, it reveals important facets of clinical governance, toxicological regulation, and the standardization of hospital formularies between the 1920s and 1940s. In doing so, it identifies pivotal moments in history that expedited the institutionalization of Western pharmacy in China.

Geographically, the spotlight is directed towards key urban centers like Hong Kong and Shanghai. Here, Western apothecaries capitalized on the narcotic trade, notably with "opium cures" and other proprietary formulations. This commercial success fuelled not just business expansion but also instigated the construction of an organized, modern supply chain within China. Equally noteworthy is the scholarly attention Chiu pays to the evolution of pharmacy education in the early 20th century, marking a pedagogical paradigm shift toward a more systematized and modernized approach.

An intriguing dimension of Chiu's narrative revolves around the coexistence and at times, contentious interaction, between Traditional Chinese Medicine (TCM) and Western pharmacology. The book enters the disputed terrains of language and culture in medical education, highlighting debates over the medium of instruction. Furthermore, the consecration of the Chinese Pharmacopoeia and the formal recognition of TCM as a standalone healthcare paradigm are treated with nuanced understanding.

What sets Chiu's work apart is its contribution to the relatively underexplored scholarship on the interaction between Western and Chinese pharmacy. Far from a simplistic account, the book adopts an interdisciplinary methodology that assimilates various cultural, economic, and sociopolitical factors. It surpasses mere chronology, offering a rich tapestry of cross-cultural adaptations, negotiations, and confrontations among an ensemble of actors including merchants, diplomats, clergy, maritime medical practitioners, and policy architects.

The book serves as a microcosm of the greater narrative of East-West interaction, epitomizing the complex interplay of awe and skepticism, engagement and restraint. From the magnanimous outlook of the Kangxi Emperor and his intercourse with Portuguese Jesuits to the persevering legacy of indigenous Chinese medicine in the face of early 20th-century challenges, Chiu's work is a crucible of insights that will satiate both academic and lay audiences.

In summary, *A History of Western Pharmacy in China* is an academically rigorous and intellectually fulfilling discourse that significantly broadens our comprehension of pharmaceutical history and Sino-Western relations. Its novelty lies in its ability to unpack two millenniums of continuous negotiation between disparate pharmacological paradigms, and in doing so, enriches our understanding of medical humanities, social history, and international relations. This is a pivotal contribution that addresses a lacuna in existing scholarship, marking it as an indispensable read for those interested in the confluence of medicine, culture, and geopolitics.

Prof. Dr. Halil Tekiner, President of the International Society for the History of Pharmacy. Head of the Department of the History of Pharmacy and Ethics, Erciyes University, Turkey

Patrick Chiu's book, *A History of Western Pharmacy in China*, effectively presents an unbiased perspective when discussing the contributions of expatriate pharmacy academics towards the development of China's pharmaceutical profession and the modern drug industry in the first half of the twentieth century. The author highlights the positive impact of formal pharmacist training, which became evident during the Second Sino-Japanese War (1937–1945). By the end of 1949, approximately

3000 pharmacists had been trained, with two thousand receiving education from local universities and colleges, and four hundred graduating from Japan's pharmacy vocational schools.

One notable example of progress highlighted in the book is the publication of the first edition of the Chinese Pharmacopoeia in 1930 and its subsequent release in 1931. However, Chiu also acknowledges the challenges faced in achieving consensus and compiling the pharmacopoeia, as senior doctors and pharmacists from various backgrounds, including British, European, Japanese, and American medical and pharmaceutical practitioners, held differing approaches to professional practice. Chiu's impartial approach and well-researched content make it a recommended resource for understanding the historical development of pharmacy in China.

Kazushige Morimoto Ph.D. D.Min, Education System-Qualified Pharmacist;
President, The Japanese Society for the History of Pharmacy

In *A History of Western Pharmacy in China* Patrick Chiu opens a new door into the complex history of the interaction between the West and East. Although concentrating on a particular scientific field, the story Chiu tells is in many ways paradigmatic of the encounter between China and the Western world: a tale of fascination and suspicion, of enthusiasm and caution. From the experience of the Kangxi Emperor, perhaps the most open of all Qing Dynasty rulers to the outside world, and his interaction with the Portuguese Jesuits, to the survival of Chinese medicine through the challenges of the early twentieth century, Chiu offers insights that should interest scholars and general readers alike.

Prof. Stephen Morgan, Rector, University of Saint Joseph, Macao

Patrick Chiu's book, *A History of Western Pharmacy in China*, thoroughly examines the journey of exotic elements of materia medica and modern drugs from the West to China. In contrast to the extensive research conducted by academics on the history of medicine, public health, and diseases, the study of modern drugs and pharmacy practice in China is still in its early stages. Chiu's book faithfullly traces the historical process of offering exotic materia medica as tributary gifts from diplomats and traders hailing from Arabia, Java, and South Asia to the imperial courts of China via the Silk Roads. With a focus on the intricate relationship between commerce, trade, culture, and science, Chiu uncovers pivotal moments that accelerated the transition of Chinese medicine and materia medica into biomedicine and modern drugs in the modern period. The book provides a comprehensive and informative account through a wealth of historical events, supplemented by images, charts, and tables. For those interested in delving into the history of Western medicine and pharmacy in China, this research reference guide comes highly recommended.

Daqing Zhang, Ph.D., Director, The Center for History of Medicine,
Peking University

The exchange of medical knowledge between the East and the West, particularly the transmission of Western medicine to the East and Chinese Medicine to the West, has been extensively debated within the international academic community. However, the exploration of the history of pharmacy in the context of interactions and exchanges between China and the West is still in its nascent stages. Addressing this gap, Patrick Chiu's latest publication, *A History of Western Pharmacy in China* offers a comprehensive examination of the assimilation of foreign elements of materia medica, including the discovery of the silver Persian medicine box, introduction of poppy, leading up to the development of domestically produced drugs like neo-arsphenamine, throughout two millennia.

Chiu's work goes beyond mere documentation to analyze the gradual adjustment of diverse cultures, ideas, and behaviours that occurred as a result of contact, often leading to collision or even conflict, among key stakeholders such as merchants, diplomatic delegations, missionaries, ship doctors, western chemists, and policy makers. By adopting a unique research perspective, the book holds significant importance for studying pharmacy history, medical and social history, and exploring the historical dynamics of foreign relations and mutual learning between China and the West.

Yongan Zhang, Ph.D., Professor, Department of History, Shanghai University

This book is written by an eminent pharmacist and pharmacy historian Patrick Chiu. He covers the period from 200 BCE when western influence on China began and was manifest in all aspects including medicine and pharmaceuticals, up to 1800 CE. Western influence includes Indian as well since coming via silk route India is towards China's west. Medicine has always been a tool for the Buddhist missionaries since it went well with their benevolent spirit and expansion goals. When it came to western medicine and pharmaceuticals it became a tool for moneymaking and power too. Chiu's initial focus is on the times when the Europeans and Americans brought opium and opium cures to Chinese southern shores and established them on the coastal region. It is a story of exploitation although Chiu does not say it in as many words. He impartially judges what came out of it, how Chinese pharmaceutical industries evolved through these habit-forming opiate drugs; how a pharmaceutical movement took a turn through it and how western biomedical and alkaloid based medicines were introduced through this channel. Leaving temporary dislike for the westerners for their politics and western medicine that came through opium and opium cures; the author reviews how Chinese were introduced to modern science of biology and how in long run it was beneficial, ending in the grand finale of the Nobel laureate Chinese pharmacist Dr. Tu Youyou. The Japanese also played a role in teaching modern pharmacy and establishing medical and pharmaceutical institutions in China. Thus politics and medicine and pharmacy went hand in hand in their efforts to win over the Chinese.

Chiu narrates this fascinating story in very scholarly manner. He has made analytical study of a wide range of sources that provides the reader with quantitative data as well. Among the books published in this field; he has, for the first time, explored the role played by all the stakeholders, such as opium traders, ship surgeons, chemists and druggists, medical missionaries, pharmacy educators, philanthropists, politicians, and public health policy makers and the interactions between them. He discusses in details the transition from sole use Chinese traditional medicine to the useful integration of the two. This book will be of paramount interest for those interested in political and medical/pharmaceutical history and reveal how they influenced each other. I recommend this book to Indian scholars in particular since Indian medical and political history traversed a similar path.

Vijaya Jayant Deshpande, Ph.D., Historian of Science, and Life Member,
Bhandarkar Oriental Research Institute, Pune, India

Reading *A History of Western Pharmacy in China* by Patrick Chiu is truly an enlightening experience. The author's extensive research on the history of modern Chinese and Western medicine, coupled with the accumulation of new historical materials and perspectives, serves as the foundation for this remarkable book. It can be considered an outstanding piece of work within this specialized field, offering a comprehensive overview of the transformations in Chinese pharmacy throughout history, particularly with a global perspective on the modern era.

Previously, academic research predominantly focused on describing Chinese Medicine or the prevalence of Western medicine in modern Chinese society. However, there was a lack of books specifically analysing the contributions made by pharmaceutical knowledge and modern drugs exported from Europe, the United States, Japan, and other regions to the development of modern Chinese pharmaceutical material culture and manufacturing technology. The ability of this book to shed light on these connections and elucidate the transformations is a testament to its groundbreaking nature.

Pi Kuo-li, Ph.D., Director, Graduate Institute of History,
National Central University, Taiwan

Conventions

Hanyu Pingying romanization is used throughout this book which has been adopted nationally in China since 1958. The previously used Anglicised or commonly known as the Wade–Giles names and terms are listed in the open and closed brackets when used the first time such as Beijing (Peking), Qingdao (Tsingtao), Dr. Zhang Chang-shao (C. S. Jang) and Zhao Chenggu (T. Q. Chou). Notable exceptions included Anglicised historical names and terms still used commonly or currently in the English media or publications: Canton Dispensary, Chiang Kai-shek, Convention of Peking, Treaty of Nanking, Shun Pao, Dr. Sun Yat-sen, Chiang Kai-shek, Dr. Heng J. Liu, Moody Meng etc. While the names of the national and provincial capitals of Beijing, Nanjing, and Tianjin will follow the established Hangyu Pingyin system, the Angli-cised geographical names of Canton, Hong Kong, Kowloon, and Macau have been used instead of Guangzhou, Xianggang, and Aomen throughout the book. Some geographical words, such as *Canton*, in the local dialect, pronounced as *Kwangtung*, could be dated back to the 16th century when first used by the Portuguese traders to denote the province of *Guangdong* as in the Hanyu Pingying. Earlier western traders used the word *Canton* interchangeably for both the city of *Guangzhou* and the region of *Guangdong*. As referred to in the Treaty of Nanking in 1842, Hong Kong grew to include the Kowloon Peninsula in the Convention of Peking in 1860 and grew to more than ten times its original size in the subsequent Second Convention of Peking in 1898. The name Peiping (Beiping, "Northern Peace") was used from 1928 to 1949 when China's capital was relocated from Peking (Beijing, "Northern Capital") to Nanking (Nanjing. "Southern Capital") during that period under the Nationalist government on the mainland. The original English names of Peking Union Medical College and Peking University, not *Beiing Xihe Yiyuan* or *Beijing Daxue* in Hanyu Pingying, have been used in the book.

The book utilizes the term "Chinese Medicine" instead of "Traditional Chinese Medicine" (TCM) to encompass a wide array of medical practices and systems orig-inating from China. This term is commonly used by scholars residing in mainland China, Hong Kong, Macau, Taiwan, and the Chinese diaspora in Southeast Asia and other parts of the world. Chinese Medicine has been employed for thousands of years and encompasses various practices, distinguishing it from Western Medicine.

The term "TCM" was initially introduced by certain Western academics, such as the late Professor Joseph Needham, to differentiate it from biomedicine and make it more accessible to Western readers. The term "*bencao*, 本草" has two meanings: as a description of native i.e., Chinese materia medica, and as a description of compilation of drug compendiums, dispensatories, formularies, or pharmacopoeias in ancient China. The term Non-Chinese materia medica is used for "海药, *haiyao*", referring to materia medica sourced from overseas markets. To ensure clarity and facilitate understanding for non-Chinese readers, whenever the Hanyu Pinyin form of the Chinese terms are mentioned for the first time, the original Chinese characters and their Hanyu Pinyin terms, such as "唐本草, *Tang Bencao*", "本草拾遗, *Bencao Shiyi*" are provided in brackets. Additionally, a conversion table containing the English or commonly used names of these technical books, is included at the end of the book and in the index for quick searching of related topics.

Lastly, the initials BCE (Before the Common Era) have been used throughout the book, whereas the CE (Common Era) initials have been excluded in the text, except in tables when referring to a specific timeframe that falls entirely within the Common Era. The initial r. in the brackets refers to the "reign" of an emperor, empress, king, queen, or Pope. Unless otherwise specified, the initials of EIC. denote the British East India Company for simplicity's sake.

Chronology of Key Events in China: 600 BCE to 1949 CE

Year (s)	Major event	Key character	Remarks
600 BCE	Yin and Yang Theory	Lao Zi	*"Book of Changes"*—philosophical basis of Chinese medicine.
500 BCE	Confucianism	Kong Fuzi	*"The Analects"*—basis of ethics and social values
Han Dynasty (206 BCE–220 CE)			
138–115 BCE	Opening of the Silk Roads	Zhang Qian	Two expeditions of 138-125 BCE and 119–115 BCE to Central Asia
Sixteen Kingdoms (304–420 CE)			
344–413 CE	"The Nirvana Route"	Kumarajiva	Buddhist monk from Kucha Kingdom settled in China
399–412 CE	First Chinese pilgrimage to India	Fa Xian	Returned to Qingdao by sea route in 412 CE
Sui and Tang Dynasties (581–907 CE)			
581–649 CE	Active transmission of Buddhism and medical literature from South Asia		
741 CE	Canton designated as the port for foreign trade	Emperor Xuan Zhong	A Maritime Administration was setup for commerce with Arabs, Indians, and Javanese
755–763 CE	Anshi Rebellion	An Lushan	Political turmoil resulted in the emergence of the Tibetan and Uyghur Kingdoms disrupting the once vibrant trade of the Silk Roads
10th C.	The collapse of the Tang dynasty in 907 CE led to blockade of the land routes of the Silk Roads by the three Persianate Sunni Muslim states		

(continued)

(continued)

Song Dynasty (960–1279 CE)

1069–1082 CE	Reform law	Wang Anshi	Wang Anshi, the chancellor, initiated tax reform and subsidy of medicines by the state to the public

Mongolian Yuan, and Ming and Manchurian Qing Dynasties (1279–1644 CE)

1279–1368 CE	Reopening of the land routes of the Silk Roads		
1513–1999 CE	Arrival of first European diplomat	Jorge Álvares	Portuguese explorer reached China by sea in the Age of Discovery. Lease of Macau as a trading post by Portugal in 1557 for 443 years until 1999
1602–1640 CE	Arrival of Jesuits in Beijing	Matteo Ricci and others	Roman Catholic Church, the Cathedral of the Immaculate Conception, was built in 1605

Manchurian Qing Dynasty (1644–1911 CE)

1757 CE	Canton system	Emperor Qianlong	Canton was designated as the only port city open for trade with foreign businesses
@ 1775 CE	Opium trade	British traders	Illegal shipments of opium from India to China by British traders
1793, and 1813 CE	First and Second British trade embassies to Beijing	Emperors Qianlong, and Jiaqing	Lord Macartney, and Lord Amherest, representing the British Crown to seek export opportunities with the Manchu Qing court in 1793 and 1813
1839–1842, and 1856–1860 CE	1st and 2nd Opium Wars	China and Britian/France	The Treaty of Nanking Peking ceded Hong Kong to the UK and five treaty ports opened for traders and missionaries to settle in 1842, and more concessions in the Convention of Peking in 1860

Republic of China (1911–1949)

Adoption of Western medicine as the model of modern health care system

People's Republic of China (1949-)

The People's Republic government pursues a hybrid of Chinese and Western medicine and pharmacy systems to serve its massive population which grew from 540 m to 1.4 b in 2023 or over 74 years

Contents

About the Author

Patrick Chiu also known by his Manchu name Irgen Gioro, was born in Canton and grew up in Hong Kong. However, his ancestral roots can be traced back to the Bordered Yellow Tribe near Kirin, Manchuria, which is now Xiping City in Jilin Province, Northeast China. He obtained a B.Sc. Pharmacy degree from De Montfort University in Leicester and pursued an MBA at the University of Hull. He also attended the Global Management Programme at IMD in Lausanne.

Throughout his career, Patrick has worked in various sectors of pharmacy, including community, hospital, and industrial pharmacy. He has held senior leadership positions with global biotech and health care companies and NGOs, such as BD, Chi Heng Foundation, Monsanto, Molnlycke Health Care, Nature's Bounty, and Roche, primarily in Greater China and the Asia Pacific region.

Since 2000, Patrick has dedicated himself to independent research in the history of exotic elements of materia medica including hulu originating from the ancient Silk Roads. Over the past decade, he has focused on scholarly research concerning Western pharmacy in China's treaty ports and Colonial Hong Kong. His first original research article, titled "*The First 100 Years of Western Pharmacy in Hong Kong*" was published in the *Pharmaceutical Historian* in June 2016. Additionally, his book titled *A History of Western Pharmacy in Colonial Hong Kong* achieved recognition as a Top 10 bestseller at Beijing's Autumn 2017 Commercial Press Book Fair. His most recent book, "*Transformation from Colonial Chemist to Global Health and Beauty Retailer: A.S. Watson*", also became a bestselling book in Hong Kong in 2022. A play on the three main characters of the Humphreys family of John, Henry, and David of the A. S. Watson will be on stage in Hong Kong and the mainland theatres from 2025 onwards.

Inspired by the work of KC Wong and Wu Lien-Teh's *Chinese History of Medicine*, published ninety-two years ago in 1932, Patrick is collaborating with academics and practitioners from mainland China, Taiwan, Hong Kong, Macau, and overseas on a five-section reference book titled "*Chinese History of Pharmacy: From Shennong to Tu Youyou*". This complete guide on the social history of pharmacy from ancient to contemporary China, highlighting the key events and milestones across two millennia is the first of its kind and is anticipated to be published online starting in the last quarter of 2024.

Patrick is the founder and president of the Hong Kong Society for the History of Pharmacy. He is a regular contributor to the Pharmaceutical Historian and serves as a senior non-resident fellow at Shanghai University. He is a keen promotor of history of pharmacy education and frequently speaks at universities and colleges in Beijing, Hong Kong, Macau, Shanghai, Singapore, and Taiwan.

Patrick is married and currently resides in Hong Kong.

Chapter 1
The Beginnings of Western Influence on Chinese Medicine

The primary objective of this opening chapter is to trace the origins of China's adoption of ancient medical and pharmaceutical technology. As China has an abundance of natural resources, what were the drivers to import exotic elements of materia medica into the country for healthcare purposes? Throughout the course of this extensive journey, knowledge and practices were disseminated by various groups, including Buddhist monks, Muslim imams, and Jesuit missionaries. Additionally, traders from Arabic, Indian, Javanese, and European backgrounds have contributed to the development of Chinese medicine by introducing exotic elements of materia medica. This enriching process has unfolded over a span of two millennia from 200 BCE to 1800, further expanding the armamentarium of Chinese medicine.

The early beginnings of western medicine can be traced back to Pedanius Dioscorides (c. 40 CE–c. 90 CE), born in southwestern Turkey circa 40 E in the Greek-speaking part of the eastern Mediterranean. His work on medicine would change world history. He lived in an age when two world powers were rising— the Roman Empire in Europe, Asia Minor and North Africa and the Han dynasty in China. Within the rising Roman Empire and Greco-Roman realm, Dioscorides would come to serve as a soldier under Emperor Nero (37 CE–68 CE). Through his early life training and travels with the Roman army, Dioscorides composed a five-volume text known in Latin as *De Materia Medica*. It became a core cannon of medicine shared across numerous cultures for over sixteen centuries.

In China, the Divine Farmer's Classic Materia Medica (神农本草经，or *Shennong Bencao Jing*), an early record of 365 Chinese materia medica (medicinal substances), began to connect with The Masters of Huainan (淮南子，*Huainanzi*), the Chinese philosophical classic from the Western Han dynasty in 122 BCE.[1] The adoption of exotic (or non-Chinese) elements of materia medica, (海药, *haiyao*), originated from the Silk Roads, by imperial apothecaries from faraway lands and oceans in ancient China, could be traced back to Zhao Mo (赵眜, r. 137–122 BCE) in his imperial tomb in the early Han dynasty (汉朝, 202 BCE to 220 CE) (Fig. 1.1). Widespread use of non-Chinese materia medica occurred millennia later in the Song

P. Chiu, *A History of Western Pharmacy in China*,
https://doi.org/10.1007/978-981-99-8635-4_1

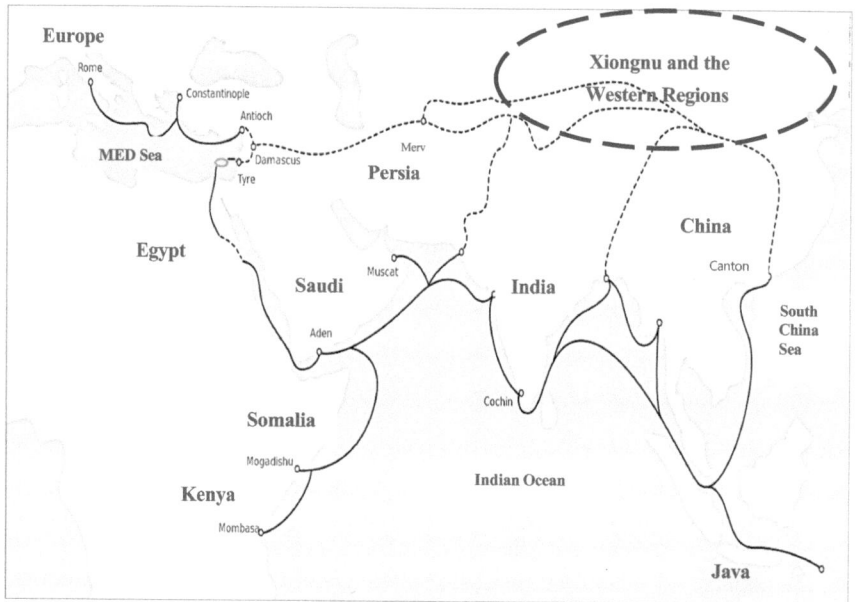

Fig. 1.1 The ancient silk roads. *Credit* Author's image bank. Key ------- land route across Euroasia from China to Syria, maritime routes ——— originated from East Africa, Europe, India, and Java

dynasty (宋朝, 960–1279). Advances in scientific discoveries, including compass design, paper making, typography, shipbuilding etc., led to quantum leaps in navigation and maritime trade with Japan and Korea in the east, Java and Vietnam in southeast Asia and India in the South West. The Silk Road trade in the Song dynasty was the first wave of large volumes and varieties imported from the Korean peninsula, Southeast Asia, Arabia and West Asia from the mid-eleventh to the late sixteenth century. Emperor Shenzong (神宗, r. 1067–1068) legitimized the medical profession and the pharmaceutical trade for the first time in the history of ancient China by authorising and publishing national pharmacopoeias. The state-owned dispensaries sold and distributed standardized prepared materia medica, including Chinese and non-Chinese origins, at affordable prices to the public.

Why were these non-Chinese materia medica that traders became enthusiastic about?

It is widely acknowledged in academic circles that numerous non-native plant species were initially introduced into China as everyday necessities like food and fiber by ancient travelers. Over time, resourceful individuals who effectively explored agricultural by-products discovered their medicinal properties long after their introduction. Notable examples of such plants include black sesame, cannabis seed, hyacinth bean, and radish.

China's geographical location and general climatic conditions impose limitations on the cultivation of certain source species that require humid tropical or warm or extreme environments. These products, such as borneol, cloves, frankincense, and rhinoceros, find application in treating acute illnesses, including convulsions in children, epilepsy, heatstroke, loss of consciousness, and delirium. Notable instances of this trend include the cultivation of cinchona in the southwest province of Yunnan since the 1920s for its anti-malarial properties and the production of santonin in the 1950s in the Shandong province for its anthelmintic uses.[2] Minerals in the form of mercuric and zinc salts would also become incorporated into Chinese medicine and some of the more exotic ones such as aconite and cinnabar had been used for longevity as prescribed by Daoist practitioners as *du* (or "poisomedicine"), though with many fatalities in ancient time due to overdose.[3]

With the increasing opium trade from India to China with the British East India Company (EIC) as the carrier, the second wave of progressive penetration of western medicine began with the Jennerian smallpox vaccination on a mass scale. Alexander Pearson, a ship surgeon to the EIC, introduced the inoculation of calf lymph in young children's arms in Macao and Canton in 1805.[4] After the two Opium Wars (1839–1842 and 1857–1860), subsequent treaties signed between China and the military powers of the United Kingdom, France, the United States, and others invariably resulted in settlement of medical and pharmaceutical missionaries and western chemists in the designated treaty ports. During the 1929–1936 period, state health policies, including those relating to drugs and pharmacy, were formulated, which laid a strong foundation for western pharmacy in modern China.

Sinification of Ayurvedic Medicines from the Ancient Silk Roads

Philosophers of ancient China, Greece and Sindhu, the region of the ancient Indus Valley civilization, shared the same views on life in seeking a balance between the body, mind, and nature.[5] As a result, they hold the same three elements as being the origins of life, "water, fire and earth", without which, understandably, humans could not survive. Dhanvantari (@ 1000 BCE), an Ayurvedic priest doctor of Sindhu, had two additional "wind and space" elements other than "water, fire and earth" as the basis of Ayurvedic medicine. A combination of two elements, will yield the three *dhatu* or "humors": *Vata* (wind and space), *Pitta* (fire and water) and *Kapha* (earth and water).[6] An imbalance of the three *dhatu* causes illnesses. Restoration of each person's unique balance of *dhata* will ensure good health and well-being.[7]

Empedocles (494–434 BCE), an ancient Greek philosopher, proposed the "Four-Element" theory with "air" as the fourth element. Hippocrates (@ 460 BCE–370 BCE), another Greek physician, further elaborated with the "Four-Humor" theory of "blood, yellow bile, black bile, and phlegm" to articulate its influence on human health. Finally, Pedanius Dioscorides (40 CE–90 CE), the renowned Greek physician, pharmacist, and botanist, documented the use of the opium poppy as an analgesic and hypnotic in his *De Materia Medica*, a five-volume Greek compendium of materia medica (or medicinal materials), dating back to the first century.[8] In ancient China, philosophers developed the concept of "energy" or *qi*, the "five-element" of "metal, wood, water, fire and earth", and the "positive" *yin* and "negative" *yang* opposite forces, over 500 years between 200–600 BCE. Chinese medicine consists of the three primary regimens of acupuncture, materia medica and medical massage (按摩 *anmo*) to restore the free flow and balance of energy.

Archaeologists found the Mausoleum of King Zhao Mo, the earliest site discovered so far with evidence of overseas pharmacy, materia medica and fragrances and scents, in China in 1983. Arab and Sindhu traders transmitted these non-Chinese materia medica from the distant Sindhu and West Asia along the ancient maritime Silk Road. A silver Persian medicine box with an almond-shaped mosaic pattern and a lacquer box containing olibanum were found among the unearthed treasures in King Zhao's burial site, built in the first century BCE (Fig. 1.2). King Zhao was the second grandson of General Zhao Tuo (Trieu Da in Vietnamese), who declared the independence of the Nanyue Kingdom (240–137 BCE) at the collapse of the Qin Empire (221–206 BCE) in 204 BCE. Nanyue Kingdom's territories encompassed parts of today's southern provinces, Guangdong, Guangxi, Jiangxi, Fujian, and Northern Vietnam.

Sandalwood burners were discovered in the Mausoleum. Sandalwood, originated in India and is widely available in Timor, is an expensive fragrance first imported into China a couple of millenniums ago. At the Yonghe Temple (the former Palace of Peace and Harmony), sandalwood was used as the trunk of the Maitreya Buddha's statue. The Tibetan Buddhist temple was converted from the former residence of Prince Yong before he became Emperor Yongzheng (1678–1735). Myrrh, a similar aromatic medicinal herb from the same continent, also entered the Chinese medicine. Olibanum, known as frankincense, is an aromatic resin originating in Arabia and North-eastern Africa (Somalia, Ethiopia and Kenya). It has also been used externally as a local stimulant in a paste form to simulate blood circulation by Chinese medicine practitioners for orthopaedic cases.[9]

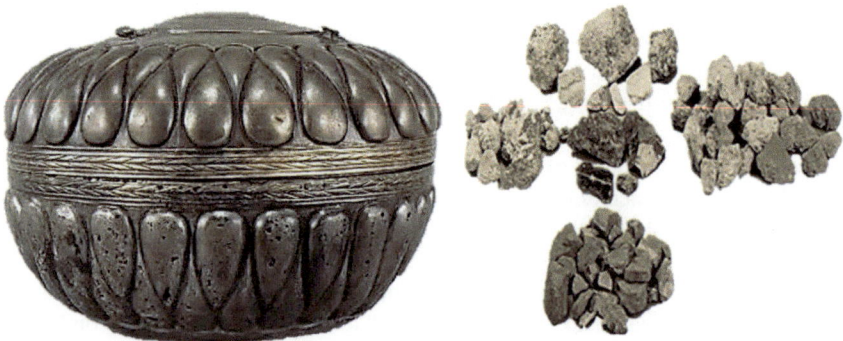

Fig. 1.2 Left: Silver Persian medicine box (Left); Right: Five colour minerals. (Left, *Sulphur*, top, *Turquoise*, Centre, *Amethyst*, Right, *Realgar*, Bottom, Ocher). *Credit* Mausoleum of the Nanyue King, The Museum of the Western Han Dynasty, Guangzhou

China's interactions with its neighbours in the Western Regions, today's Xinjiang Uyghur Autonomous Region, can be traced back to Zhang Qian (张骞, Chang Chien, 164–114 BCE), a Western Han dynasty official who conducted two expeditions to Central Asia from 135 to 115 BCE. The Western Region is also used to refer to the ancient states in Bactria, Fergana, Sodgiana and Transoxiana in Central Asia, Seleucid in Mesopotamia, and India in South Asia in the Records of the Great Historian (史记, "*Shiji*") by Sima Qian (司马迁, 145–86 BCE) in 90 BCE.

Emperor Wu (武帝, 141–87 BCE) sent Zhang Qian to the nomadic Yuezhi (now Gansu province) in Central Asia to form a military alliance against the hostile Huns (匈奴, "Xiongnu"), who controlled most parts of the Western Region). Zhang's two long trips of 138–125 BCE and 119–115 BCE to Central and South Asia led to the opening of the land routes of the ancient Silk Roads. His passages along the Xian (Changan)—Tianshan corridor ran from Xian in the Shaanxi province of northwest China, westwards through the Hesi corridor, passing through Tianshan (the "Heavenly Mountains" or Tengri Tagh in Uyghur) and the valleys of Kazakhstan and northern Kyrgyzstan. Zhang brought back functional foods with therapeutic uses, such as alfalfa, pomegranate, walnut, and coriander, which enriched the armamentarium of Chinese medicine.

The ancient Silk Road also served as the "Nirvana Route", a highway of ideas between India and China that took Ayurveda and Buddhist medicine to China in the Eastern Han period (23–220).[10] Kumarajiva (344–413) was an early Buddhist monk from the Kingdom Kucha (库车, now 龟兹, Qiuchi, Xinjiang Uyghur Autonomous Region) who travelled to Changan (长安, now "Xian") in 401. He was the missionary who transmitted the Mahāyāna school of Buddhist philosophy to China. Kumarajiva translated many sutras, including the most important ones of Vajracchedika Prajnaparamita Sutra ("Diamond Sutra"), Shorter Sukhavati-vyuha Sutra (one of the two Indian Mahayana sutras that describe the "Pure Land of Amitabha"), and Saddharma Puṇḍarika Sutra ("Lotus Sutra"). In the early fifth century, Chinese junks made annual trips to Java, one of the largest islands of modern-day Indonesia, and India based on the southwest and northeast monsoon sequence. Master Fa Xian (法显, "Fa Hsien", 337–422) was the first known Buddhist master who paid a long pilgrimage visit to India. Master Fa travelled across the Western Region and returned by sea route via Sri Lanka, Java, reaching the shores of Qingdao (青岛, "Tsingtao") in 412.

An Indian monk, Bodhidharma (菩提达摩, 470–532), born as a prince in the Pallava Kingdom in South India, became a fully enlightened Zen master at age 22. He answered the calling of Buddha by going to China and arriving in Canton by the sea route. He continued to Luoyang in Central China and built the Shaolin Temple in 495. Based on these travel records, the maritime route of the Silk Road had become an established shipping line between China and India from the early fifth century. Dating back to the Northern and Southern dynasties (420–589), three out of the seven Sanskrit treatises, known as the Bower Manuscripts, relating to Ayurvedic pharmacy, were discovered in a Buddhist stupa in Qiuci by Lieutenant Hamilton Bower, a British army officer, in 1890. Also, during this period, a hybrid of Confucianism and Daoism (Taoism) philosophy (modern term, "metaphysics") emerged as the mainstream religion. It influenced the practice of Chinese medicine in the Central Plains.[11]

Daoist Chinese medicine practitioner Tao Hongjing (陶弘景, 456–536) compiled The Collection of Commentaries on the Classic of Materia Medica (本草经集注, "*Bencao Jing Jizhu*") between 480 and 489 during the Qi dynasty (齐朝). The Collection contains seven hundred and thirty materia medica, almost double the number of three hundred and sixty-five recorded in the Divine Farmer's Classic Compendium of Materia Medica after a 500-year lapse. Unfortunately, there were many inaccuracies in Tao's work under the influence of the metaphysics school of thought. In the sixth and seventh centuries of the Sui (隋朝, 581–618) and early Tang (唐初, 598–649) dynasties, active transmission of religious and medical literature in Buddhism occurred. Bodhidharma in the late fifth and early sixth century, and Xuan Zhuang's in the mid-seventh century were the most acclaimed Buddhist masters who translated many sutras and treaties like his predecessors of Kumarajiva and Fa Xian.[12]

Auriel Stein and Paul Pelliott, in their archaeological expeditions, unearthed many rolls of manuscripts in Dunhuang, an ancient entrepot of trading and religious activities on the Silk Road, in today's Gansu province, China in 1907 and 1908, respectively. These documents contain detailed pharmaceutics in Sanskrit, Sogdian, Uyghur, Kucha and other languages of the tenth century in the Mogao Caves (千佛洞, "the Seventeenth Cave of Thousand Buddhas").[13] Of great significance, Jivaka Pustaka ("*Jivaka's Book*") is a bilingual medical text containing a collection of Indian Ayurvedic prescriptions written in Sanskrit and Khotanese, now kept in the India Office and Oriental Collections of the British Library.[14] Persian traders introduced Triphala, a medicinal wine containing black myrobalan, beleric myrobalan and Indian gooseberry, to relieve cough and diarrhoea during the mid-Tang (762–827) dynasty.[15] Today, Triphala is a popular Ayurvedic health supplement in drug stores globally.

Sun Simiao (581–682), known as the "Master of Medicines", was a Daoist (Taoist) apothecary with expertise in alchemy and medicines of longevity. Based on his earlier 30-volume medical encyclopedia of Essential Prescriptions Worth a Thousand in Gold for Every Emergency (备急千金要方, *Beiji Qianjin Yaofang*) published in 652, Sun authored A Supplement of the Essential Prescriptions (千金翼方, "*Qianjin Yi Fang*") with 800 materia medica in 682. Sun's work was a dispensatory, not an official pharmacopoeia or formulary, which consisted of prescriptions used by Chinese medicine practitioners of his time. The most remarkable Ayurvedic formulation recorded by Sun was indeed a theriac, named the "Jiva Pill" (耆婆丸) for treating epilepsy, jaundice, cough, deafness, and malaria.[16]

Incorporation of Overseas (Non-Chinese) Materia Medica

In 657 CE, Emperor Gaozong (高宗, r. 649–683) of the Tang dynasty authorized and funded a court official, Su Jing (599–674), to standardize the descriptions of commonly used Chinese materia medica. Under Li Ji's (李绩, 594–669) editorial direction, Su completed the compilation of China's first national pharmacopoeia: *Xin Xiu Bencao* (新修本草, the "*Newly Revised Materia Medica*"), better known as the Tang Pharmacopeia (唐本草, "*Tang Bencao*") within 2 years in 659. The objectives of the Pharmacopoeia were to correct the inaccuracies in the Daoist Master Tao's *Bencao Jing Jizhu*. Supported by a team of twenty-three medical and pharmaceutical experts, the Tang Pharmacopeia was completed with 850 drug monographs of which 142 were new Chinese materia medica, on schedule.[17] Eighty years later, Chen Zangqi (陳藏器, 687–757), a court official who was also an apothecary, revised the Pharmacopoeia with the long overdue *Bencao Shiyi* (本草拾遺, the "Tang Pharmacopoeia" Supplement) in 739. An exotic Non-Chinese materia medica, poppy seeds, were included for the first time among the 692 new drug monographs in the Supplement.

With foreign trade vibrant, Emperor Xuan Zong (玄宗, r. 712–756) designated an area in Canton and set up a Maritime Administration responsible for commerce with Arabs, Indians, and Javanese merchants in the foreign community in Canton in 741. It was indeed a visionary move by the Tang imperial court. The 8-year "An Lushan Rebellion" (安史之乱, 755–763) and its subsequent dominance of Tibetan and Uyghur kingdoms in Central Asia halted the flow of the bustling trade on the land route of the Silk Road to the Central Plains. A shipwreck on Belitung Island in the Java Sea in the ninth century was evidence of Arab-China trade. Sixty thousand pieces of merchandise were recovered from an Arab dhow of 18-m length consisting of jars filled with valuable commodities loaded in Canton and destined for Baghdad around 830. The same merchandise displayed in the Asian Civilization Museum in Singapore recently consisted of jars filled with valuable herbs, teas and spices, and gold and silver vessels.

Li Xun (李珣, 855–903), a third-generation Persian and an apothecary by profession living in the Lingnan region compiled a dispensatory containing one hundred and twenty-eight monographs of materia medica from overseas (海药, "*Haiyao*") known as the Compendium of Non-Chinese Materia Medica (海药本草, "*Haiyao bencao*"), in the late ninth and early tenth centuries.[18] These include eleven minerals, thirty-nine herbs, forty-nine resins, fifteen animals, ten fruits and four others imported by the maritime Silk Road, many originating from Sindhu, Persia (波斯, "*Bosi*"), and the Arabian coast.[19] After the collapse of the Tang dynasty in 907, the Silk Road was blocked by the three Persinate Sunni Muslim states of Samanid Iranian, Seljuk Oghuz Turks, and the Khwarezmid Turkic mamluk tribes in the tenth and eleventh centuries. Hence, importing non-Chinese materia medica as tributary presents from far-away kingdoms and states in the Arabian Peninsula, the Persian Gulf, the Indian Ocean and the East and South China Seas relied primarily on the maritime routes. Since the tenth century, the increasing import of materia medica from overseas has enriched the domestic cultivated or grown materia medica portfolio. As a result, non-Chinese materia medica has become an integrated part of the Chinese medicine therapeutic regimen.

In the mid-Northern Song dynasty (北宋, 960–1127), Wang Anshi (王安石, 1021–1086) was appointed as the state chancellor by Emperor Shenzong (神宗, r 1067–1085) in 1070. Wang introduced new policies to improve defence, public health, social order, education and governance by raising landowners' tax revenue. One of Chancellor Wang's long-lasting impacts on public health was to provide affordable medicine to the masses through the state-owned dispensaries. Chinese medicine practitioners and dispensers were to provide medical treatment and compounding and mixing at these People's Pharmacy's retail outlets. As a result, ready-made finished dosage forms of medicinal herbs and minerals in pills, pastes, and powders appeared for the first time.

In 1077, the first state-owned Compounding Dispensary (熟药所, "Shu Yao Suo") was opened in Kaifeng (开封)—the capital of the Northern Song dynasty.[20] A year later, Emperor Shenzong (神宗, 1048–1085) funded the publication and distribution of the National Formulary (太平惠民和剂药方, Taiping Huimin Hejiyaofang). The Formulary comprised 788 formulations for general medicine, paediatrics and gynaecology, which the Imperial Dispensary (太医局 "Tai Yi Ju") developed as the standardized pharmaceutical formulations of what had evolved over the past centuries. Only those indigenous and imported materia medica that met the standards and specifications of the Formulary were sold in the Dispensaries, which had increased to 5 by 1106. With one third less in retail pricing for standardised materia medica, this policy change and the elevation of professional status of Chinese medicine practitioners serving the public in the Dispensaries opened a new chapter of social medicine in China in the eleventh century. By 1152, the imperial court set up seventy of these Dispensaries, now renamed as State Municipal Dispensary Stores (太平惠民局, "Taiping Huiminju") to provide out-patient clinical service and dispensing of prepared materia medica at affordable prices to the public.[21] In the same period, advances in block printing, shipbuilding and compass design in navigation in the Song dynasty (960–1279) boosted the transmission of medical knowledge, science and religion between China, India, Southeast Asia, Persia and Arabia using the maritime Silk Roads. The public health policy implemented by Chancellor Wang Anxi in 1072 not only thrived but continued to flourish from the Mongolian Yuan dynasty until the mid-Ming dynasty (1368–1644). However, it gradually declined starting in the early sixteenth century. By 1560, all the Dispensary Stores had closed, leaving behind a rich legacy of social pharmacy.[22] Nevertheless, this concept experienced a remarkable revival nearly 400 years later when Communist China, on its path to modernity, embraced it once again in 1949.

Ten years after the first Compounding Dispensary was established, the Quanzhou (泉州, Quanzhou, Zayton) Maritime Administration was inaugurated in 1087. Located in the southern coastal Fujian region, Quanzhou soon succeeded Canton to become the major port of entry for ships arriving from overseas markets with traders from Arabia, Persia, and East and Southeast Asia. Zhao Rugua (赵汝适, Chao Ju-kuo) 1170–1231, a late Song dynasty court official, became the Administrator of Quanzhou Customs in 1224. The following year, he compiled a two-volume compendium, Zhu Fan Zhi (诸藩志 A Chinese Gazetteer of Foreign Lands). Volume one of the Gazetteer contains monographs describing 158 countries and states and customs of its peoples (Table. 1.1). The inflow of materia medica from aboard enrich the armamentarium of Chinese medicine practitioners' choice of

Table 1.1 Selective countries listed in Volume 1 of Zhu Fan Zhi: *A Gazetteer of Foreign Lands.*

Era/Country					
Year in CE	Anglicized name	Geographical name			
		Chinese	Pinying	Local language	Location
1862–1945 CE	Cochinchine	交趾	Jiaozhi	Nam Kỳ	Southern tip of Indochina
137–1695 CE	Champa Kingdom	占城	Zhancheng	Chiem Thanh	A kingdom situated in Central and Southern Indochina
68 CE	Cambodia Kingdom	真里	Zhenla	Kâmpǔchéa	Western Indochina
7th–13th C	Samboja Kingdom	三佛齊	Sanfoqi	Srivijaya	Malaya and Indonesia
632–1258 CE	Roman Byzantine Empire	大食	Dashi	Arabia	Mediterranean Sea
1130–1816 CE	Kingdom of Sicily	西西里	Xixili	Sicilianu	Southern Italy

Source Zhu Fan Zhi

therapeutics. The Imperial Dispensary selectively included the clinically efficacious materia medica in its formularies for sale in the Compounding Dispensaries.

The Canon of Medicine and Islamic Formulary in the Mongolian Yuan Era

The Yuan dynasty (1271–1368) succeeded the Song dynasty and had a vibrant inland trade across the member states of the Mongolian Empire. During the reign of the Mongol emperors, China set up two major ethnic and religious medical systems addressing the needs of the Han Chinese and Muslim subjects by separate administration of the Chinese medicine and Islamic disciplines instead of a fully integrated health system for all. Kubli Khan (Emperor Shizu, first Mongolian Emperor, r. 1264–1293), decided to compile a unified Great Yuan Pharmacopoeia (大元本草, *Da Yuan Bencao*) as an official pharmacopeia towards a unified medical system using both Chinese and non-Chinese materia medica. Kublai Khan appointed Xu Guozhen (许郭祯) as a minister in charge of medical affairs and the Great Yuan Pharmacopoeia's compilation. A team of twenty medical and pharmacy scholars under the leadership of Minister Xu completed the work in 1288, the 25th year of Emperor Shizu's reign. Unfortunately, the intended *Great Yuan Pharmacopoeia* was never published.

Dr. Fan Ka Wai, an authority on the medieval and pre-modern history of Chinese medicine, shared his views in a recent history of pharmacy workshop:

> Medical scholars conducted reviews of Chinese and non-Chinese materia medica in the Tang and Song dynasties. Only those with substantive evidence of efficacy and safety would be listed with a drug monograph in the National Pharmacopoeia or National Formulary. However, they were reluctant to include exotic elements of materia medica from overseas if similar Chinese materia medica were already available in the previous national pharmacopoeias and formularies. The political forces of the Yuan court encouraged competition between the Han medical and pharmaceutical scholars and those from the Islamic world. As a result, Han medical and pharmaceutical scholars would alienate those from the Western Regions. The Yuan emperors missed an excellent opportunity to integrate non-Chinese materia medica of Arabic/Persian origin with that of Chinese materia medica early in their rule.[23]

A century later, towards the end of the Yuan dynasty in the 1360 s, Chinese Muslim medical and pharmaceutical scholars translated Ibn Sina's (Avicenna, 980–1037) *The Canon of Medicine* of 1025. As a result, *Hui Hui Yaofan* (回回药方, "The Islamic Formulary"), though not as an official pharmacopoeia, was a complete medical manual containing 650 formulations of popular Arabic and Persian medicines used by the Muslim population residing in China. It was, therefore, a drug formulary for the ethnic minority.[24] However, as the *Da Yuan Bencao* (大元本草, "*Great Yuan Pharmacopoeia*") was not released as a national pharmacopoeia like the *Xinxiu Bencao* (新修本草, "Tang Pharmacopoeia") or the National Formulary like the *Taiping Huimin Hejijufang* for the Han population, it had a negligible impact on the practice of Chinese medicine.

The Yuan State implemented sea embargoes four times; each prohibition was for about 11 years. Moreover, China was self-sufficient with a vibrant economy, and there was little, if any, adverse impact on overseas trade. The gradual decline of the land and maritime routes of the Silk Road was, to a greater extent, due to the isolation policy put in place by the Ming Emperors. Nevertheless, Admiral Zheng He ((郑和, Cheng Ho, 1371–1433) temporarily revived the maritime Silk Road with his seven naval expeditions to the Arabian Peninsula, East Africa, and South and Southeast Asia from 1405 to 1433. Admiral Zheng was a Persian descendant of the Islamic faith who came from a military family of the previous Yuan dynasty.[25] Zheng's religious faith and knowledge of Arabic culture helped his exploration of the thirty-odd countries and territories with many Islamic states in the Indian subcontinent, Western Asia, and as far as Zanzibar, an island off the coast of East Africa (now part of Tanzania). His overseas expeditions brought back the common folk medicines of Arabic, Indian, Malay/Indonesian and Persian origins. In the seventh and his last overseas expedition, Zheng He died in Calicut (Kozhikode) on the Malabar coast in Kerala, India, in 1433. As a eunuch, the Admiral did not leave any descendants.

During this period, Prince Zhu Su (1370–1425), a renowned apothecary and botanist and a sibling of Emperor Yongle (永乐 r. 1402–1424), compiled the "Formulary of General Medicine" (普济方, *Puji fang*) in 1390 with chaulmoogra oil included for the first time for the treatment of leprosy. Due to continuous intrusions by organized Japanese pirates, the restriction of maritime trade in the Ming dynasty was the longest and was close to 200 years.[26] When the rulers of the Ottoman Empire (1299–1922) blocked the land trade to India across the Mediterranean after they seized the city of Constantinople in 1453, maritime trade was the only option.

Portuguese Navigators, Jesuits, and Cinchona Bark

China was in total isolation from 1473 to 1567. For nearly a century, the Ottoman rulers in the west and the Japanese in the east sealed off the land and the maritime routes of the Silk Road. From Europe, Portuguese explorer Vasco de Gama (1460–1524), the first European navigator who discovered the maritime route to reach India via the Atlantic Ocean, arrived in Calicut in 1499, sixty years after Admiral Zheng He was buried there. De Gama's trip to India was continued eastward by his compatriot, Tome Pires (1465–1540), a respectable apothecary and merchant who led Portugal's first embassy to China in 1517.

Forty years later, the Portuguese leased Macau on the South China coast, as a trading post from the Ming government (1368–1644) in 1557. Twelve years down the history path, the first bishop, and founder of the Holy House of Mercy of Macau, Belchior Carneiro (1516–1583), set up Asia's first western hospital—St. Raphael Hospital or, as called by the locals, the "Temple of Cures" (医人庙, *Yi Ren Miao*, Cantonese *Yi Yan Miu*) in 1569.[27] Around this time, Li Shizhen (1518–1593), a great apothecary and botanist, completed the Compendium of Materia Medica (本草纲目, *Bencao gang mu*), in 1578. He took 27 years to review and compile the largest non-official dispensary in the history of Chinas. After 18 years, the publication of *Bencao Gangmu* eventually happened in Nanking in 1596. Based on Chen Zangqi's Supplement of 739, the contents of *Bencao Gangmu* vastly increased the drug monographs from 692 to 1892, or an increase of a thousand Chinese materia medica items. Li included a formal description of Afun, "opium tears" or dried latex obtained from the opium seed capsule, medicinal uses in angina, dry cough, emesis, pain, spasms, and vasodilatation (Fig. 1.3). Li's Compendium recorded prepared opium resin's therapeutic use for the first time. Previous dispensatories or pharmacopoeias only mentioned poppy seeds, which had insignificant therapeutic or habit-forming effects.

The first Portuguese official arrived in Macau in 1557, Spanish, Dutch, English, French, American, and other traders soon followed in the next 200 years. The St. Paul's College of Macau, also known as the College of Madre de Deus, was established in 1594 and held classes in medicine, with a clinic soon opened. Alessandro Valignano (1539–1606 CE), Visitor of the Eastern Missions of the Jesuits, drew up the "Résolutions and Cérémonial" policy and sought the Vatican's approval to accommodating local customs and cultural practices of the Japanese during his tour of Japan from 1579 to 1582.[28]

Decades later, the Jesuits of the Roman Catholic Church, with Italian priest Matteo Ricci (1552–1610), led a religious mission and arrived in Beijing in 1601 (Fig. 1.4). The Jesuits soon constructed St. Paul's Church in Macau from 1602 to 1640, making it the gateway of the Roman Catholic Church to China and Japan. Upon approval by

Fig. 1.3 Afun (Opium
poppy, (Papaver
somniferum) capsule, 1853.
Credit M.A. Burnett, 1851,
Wellcome Collection

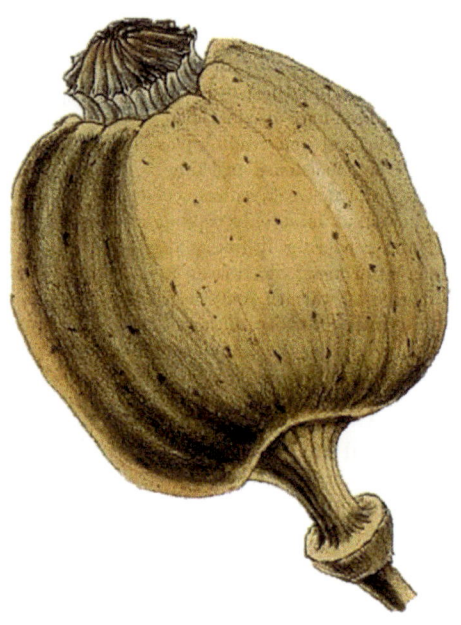

Emperor Wanli (万历 r. 1572–1620) in the 23rd year of his reign in 1605, Matteo
Ricci (利玛窦, 1552–1610) built the first Roman Catholic Church, the Cathedral
of the Immaculate Conception (南堂, "the *South Chapel*", *Nantang*) in Beijing
in 1605. He and his successors followed the Résolutions and Cérémonial policy
and gained acceptance by the upper echelon of the imperial court of the late Ming
(1601–1644), and the Manchu Qing dynasty (1644–1911). In the 10th year of his
reign, Emperor Shunzhi (顺治 r. 1643–1661), the second emperor of the Manchu
Qing Empire, approved the Imperial Hospital's expansion with a completely new
Imperial Pharmacy in 1653, The latter's role was to dispense finished dosage forms
of Chinese medicine in pills, powders, liquid concentrates for oral use, ointments for
external use, and unique formulations for the emperor and the empress.

The pharmacy's staff followed stringent dispensing procedures to ensure the
utmost quality and safety of such dispensed concoctions. After 8 years in operation, the Imperial Pharmacy was closed for renovation in 1662 and reopened 5 years
later in 1667 (the 6th year of Emperor Kangxi's reign). Finally, in 1684, the Imperial
Hospital management agreed to transfer the Imperial Pharmacy to the Ministry of
Interior. Successors of Emperor Kangxi (康熙 r. 1661–1722), Emperors Yongzheng
(雍正 r. 1722–1735) and Qianlong (乾隆 r. 1735–1796) were all keen to stock up
the Imperial Pharmacy with an abundant inventory of Chinese materia medica and
non-Chinese materia medica for use by the royal court and the military during their
reigns.[29]

Pope Alexander VII (r. 1655–1667) issued a proclamation officially allowing
the practice of Confucian rites in converting non-believers in China in 1656. With a
positive gesture extended to the Chinese by the Roman Catholic Church, the Governor

Fig. 1.4 Matteo Ricci
(1552–1610), Jesuit
Missionary, oil on canvas.
Credit Emmanuel Pereira
(Chinese Jesuit Yu Wen-hui,
1610)

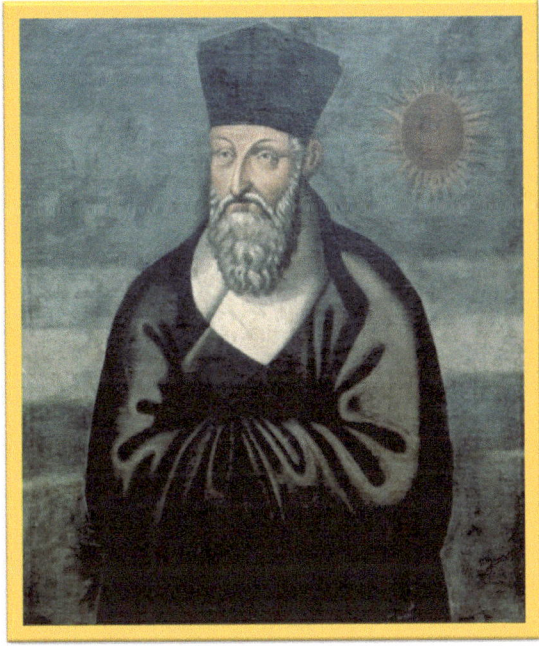

General of Batavia of the Dutch East Indies dispatched the Dutch East India Company on behalf of the Kingdom of Netherlands to the "Middle Kingdom" in July 1656.[30,31] Tributary gifts to Emperor Shunzhi (1638–1661) included cloves, cinnamon, and sandalwood, and to the Empress, rose water. From time immemorial, the Chinese emperors had received these exotic elements dispatched from the ancient Silk Road. The Manchu Qing emperors and the noble class extensively used aromatic (essential or volatile) oils. The regularly stocked items included oils of cardamon, balsam, ambergris, musk, peppermint, cinnamon, sandalwood, clove, citron, tangerine, and rose in the three locations of the Imperial Pharmacy stores (Figs. 1.5, 1.6, 1.7 and 1.8).

Essential oils of these herbs and spices have been used as incense sticks to worship ancestors and gods, holy smoke to dissipate evil spirits, scent sachets for gentries and nobilities and as Chinese medicine to treat illness. Improving the relationship between the Roman Catholic Church and the Qing court led Emperor Kangxi to approve the practice of Christianity in 1692. France soon followed up with King Louis XIV (r. 1643–1715) dispatching Jesuits to be stationed in China. Father Jean de Fontaney, a Jesuit and scholar in mathematics and astronomy, brought Quinquina (aka Cinchona), a Peruvian bark named after Countess Cinchona, from the Church's medical stock in Puducherry (Pondicherry), India to cure Emperor Kangxi's intermittent fever in July 1693 (Fig. 1.9). His Majesty's interest in medicine had motivated foreign missionaries and diplomatic missions to collect and present clinically proven remedies, including Cinchona bark, from reliable sources for the Manchu Imperial

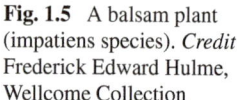

Fig. 1.5 A balsam plant (impatiens species). *Credit* Frederick Edward Hulme, Wellcome Collection

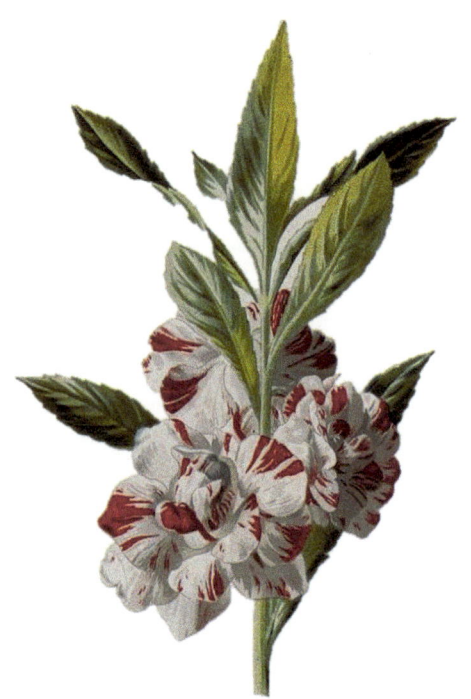

Pharmacy. (See Chap. 2). In 1715, in the 61st year of the reign of Kangxi, the Hall of Martial Valour (the Hall, *Wuyingdian*), previously used as a book mending and printing workshop of the imperial palace, was converted into a dispensing room of the Imperial Pharmacy.

The Hall was the primary site of storage of non-Chinese materia medica. Three other satellite pharmacies included the Palace of Heavenly Purity (乾清宫, *Qian-qing Gong*), the Hall of Mental Cultivation Workshop (养心殿, *Yangxin Hall Work-shop*), and the Old Summer Palace (圆明园, *Yuanming Palace*) were the other three locations. The Hall prepared herbal distillates and essential oils of non-Chinese materia medica presented by overseas delegations or Manchu Qing officials. These premises were close to the imperial residences of the empress, the emperor's mother, and the next-in-line to the imperial throne, which also kept a smaller inventory of non-Chinese materia medica. Moreover, they did reinforce the views of the imperial family that aromatic oils such as balsam oil were a unique class of non-Chinese materia medica and were held in high regard for hunting and war injuries.

Balsamic oil was well known for its antiseptic properties for wounds. It was used as an emergency military pharmacy in the pacification war against Khoshud's rebellion in Qinghai, Northwest China, in 1723.[32] An inventory count conducted in the Hall in August 1814, the nineteenth year of the reign of Emperor Jiaqing (嘉庆 r. 1796–1820), revealed that the Imperial Pharmacy stocked one hundred and twenty

Fig. 1.6 Peppermint
(*Menthe piperita*). *Credit*
Rowan McOnegal,
Wellcome Collection

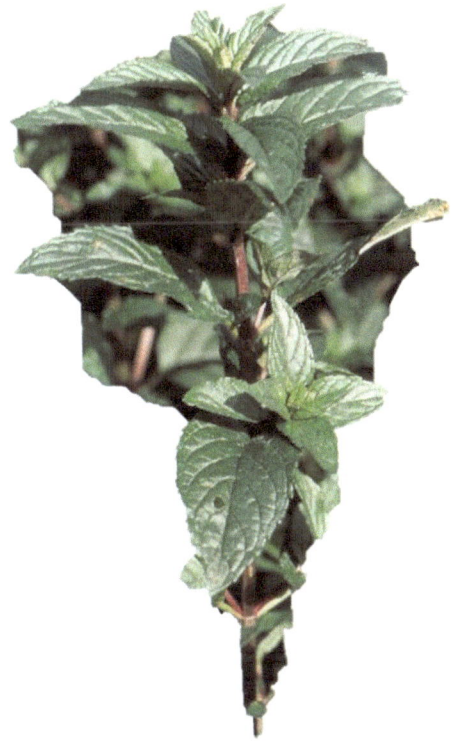

Fig. 1.7 Sandalwood
(*Sanalum album*). *Credit*
Francis Sinclair, Wellcome
Collection

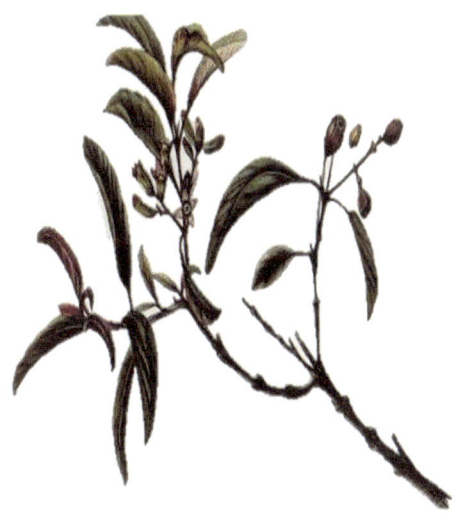

Fig. 1.8 Clove plant
(*Syzygium aromaticum*).
Credit Wellcome Collection

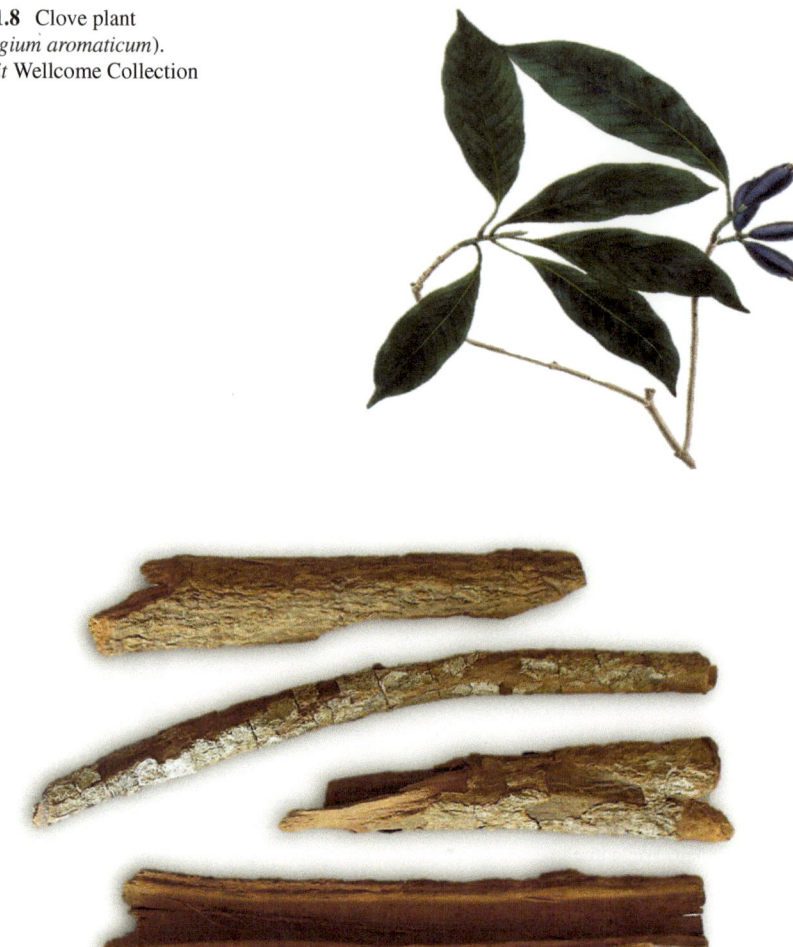

Fig. 1.9 Cinchona bark, Europe, 1601–1700. *Credit* Science Museum, London

two types of non-Chinese materia medica. Most were for oral consumption, and a few aromatic oils or preparations were for external use.

Pope Clement XI (r. 1700–1721) sent Charles-Thomas Maillard de Tournon as papal legatel to the East Indies and China to meet Emperor Kangxi in 1705. De Tournon informed Emperor Kangxi that Confucian rites and rituals in paying respect to the deceased ancestors were against the Roman Catholic Church's practices of idol worship. In total dismay, Emperor Kangxi swiftly reversed his 1692 edit. The Manchu Qing emperors and the imperial court officials viewed Christianity with suspicion of destabilizing the Manchurian minority-led Confucian state, and missionaries were not allowed to evangelise. The saga of on and off permission for Chinese Catholics to observe Confucian and Daoist cultural practices and customs by the Vatican's successive popes was termed the "Chinese Rites Controversy". Pope Clement XI's decision delayed the re-entry of Christian missionaries by 150 years until China lost the First Opium War by signing the Treaty of Nanking in 1842.[33]. The transition from Chinese medicine to Western pharmacy took place gradually over a period of 2000 years, as indicated by the compilation of pharmacopoeias and formularies until the publication of The Chinese Pharmacopeia of 1930. (Table 1.2).

Table 1.2 Key Classics of Pharmacopoeias and Formularies

Dynasty	Year(s) of publication	Major compendium, formulary and pharmacopoeia of materia medica	Drug monographs/formulary prescriptions	
			Total	Remarks
Eastern Han	25–220 CE	神农本草经, *Shennong Bencao Jing* The Divine Farmer's Classic of Materia Medica	365	Linseed and rock salt are exotic elements from the Western Regions
Qi	479–420 CE	本草经集注, *Bencao Jing Jizhu* Collection of Commentaries on the Classic of Materia Medica	730	Twice the drug monographs of *Shennong Bencao Jing*
Tang	659 CE	新修本草(唐本草), *Xinxiu Bencao* (Tang Pharmacopoeia) Newly Revised Materia Medica	850	1st National Pharmacopoeia of Tang dynasty with 142 newly added drug monographs
	682 CE	千金翼方, *Qianjin Yifang* A Supplement to the Essential Prescriptions Worth a Thousand Gold for Every Emergency	5300	1st Formulary of 800 drug monographs including Ayurvedic and Persian medicines for all medical conditions
	739 CE	本草拾遗 *Bencao Shiyi* Newly Revised Materia Medica Supplement	692	692 supplementary drug monographs of the *Xinxiu Bencao* inlcuding the exotic poppy seeds imported from Central Asia
Song	@900 CE	海药本草, *Haiyao Bencao* Compendium of Overseas Materia Medica	128	First drug compendium complied with exotic materia medica originating from originating from Sindhu, Persia and the Arabian coast

(continued)

Table 1.2 (continued)

Dynasty	Year(s) of publication	Major compendium, formulary and pharmacopoeia of materia medica	Drug monographs/formulary prescriptions	
			Total	Remarks
	1078 CE	太平惠民和剂局方, *Taiping Huiming Heji Yaofang* Formulary of the Taiping People's Pharmacy	788	*Taiping Huiming Heji Jufang* is the first official National Formulary containing 788 formulary prescriptions with standardized Chinese and imported materia medica for sales at the state owned people's pharmacies
	1108 CE	证类本草, *Zhenglei Bencao* Classified Materia Medica	1476	A most praiseworthy National Pharmacopoeia of the Song dynasty
	1125 CE	诸藩志, *Zhu Fan Zhi* A Chinese Gazetteer of Foreign Lands	54	A two-volume gazette which documents 158 countries and their customs in volume 1 and 54 commonly used exotic materia medica imported for sale
Yuan	@1360 CE	回回药方, *Hui Hui Yao Fang* The Islamic Formulary	650	Compiled by Chinese Muslim medical scholars based on The Cannon of Medicine of 1025 collated by Ibn Sina (Avicenna)
Ming	1596 CE	本草纲目 *Bencao Gangmu* Compendium of Materia Medica	1892	An Extra Pharmacopoeia containing 1892 drug monographs with an increase of 374 newly discovered materia medica, 1109 illustrations of materia medica and 11096 formulary prescriptions

(continued)

Table 1.2 (continued)

Dynasty	Year(s) of publication	Major compendium, formulary and pharmacopoeia of materia medica	Drug monographs/formulary prescriptions	
			Total	Remarks
Qing	1765 CE	本草纲目拾遗, *Bencao Gangmu Shiyi* Supplementary Compendium of Materia Medica	921	Newly added 716 drug monographs including manyexotic materia medica e.g., American ginseng, cinchona, common rue, Japanese ginseng, opium, tobacco etc. imported
Republic	1930	中华药典 *Zhonghua Yaodian* Chinese Pharmacopoeia	718	The first National Pharmacopoeia of the Nationalist government published in May 1930 with 10% of the drug monographs originated from Chinese materia medica

Notes and References

1. Divine Farmer (Shennong, "神农") was a mythological "god of agriculture" dating back to the pre-dynasty time of 4700 years ago in today's Baoji area of Shaanxi province. The book *Divine Farmer's Classic Materia Medica* (Shengnong Benaco Jing, "神农本草经") was compiled by ancient apothecaries at the turn of the Common Era @ the first century in honour of Shennong's divinity of healing power.
2. Hu, Shiu Ying, "History of the Introduction of Exotic Elements into Traditional Chinese Medicine", *Journal of the Arnold Arboretum',* 71, no.4 (October 1990): 487–526.
3. Liu, Yan, *Healing with Poisons: Potent Medicines in Medieval China,* (Seattle: University of Washington Press, 2021), 10–15, 173–174.
4. The word *Canton,* in local dialect pronounced as *Kwang-tung,* was first used by Portuguese traders to denote the province of Guangdong ("广东"). Earlier western traders used the word *Canton* interchangeably for both the city of *Guangzhou* ("广州") and the province of *Guangdong.*
5. Shendu ("身毒") is a Chinse transliteration of the Sindhu Kingdom on the modern Indian subcontinent from the pre-Qin period (前秦, Paleolithic age—221 BCE) to the Sui (隋朝, 581–618 CE) and Tang (唐朝, 618–907 CE) dynasties. Its scope mainly refers to the present-day Indus River Basin with two third of the territories located in the state of Pakistan.
6. Deshpande, V, Glimpses of Ayurveda in Medieval Chinese Medicine, *Indian Journal of History of Science,* 43.2, 2008: 137–161.
7. V. Deshpande, a Sanskrit and Ayurveda scholar, explained the 'Tridosa theory' that the body is sustaintianed by the three *dhatu.* When a dhatu is rendering an adverse effect due to its deficit or excess, it is called a "dosa". Some-times all of the dosas together cause a disease in which case it is called as due to *sannipata* or concurrence of the doasa.
8. Laios, K et al., "Drugs for Mental Illnesses in Ancient Greek Medicine", Psychiatriki 30, no.1 2019: 58–56. https://www.psychiatriki-journal.gr/documents//30.1-EN-2019-58.pdf.

9. In religious ceremonies, olibatum is used alone or mixed with wood scraps, rolled into long thin incense sticks or coils, and burnt as offerings in the names of the ancestors and gods in homes and in the Buddhist, Confucius and Daoist temples.

10. In Indian religions (Buddhism, Hinduism, Jainism, and Sikhism), *Nirvana* is the ultimate state of Salvation with freedom, happiness and peace.

11. Central Plains (Zhongyuan, "中原"), in modern day in Henan province, commonly refers to the region below the lower and middle reaches of the Yellow Reiver with two major cities of Luoyang and Kaifeng. *Zhongyuan* has been perceived as the cradle of Chinese civilization.

12. Xuan Zang ("玄奘", 602–664) was the monk in the early Tang dynasty famous for his pilgrimage to India who travelled the forward route on land and the return route by sea.

13. The Mogao Caves ("莫高窟") in Dunhuang, Gansu Province, is a former oasis town located in the furthest western part of the Hexi corridor of the ancient Silk Road.

14. Yoeli-Tlalim, R, *ReOrienting Histories of Medicine Encounters Along the Silk Road*, (London: Bloomsbury Academic, 2021), 1–24.

15. Chen, M 陈明, 'Method from Persia': Study on the Origins of the "Three Myrobalan Decoction", translated by Jack Hargreaves, *Hualin International Journal of Buddhist Studies*, (New York: Cambria Press, 2021), 4. no.2:1-78. 29 September 2023. https://buddhism.lib.ntu.edu.tw/FULLTEXT/JR-MAG/mag640001.pdf.

16. The *Jiva Pill* reportedly originated from the *Compendium of Charaka*, one of the three ancient Sanskrit foundational texts of Ayurveda. Charaka was born in Kashmir around the first century CE.

17. During the period of Northern and Southern dynasties (420–589), a hybrid of Confucianism and Taoism philosophy (modern term as "metaphysics") became the mainstream and influenced the practice of Chinese Medicine. "Xinxiu Bencao" 新修本草 [The Newly Revised Pharmacopoeia] of 659 was complied with the objective to correct the inaccuracies reported in the *Bencao Jing Jizhu* 本草经集注 [Collected Commentaries to the Materia Medica] which were published by the Taoist alchemist and pharmacologist Master Tao Hongjing 陶弘景 (456–536) @ early sixth century. Tao Hongjing's *Bencao Jing Jizhu* doubles the number of bencao from 365 recorded in the *Divine Farmer's Classic Materia Medica* to 730 over a 500-year period with many inappropriately recorded under the influence of the metaphysics school of thought.

18. The Lingnan 岭南 region was a geographic area encompassing the lands in the south of the Nanling Mountains which included the modern-day provinces of Guangdong, Guangxi, Hainan, Hong Kong, Macau and Northern and Central Vietnam. Ngo Quyen 吳權, a Southwest regional warlord, declared separation from the Southern Han dynasty to form the Ngo dynasty in north and central Vietnam, in 938.

19. "Bosi" 波斯 in Chinese or Pars in Farsi is the anglicized term of Persia on modern Iran.

20. Leung, AK, "Song-Yuan-Ming di difang yiliao ziyuan chutan" (A preliminary study on local medical resources of the Song-Yuan-Ming dynasties), *Zhongguo shehui lishi pinglun* (Review of Chinese Social History), 3, Beijing: Zhonghua shuju, 2001: 225.

21. Goldschmidt, A, *The Evolution of Chinese Medicine: Song Dynasty, 960–1200*, (London and New York: Routledge, 2009), 130-131.

22. Leung, AK, "Organized Medicine in Ming-Qing China: State and Private Medical Institutions in the Lower Yangzi Region", *Late Imperial China*, 8/1, 1987: 140–141.

23. Fan, K 范家伟, "Yuandai Guangxiu Bencao yu Zhongxi Yaowu Ronghe" 元代官修本草与中西药物融合 [Great Yuan Bencao and the Integration of Materia Medica Ex China], "Zhongxi wujian: xiyaoxue di chuanru yu zhongguo yaoxue di liubian gongzuofang" 中西互鉴: 西药学的传入与中国药学的流变工作坊 [Workshop on Mutual Learning between China and the West: the Introduction of Western Pharmacy and the Evolution of Chinese Pharmacy], Department of History, Shanghai University, 11 February 2023.

24. Of China's 1.4 billion in 2023, there are fifty-six nationalities of whom ninety-two percent are of the Han ethnic group originating in the Central Plains (modern Henan province) which the two main rivers of Yangtze and Yellow River pass through. The other five minorities with over ten million population are Zang 藏 (Tibetan, 20 million), Uyghurs 维 (12 million), Hui 范 (Chinese Muslim, 11 million), Miao 苗 (Hmong, 11 million) and Manchurian 满 (10 million).

25. Admiral Zheng He's 郑和 expeditions brought back the *non-Chinese materia medica* 海药 including: rhino horn, antelope horn, asafoetida, frankincense, clove, cardamon, aloe vera, momordica, styrax oil, amber, hematoxylin, amomum, Malus micromalus, Psoralea corylifolia, benzoin, ambergris, Acronychia pedunculata, Philippine mahogany, rosemary, agarwood, styrax, Pistacia terebinthus, jackfruit, and cassia pods, myrobalans.

26. Trade with neighbouring countries halted when the Customs Administration in Quanzhou 泉州, Ningbo 宁波 and Guangzhou 广州 ports closed for business for almost two centuries from 1374 to 1567.

27. The St. Raphael Hospital and Garden or locally called the 医人庙, *I Yan Miao*, "Temple of Cures" 医人庙 was originally located on Rua de Pedro Nolasco da Silva. The current building was constructed in the early twentieth-century and is now used by the Consulate General of Portugal for Hong Kong and Macau.

28. Hoey, JB, *"Alessandro Valignano and the Restructuring of the Jesuit Mission in Japan, 1579–1582"*, Eleutheria 1, no. 1 (2010): 23–42. Accessed 29 September 2023. https://digitalcommons.liberty.edu/eleu/vol1/iss1.

29. When compounding and dispensing herbal preparations, an apothecary of the imperial hospital and a eunuch assistant of the imperial pharmacy would monitor the whole process. Each dose was prepared in double portions, with one taken by the imperial apothecary or the eunuch as the assistant before the other portion was presented to His Majesty and Her Royal Highness.

30. The term *"Middle Kingdom"* is a translation of the Chinse term *Zhongguo* when first used by the Portuguese in the sixteenth century. *"Zhong"* means *"Central"*, and *"Guo"* means *"Country"*. China was under imperial rule until 1911 so westerners interpreted and used the term *"Country"* as *"Kingdom"* in the nineteenth century.

31. The Dutch succeeded the Portuguese and Spanish as the major trader for commodity trading in pottery and silk in the East Asia in the early seventeenth century. The Dutch East India Company was founded in 1602 to conduct trade with India, and Asia on behalf of the Dutch government.

32. "Qinggong neiwu fu zaoban chu dangan zonghui" 清宫内务府造办处档案总汇, [A Collection of Archives of the Ministry of Interior of the Qing Dynasty], Zongguo di yi lishi dangan guan, xiānggǎng zhongwwn daxue wenwu guan he bian, 中国第一历史档案馆、香港中文大学文物馆合编, [A Joint Publication of The First Historical Archives of China and the Art Museum of the Chinese University of Hong Kong], (Beijing, People's Publishing House 2005), no. 3: 410.

33. Mungeloo, DE, *The Great Encounter of China, 1500–1800* (Langham, Rowman & Littlefield 2005), 27–39.

Chapter 2
Trade Wars and the Emergence of Western Pharmacy

This chapter covers the key actors who played pivotal roles in opening China by force while spearheading change within a Confucian society known for its proud traditional values and cautious attitude towards embracing new advancements in science and technology. It also delves deeper into the rapid transformation of the European pharmaceutical industry which was turned from a lack of materia medica in pain relief to become the leader in innovation and manufacturing powerhouse by the end of the nineteenth century.

Britain's trade with China reportedly began in the 1620 s, with a merchant ship, Unicorn, sinking near Macau, where the Portuguese had landed seventy years earlier in 1557.[1] The English (later called British) East India Company (EIC) was the largest tea trader among the European East India companies from the seventeenth to the early nineteenth century. EIC set up its office, warehouse, and residential quarters called the British Factory within the "Thirteen Factory" trade zone in the Southern province of Canton (Guangdong, previously called Kwangtung) to conduct business in 1751.[2] From 1760 to 1833. China recorded a sixfold increase in tea shipments to Britain, resulting in an increasing trade deficit, until about the 1820s (Chart 2.1). The two British diplomatic delegations led by Lord George Macartney and Lord William Amherst in 1793 and 1816 respectively, to seek a trade balance with China, failed. This sowed the seeds of future military conflicts between the two imperial powers. What could the western world offer China in the eighteenth and nineteenth centuries? Sir Robert Hart (1835–1911), the Inspector-General of China's Imperial Maritime Custom Service 1863–1911, said:

> The Chinese have the best food in the world, rice, the best drink, tea, clothing, cotton, silk, and fur. Possessing these staples and their innumerable native adjuncts, they do not need to buy a penny's worth elsewhere.[3]

British India's opium trade with China, under the administration of EIC, rapidly reversed the trade imbalance and the net outflow of silver from the trading seasons of 1820 onwards until 1839 in the UK's favour. When EIC's monopoly of trade in China was ended by the British Crown at the end of 1833, British traders and supercargoes

© The Author(s), under exclusive license to Springer Nature Singapore Pte Ltd. 2023
P. Chiu, *A History of Western Pharmacy in China*,
https://doi.org/10.1007/978-981-99-8635-4_2

Chart 2.1 British East India
Company tea export from
China to Britain 1760–1833
CE. *Source* Yan Z.P. Ed.,
Economic History of
Modern China, 2012: 15

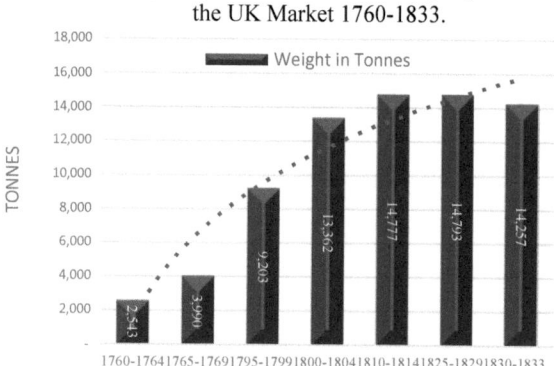

An Eighty-Sevenfold Increase in Tonnage
of Opium Trade by China, 1650-1880

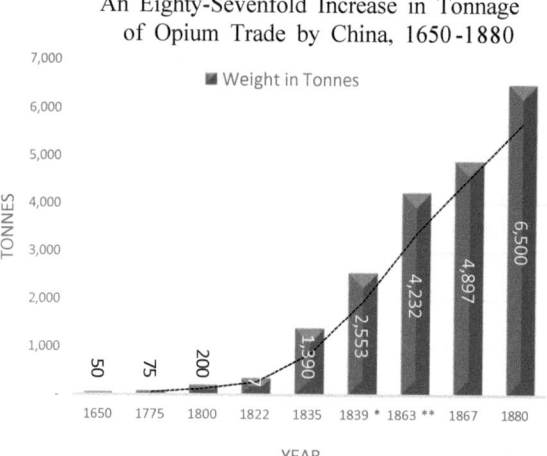

Chart 2.2 Opium Imports into China, 1650–1880. *Note* *When the British EIC monopoly in trade with China was ended by the British Parliament in 1833 in favour of the free traders, the volume of opium imports double from 1835 to 1839. **The loss of the two Opium Wars (1839–1842, 1856–1860) by China with the opening of treaty ports resulting in more opium were imported from 1863 to 1880. *Source A Century of Interntaional Drug Control*, United Nations Office on Drug Control, 2008:23

who dealt with opium shipments showed a dramatic ascent from the trading seasons of 1835–1839 and continued unabated to the apex in 1880 (Charts 2.2 and 2.3).[4]

Jardine and Matheson & Co. (JM & CO.) succeeded EIC and became the leading supplier of Indian brands of opium. William Jardine (1784–1843), a founder of JM, returned to London in September 1839 and successfully persuaded the British Foreign

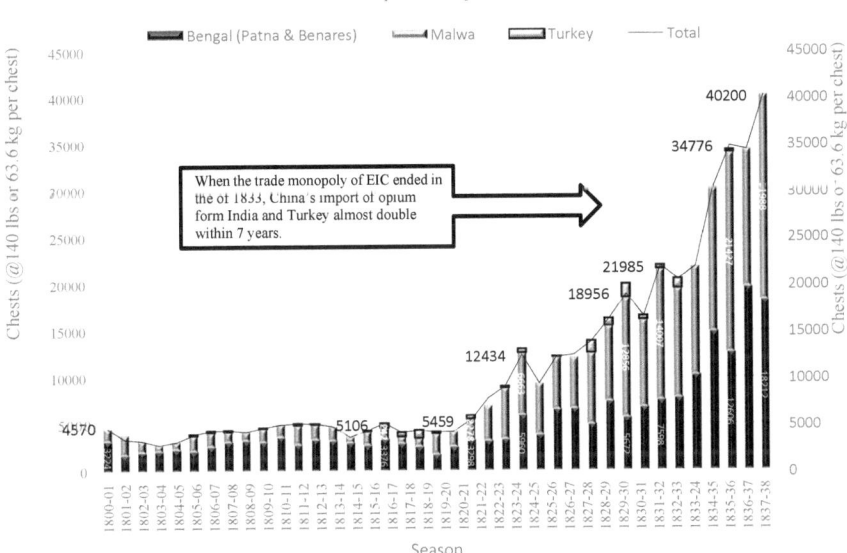

Chart 2.3 Opium Shipments to China, 1800–1838. *Source* The International Relations of the Chinese Empire, Volume 1

Minister, Lord Palmerston, to wage war on China in retaliation for the confiscation and burning of opium by Lin Zexu, a Manchu Qing official, in Bocca Tigris ("Mouth of Tiger", *Humen*) in June 1839. As a result, the British occupied Hong Kong and made excursions into other port cities, cumulatively leading to the First Opium War of 1839–1842. With the signing of the Treaty of Nanking in 1842, foreign traders and medical missionaries arrived in Hong Kong, Shanghai, and other treaty ports in droves in the 1840s, marking the beginning of western pharmacies (See Chap. 4 on The Rise of Western Chemists). Hong Kong's strategic importance in the opium trade could be reflected by its tax revenue which ranged from 15 to 50% from 1842 to 1941 and was essential to Hong Kong's treasury in the first century of its history.[5] At the end of the Second Opium War (1856–1960), many ports have been opened to foreign trade in addition to the five treaty ports of Amoy (Xiamen), Canton, Foochow (Fuzhou), Ningpo (Ningbo) and Shanghai (Fig. 2.1).

Alkaloids, Ether and Drug Discovery

1804 was the western world's watershed year in the emergence of the modern pharmaceutical industry. Friedrich Wilhelm Adam Serturner (1783–1841) of Paderborn, North Rhine-Westphalia, became the first pharmacist who developed a technique in the isolation of alkaloids from the opium poppy in 1804. Sertuner's purification of

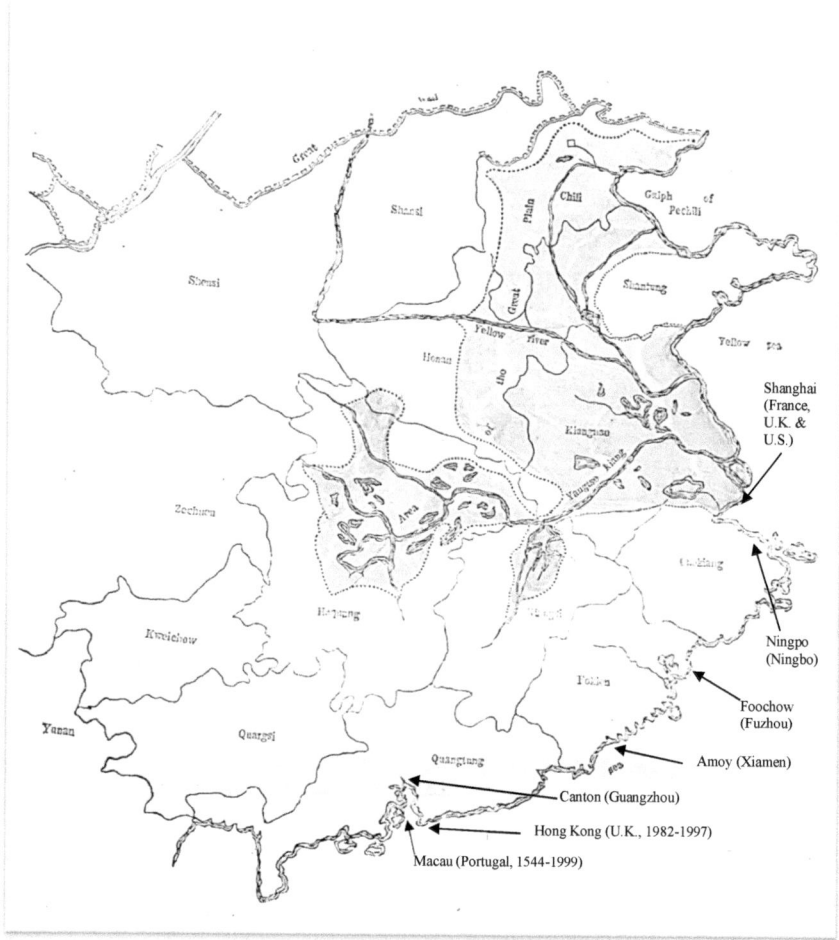

Fig. 2.1 Map of China showing the colony of Hong Kong and the five treaty ports in 1865. Shanghai had three settlements of France (1849–1943), the UK (1843), and the U.S. (1848) which the U.K. and the U.S merged their enclaves into the Shanghai international settlements in 1863 which all ended in 1943. The shaded area is the great plains, 1865. *Credit* Roy Delbyck. Original map from the Journal of the North-China Branch of the Royal Asiatic Society, new series No. II, December 1865, Shanghai, Printed at the Presbyterian Mission Press, MDCCCLXVI. *Note* Certain names appeared in the map of China have changed due to change of geographical boundary, e.g.: *Chili* was a region that corresponds to today's Liaoning province, the *Gulph of Peichili* to that of Bohai, *Haquang* to that of Huan and Hubei provinces, *Jiangnan* to that of Zhejiang and parts of Anhui, Fujian and Jiangsu province

morphine from opium poppies inspired other chemists to pursue the isolation and identification of active drugs in the nineteenth century (Table 2.1). Mass production of the alkaloid drug morphine was by Heinrich Emanuel Merck (1794–1855), who revolutionized treating pain, cough and dysentery in 1827. Merck inherited the family pharmacy business of Engel-Apotheke in 1816.[6] However, it took E Merck a decade to master extracting opium alkaloids based on a method developed by Serturner. The launch of commercial morphine in the late 1830s made E Merck of Darmstadt the leading supplier of alkaloid drugs in Europe. The extraction of cinchonine and quinine from cinchona bark in 1820 by Jean Bienaimé Caventou, a professor of the Ecole de Pharmacie in Paris, France, was the first time in human history that fever could be relieved effectively. Caventou collaborated with a fellow retail pharmacist, Pierre Joseph Pelletier, which led to the mass production and supply of quinine. The availability of quinine to front-line soldiers soon resolved the challenges of malaria faced by the troops of European colonial powers in the first half of the nineteenth century.

British soldiers, in particular; faced the deadly malaria disease in their newly colonized tropical territories of India, the Straits Settlements, Hong Kong, and the West Indies in the first half of the nineteenth century. The anti-malarial properties of quinine

Table 2.1 Drug discovery and isolation of alkaloid drugs in the nineteenth century: scientific study of medicinal plants (pharmacognosy)

Year	Compound	Investigator	Drug action/indication
1817	Narcotine	Robinquet	Also called noscapine: an anti-tussive drug
1818	Strychnine	Caventou and Pelletier	Poison: a pesticide
1819	Colchicine	Meissner and Caventou	Lowering of uric acid: gout
1820	Caffeine	Runge; Caventou and Pelletier	Vasodilation, diuresis etc.: central stimulant: mental alertness and fatigue
1820	Quinine	Caventou and Pelletier	Lowering of fever: malarial fever
1822	Emetine	Pelletier and Magendie	Anti-amoebic and to induce vomiting
1828	Nicotine	Posselt and Reimann	Central stimulant; mental alertness
1832	Codeine	Robinquet	Narcotic analgesic
1833	Atropine	Geiger and hess	Vasoconstriction
1842	Theobromine	Woskresenky	Similar to caffeine
1848	Papaverine	Merck	Vasodliation: circulatory diseases
1851	Choline	Babo and Hirschbrunn	A nutrient similar to B vitamins
1860	Cocaine	Niemann	Central stimulant
1870	Muscarine	Schmiedeberg and Koppe	Vasodilation: glaucoma, urinary incontinence and irritable bowel syndrome

Credit Adapted from Ryan Huxanle and Stephen Schwartz, Molecular Intervention, Nov. 2003: 6

soon gave rise to a colonial beverage industry with its first commercially available "tonic water" known to the military stationed in British India in 1858. Across the Atlantic, pharmacist Charles Pfizer and his cousin, Charles Erhardt, a candy maker from Germany, established Charles Pfizer and Company in Brooklyn, New York City, in 1849. They produced a dewormer (anthelmintic) bonbon containing santonin, an effective herbal anti-intestinal parasitic drug from Turkestan, Central Asia.

In the second half of the nineteenth century, the discovery of anaesthetics and antiseptics improved the survival rates of surgical operations, particularly obstetric surgeries, to an unprecedented level. In 1855, German chemist Frederick Gaedcke (1828–1890) extracted anaesthetic ingredients from coca leaves. Five years later, Frederick Gaedcke's colleague Albert Newman refined a high-purity substance he named cocaine.

Finally, Carl Koller demonstrated cocaine's use as a local anaesthetic in ophthalmology in 1884. In the same year, the famous Austrian psychologist Sigmund Freud (1856–1939) recommended using cocaine as a substitute for alcohol and morphine addiction. The German Merck chemical plant and the American Parker (now Pfizer) pharmaceutical plant quantified the production and sales of cocaine. With a dominant position in the pain relief market, *E. Merck be*came the largest pharmaceutical manufacturer in Germany and the world, with its dominant market share of cocaine, codeine and morphine, during the nineteenth and early twentieth centuries. When the US declared war on Germany in WWI in April 1917 and the Merck's US subsidiary detached from its German parent, which merged with Sharpe and Dhome to become Merck Sharpe and Dhome (aka MSD) in 1953.

Ether was successfully applied as a general anaesthetic by William T.G. Morton (1819–1868) to remove a tumour from a patient's neck at the Massachusetts General Hospital in 1846. Although the English chemist Joseph Priestly (1773–1704) discovered the anaesthetic gas nitrous oxide (known as laughing gas) in 1776, its clinical use in dentistry was only successfully applied almost a century later in the 1860s. In the following year, James Young Simpson (1811–1870), a professor of midwifery at the University of Edinburgh and the physician to Queen Victoria, searched for a colourless, non-explosive substitute for ether, something with a pleasant smell to patients, faster onset and easier to administer and found chloroform to be an effective anaesthetic. The use of chloroform in obstetrics became widespread throughout the British Empire in the nineteenth century. For example, William Aurelius Hartland (1822–1858) at the Seamen's Hospital in Wanchai, Victoria City (aka Hong Kong) recorded the use of chloroform in its first surgical operation on 18 March 1848. Queen Victoria also gave birth to her last two children, Prince Leopold, the eighth child in 1853, and Princess Beatrice, the ninth and the last child in 1857, with the chloroform anaesthetic.

In 1867, Joseph Lister (1827–1912), a professor of surgery at the University of Glasgow, extended the antiseptic theory of Ignaz Philipp Semmelweis, an obstetrician in Vienna, by applying phenol as an antiseptic to sterilize the hands of assistants, surgical instruments and their patients' incisions after operating. This antiseptic practice drastically reduced sepsis and fatalities due to childbed fevers and post-operative infections.

Many plants store chemicals as inactive glycosides, other than alkaloids, broken down into active drugs upon hydrolysis. French chemists Pierre Robiquet and Antoine Boutron-Charlard identified the first glycoside, amygdalin, in 1830. Oswald Schmiedeberg, professor at the Institute of Pharmacology in Strasburg, France, obtained a pure form of digitoxin in 1875. He used digitoxin, an important glycoside isolated from foxglove (digitalis), to treat congestive heart failure. In the last quarter of the nineteenth century, pharmaceutical houses in Germany conducted active research and development work on chemical and dyestuff's downstream products to optimise their investment returns. The rise of F. Bayer & Co. from a small dye company, which originated in Barmen in 1867, to a leading global chemical and pharmaceutical giant was a classic example.

In 1896, Bayer's director of pharmaceutical research, Arthur Eichengrun (1867–1949), with help from his laboratory assistant, Felix Hoffmann (1868–1946), synthesized two chemical drugs within a two-week interval in 1898. Both became the top-selling drug throughout the world in the early twentieth century. Acetylsalicylic acid (ASA, trade name Aspirin) is an analgesic, fever-lowering medicine and a blood thinner today. Heroin was used as a powerful cough suppressant for tuberculosis and pneumonia when first discovered. However, heroin's highly addictive effect and the tendency to be abused by its users prompted Bayer to withdraw the drug from the market in the early 1910s.[7] John Newport Langley (1852–1925), professor of physiology at Cambridge University, first published the "chemical receptor theory" in the Journal of Physiology in 1905. Professor Paul Ehrlich (1854–1915), a German physician and scientist of the Institute of Experimental Therapy in Frankfurt, verified Langley's theory with his "Magic Bullet", a significant milestone in drug discovery in the twentieth century. Paul Ehrlich (1854–1915) discovered that chemical dyes, such as arsenic compounds, could be bound onto microbes in 1907. Two years later, Ehrlich developed a drug codenamed 606 (chemical name arsphenamine, trade name Salvarsan). The latter was a highly effective antimicrobial but equally toxic arsenic drug in treating syphilis and was marketed by Hoechst GmbH (now Sanofi) in 1909. The discovery of chemical drug 606 (Salvarsan, generic drug name arsphenamine) was a godsend. It immediately replaced the ineffective mercury ointment, formulated by Swiss alchemist and apothecary, Paracelsius (1493–1541) to treat syphilis for over four centuries with mainly placebo effects. In the first half of the twentieth century, advances in the discovery of chemical drugs on both sides of the Atlantic Ocean, whether it was a targeted search like 606 or by serendipity like penicillin, led to a dramatic improvement in life expectancy to a level not seen at any time in human history.

However, the standards of chemical drugs, produced as bulk chemicals and packaged in solid dosage forms by tableting technology in factory production lines, could be better specified by the publication of drug monographs in national pharmacopoeias and pharmaceutical codex. In the nineteenth and twentieth centuries, the British and the US pharmacopoeias were gold standards for chemical, herbal and mineral drugs. With the easy availability and a lack of regulatory control of chemical drugs in Europe and North America, the free sale of pharmacopoeia narcotic drugs of cocaine, morphine, and heroin caused substantial social issues. For example, tens of millions of people abused laudanum, containing 10% powdered opium or 1% morphine, as a leisure drug in Asia, Europe, the UK and the US at the close of the nineteenth century.

In Asia, "opium cures", initially imported by western chemists in the early 1870s in the treaty ports of China and the colony of Hong Kong, soon flooded the market to substitute for opium smoking. By the 1890s, morphine injections and later heroin pills became hotly sought-after "opium cures" by tens of millions of leisure drug users. In 1900, Japanese and domestic manufacturers in China became the dominant suppliers of "opium cures" until the Second Sino-Japanese War (or the Pacific Theatre of World War II) ended in August 1945. Another milestone was erected for chemical drugs when a British Medical Research Council investigation published the double-blind cross-over drug trial of Streptomycin in the 30 October 1948 edition of the "British Medical Journal", verifying the clinical efficacy of the single-drug molecule.[8]

The East India Company, Ship Surgeons and Opium Traders

European monarchies awarded trade privileges to their respective country's East India Company, including the English in 1600, the Dutch in 1602, the French in 1664, and the Swedish in 1731. The English East India Company (EIC), granted under a Royal Charter by Queen Elizabeth I in 1600, was renamed the British East India Company a century later when the Kingdom of Scotland formed a political union with the Kingdom of England on 1 May 1707 to become the United Kingdom of Great Britain (Figs. 2.2 and 2.3). Tea, silk, porcelain, and Chinese materia medica exports to imperial British and European powers from the 1550s to 1830s generated a trade surplus in China's favour, increasing frustrations in these western countries. Moreover, the latter's agricultural or horticultural sectors could not supply the kind of medicinal herbs, fragrances and scents, and spices that the Chinese had become accustomed to with imports from Arabia, South and Southeast Asia throughout the previous two millennia. Although the Portuguese traders introduced tobacco smoking to China from South America in the mid-late sixteenth century, it was the Dutch traders who introduced opium mixed with tobacco from Java, via Taiwan, to the mainland a century later. The upper class of the Manchu Qing court picked up the habit in the mid-seventeenth century and they soon found a new way of smoking opium for enjoyment instead of mixing it with tobacco leaves. Only a small quantity of opium was imported then.

Among the western countries, the British became habitual drinkers of the first of the world's fast-moving consumer goods (FMCGs)—tea from China—until the 1830s when British imports gradually switched to India and Sri Lanka. On the other hand, tea from China produced one-tenth of the total tax revenue of England and the entire profit of the East India Company.[9] Increasing cargo of tea was being loaded onto the freighters from Europe without the export levies being paid due to rampant corruption of the officials in the three other ports besides Canton. The loss of the

Fig. 2.2 Corporate logo of
the English East India
Company in 1600s. *Source*
Author's image bank

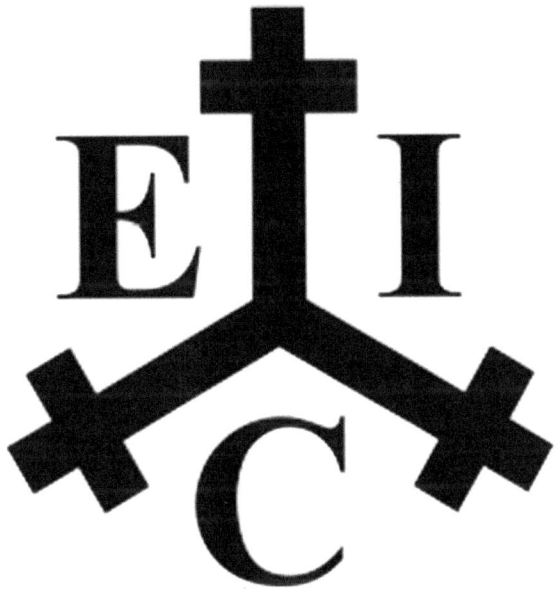

Fig. 2.3 Coats of arms, the
English East India Company
since 1600s. *Source*
Wikipedia

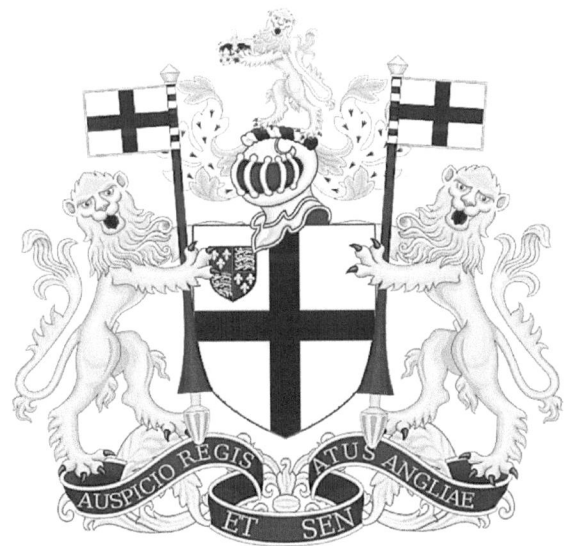

export excise tax led Emperor Kangxi to allow Canton, the only coastal city, to open
for trade with overseas merchants in 1757.

The more aggressive opium traders of the EIC teamed up with pirates using Macau
as a hub for smuggling opium in the late eighteenth century. They did it without
paying the hefty import duties imposed by the Manchu Qing government, with help

from the co-hong traders.[10] By then, a new class of opium smokers was emerging in the coastal provinces and southern China. These were the migrant workers who worked as transportation workers in the ports and turned to opium dross collected from the opium pipes of wealthy smokers or the opium dens. Opium dross was sold as second-hand smoke to the public. The EIC would allow its key employees in each voyage, such as a ship captain or surgeon, an amount of free cargo space appropriate to their rank, known as a "cargo privilege".

For example, many ship surgeons would carry medicines from animal parts or of herbal origins such as cassia, cochineal and musk as their cargo privilege for trading in the ports the EIC ships visited. As opium was the most profitable and was highly restricted, the EIC was cautious about not openly flaunting the Manchu Qing laws and regulations in the opium trade. However, the inland provinces were virtually untapped. As a result, the more ambitious employees of EIC, including ship surgeons such as Thomas Weeding, William Jardine, Robert Wigram, and others, became frustrated and could not wait. They soon left the employment of EIC and became independent opium traders.

William Jardine (1784–1843) decided to branch out as an independent opium trader in 1817 and partnered with a retired ship surgeon Thomas Wedding, and Parsi Indian cotton and opium trader Framji Cowaji Banaji (1767–1851). Jardine eventually teamed up with James Matheson to form Jardine, Matheson & Co. (JM & Co.) in 1832 (Fig. 2.4). With intensive advocacy and lobbying by the liberal trade activists in the United Kingdom, the British Parliament eventually terminated EIC's trade monopoly in India in 1813 and China in 1833.[11] During the 64 years from 1775 to 1839, the quantity of imports of opium took a quantum leap from 75 to 2553 tonnes, or 35 times.[12] Stricter laws with severe punishment by execution did not halt the smuggling of the highly profitable Patna brand of opium, equivalent to about 20–40% of the official import figures, from British India to China. This was primarily due to the high profitability of opium trade reaped by both Chinese and British merchants led to rampant corruption of middle-ranking officials who turned a blind eye to such clandestine activities. JM & Co. became the de facto 'King of Opium' in China after the British Crown withdrew EIC's trade monopoly in 1833.

JM & Co.'s official market share of opium imports was close to half the volume imported into China, with more shipments going through unofficial channels. However, a dispute on the taxing of illegal opium with the Chinese Customs Administration resulted in the opium stock of the traders, of which JM & Co. was the largest one, being confiscated and by Lin Zexu in Bogus Tigris (*Humen*) in June 1839. William Jardine arrived in London in September 1839. He successfully convinced the British government to send a large fleet of warships to China in mid-1840, which resulted in the First Opium War (First Anglo-Chinese War, 1839–1842). Benjamin Casson's recent research articulated the influence of Jardine on the First Opium War (1939–1942):

> Beyond Jardine's role in developing some of the military strategies used during the First Opium War, it is also important to understand his role as an opium importer. Since the early 1830's, Jardine & Matheson Co. had made a fortune as one of the premiere opium smugglers in China. The perfect way to expand the already growing trade was to have more Chinese ports

Fig. 2.4 Sir William Jardine
(1784–1843), opium trader,
lithograph, 1849. *Credit* T.H.
Miguire (1821–1895),
Wellcome Collection

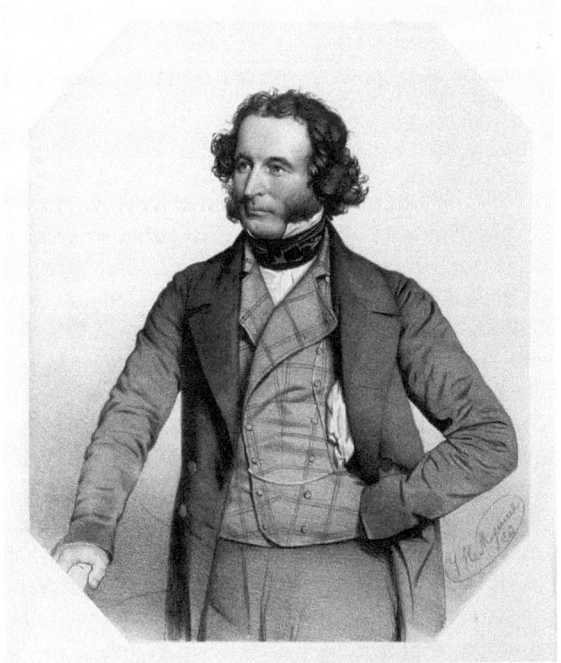

opened, and therefore accessible, to the highly addictive drug. With the Chinese hesitancy to open their Empire to further foreign influence, an open affront was the only way to increase the expansion of free trade. Recognizing this, Jardine began pushing for war as early as 1834. By the late 1830's he was a huge contributor to a media campaign that promoted the war, and by 1839 he had met with Lord Palmerston, and made his suggestions to the Foreign Office.[13]

After a protracted war, the governments of the Manchu Qing Empire and the United Kingdom eventually signed the Treaty of Nanking in 1842. Along with Hong Kong Island, ceded to the United Kingdom, five treaty ports also opened for business and missionary work (See Chap. 4). The opening of China in 1842 marked a significant turning point in Sino-British relationship. This event triggered a series of military conflicts as China sought to resolve disputes with Western powers and Japan. These conflicts persisted until the conclusion of World War II in 1945.

Adoption of Variolation, Needles and Pharmaceutical Technologies

Native civilizations have practised vaccination in Africa, Asia, and Europe since time immemorial. Master Ge Hong (283–363 CE), a Taoist alchemist and apothecary, published an eight-volume, seventy-chapter compendium of formulations to treat acute illnesses—*Zhou Hou Jiu Zu Fang* (肘后备急方, A Handbook of Formulas for Emergencies). He described ten formulations to treat rabies in the Formulary's chapter 54 of volume 7, with one using the rabies brain tissue:

> To treat patients with rabid dog bites is by variolation (applying the raw brain tissue of the freshly killed dog onto the wounds of patients) to confer lasting immunity to rabies.[14,15]

With 10% fatalities among those without vaccination in the 1790s in Britain, Edward Jenner (1749–1823), a physician in Gloucestershire, developed a variolation method using cowpox as the source material to impart smallpox immunity to children in 1796. The news of Jenner's incredible success in preventing smallpox infection in small children travelled far and fast across the continents. Dr. Alexander Pearson (1780–1874), a senior surgeon to the EIC, introduced the Jennerian vaccination in Macao and Canton in 1805.[16] Pearson published a booklet "The Extraordinary History of a New Method of Inoculation Discovered in the Kingdom of England" in 1805 and was translated by George Staunton into Chinese known as *Yingjiliiguo Xinchu Zongdou Qishu* (英吉利国新出种痘奇书) soon afterwards.[17] He subsequently taught the smallpox vaccination technique to several Chinese employees of the British Factory in Canton. One of them, Qiu Xi (邱熙), published the *Yindou Lue* (引痘略, Introduction to the Extraction of the Cowpox Vaccine) in 1817 on Pearson's application of cowpox to prevent smallpox using the meridian points of the acupuncture theory of Chinese medicine, which gained broad acceptance nationwide in the nineteenth century (Fig. 2.5).

Infectious diseases were the most debilitating ones in the rapidly industrialised countries of Europe in the second half of the nineteenth century due to poor nutrition, overcrowding and lack of sanitation facilities, including the supply of clean water at home. A French chemist and microbiologist, Louis Pasteur (1822–1895) published the "Germ Theory" in 1861. At the same time, Robert Koch (1843–1910), Director of the Prussian Hygienic Institute, halted the active use of parenteral administration, due to infections arising from the cross-use of needles, until moist heat sterilization was developed in 1881.

Koch extended steam sterilization to surgical instruments and morphine injection which soon became popular to relieve severe cough of tuberculosis and pneumonia in the industrialized towns of Europe. [18]Pasteur's theory had broad applications in vaccination, microbial fermentation, and pasteurization. Koch's research and development of the chicken cholera vaccine in 1879 laid the foundation for the newly developed immunology discipline. Koch discovered anthrax in 1876 which Pasteur subsequently verified. This led to the eventual launch of the live attenuated (weakened bacteria) cholera vaccine and inactivated (killed bacteria) anthrax vaccine in humans (1897 and 1904, respectively) demonstrating the principle of active and passive immunity through vaccination (Chart 2.4).

Waldemar Haffkine, the Ukraina-French bacteriologist, invented the plague vaccine in 1897. With help from Paul Ehrlich (1854–1915), a renowned physician and scientist at the Berlin Institute of Infectious Diseases, Emil von Behring (1854–1917), a physiologist, developed the passive immunity (or serum) therapy by using

Fig. 2.5 Summary of variolation (*Yin Dou Lue*), 1817. Block-Print in 1518. *Credit* Qiu Xi (Assisant to Dr. Alexander Perason)

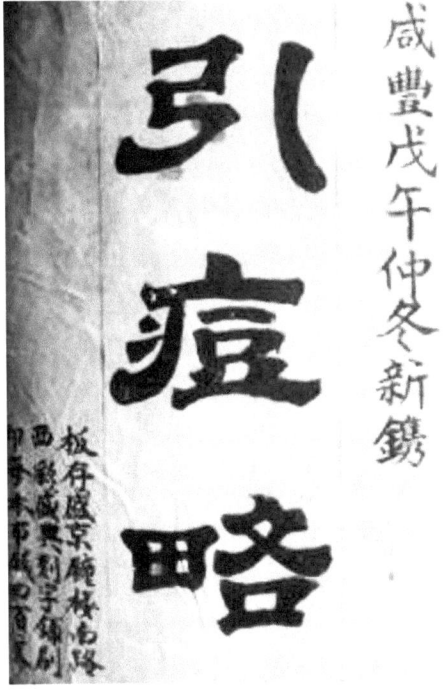

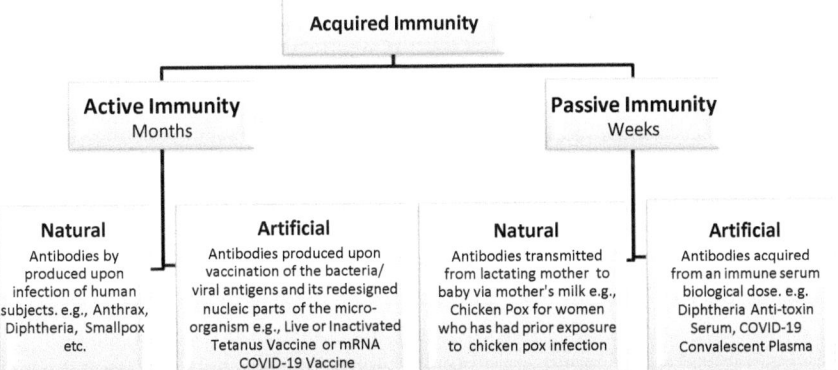

Chart 2.4 Types of acquired immunity; and their Bacteria/viral vaccines and plasma/sera. *Credit* Adapted from vaccines and immunization. Accessed May 3, 2023. https://www.who.int/health-topics/vaccines-andimmunization?adgroupsurvey

antitoxins (which contain antibodies) to treat the often fatal diphtheria infections in young children in 1894. Ehrlich further developed the standardization of diphtheria antitoxin, improving the serum therapy's success rate. Behring's research in the attenuated form of diphtheria toxoid vaccine to provide active immunity was further improved by the French scientist Gaston Gamon (1886–1963) using formaldehyde to inactivate the diphtheria toxoid. This technique has led to the low-cost production of diphtheria and tetanus vaccines. Mass immunization for children became feasible in the 1920s and 1930s, which saved millions of lives that would have otherwise been lost (Fig. 2.5). The combined pertussis, diphtheria, and tetanus vaccine to immunize children, produced in 1948, was another success in preventing these infections. Between 1890 and 1950, bacterial vaccine development increased, including the Bacillis–Calmette–Guerin (BCG) vaccination, which is still used today.

The liquid dosage form has existed as a medicinal soup in traditional medicine for centuries. A mixture of syrup in the modern era has been a popular oral drug administration method since the nineteenth century for the young and the senile. Suppositories, administered through the other end of the gut to bypass the gastric acid and enzymatic destruction in the duodenum and small intestines, remain a popular pharmaceutical dosage form in continental Europe, particularly France. Other oral dosage forms, such as the one-piece soft gelatin capsule, were developed by two French men; a pharmacy assistant, Francois Achille Barnabe Mothes, and pharmacist Joseph Gerard Auguste Dublanc, in 1834. Twelve years later, another French pharmacist, J. C. Lehuby, patented the two-piece empty hard gelatin capsule by dipping metal pins into glycerogelatin.[19]

Innovation in drug administration by parenteral means in the form of glass syringes and metal needles was a breakthrough. Intravenous drug administration of antibiotics is the only way to treat life-threatening acute infections, as the oral route takes half an hour through the gut before absorption into the bloodstream. Alexander Wood (1817–1884), a Scottish physician who graduated with an MD at the University of Edinburgh in 1832, was inspired by Simpson's anaesthesia technique to relieve pain during operations. Wood injected morphine into the discomfort area where the patient complained of neuralgia. As pharmacies were not under regulatory control in Europe, North America or the treaty ports of China, western medical missionaries led by Dr. John Glasgow Kerr (1824–1901) at the Canton Hospital used morphine injection as an "*opium cure*" in late 1892. Western retail chemists such as A.S. Watson promptly found that morphine injections could replace the opium smoking of tens of millions of labourers. Watson's brand of "opium cures" became a star product in the next 40 years.

Medical technology was elevated to the next quantum in the late nineteenth century when Wilhelm Conrad Rontgen (1845–1923), a German physicist and mechanical engineer, produced and detected electromagnetic radiation in a wavelength range called X-rays or Rontgen rays in 1895. The discovery of X-rays broadened diagnostic radiography in viewing the internal organs, such as the lungs of tuberculosis patients with scarry tissue, and the prognosis of chronic and fatal diseases such as malignant tumours. Ten years later, Pierre and Marie Curie received the Nobel Prize in Physics for their pioneering work in developing the "radioactivity" theory.[20]

Notes and References

1. O'Connor, Daniel, *Chaplains of the East India Company, 1601–1858* (London, Continuum 2012), 26.
2. The Thirteen Factories or "Hongs" 十三行 were western trading houses from Europe and the United States allowed to set up an office and warehouse by the Manchu Qing government of China in the late eighteenth century in the designated area of Canton 广东. Each of the "Thirteen Hongs" conducted their import and export business via their respective Chinese agents known as "Co-Hongs" 公行 who also served as the guarantors of their foreign principals should a trade dispute arisen.
3. Leigh, Denis, Medicine, The City and China, Medical History, 18 (1974):51-67. Accessed 29 September 2023. https://www.ncbi.nlm.nih.gov/pmc/articles/PMC1081522/pdf/medhist00 120-0056.pdf.
4. As owner representative for the goods carried on board of the English (later as British) East India Company fleet, the supercargoes on board of the English (later as British) East India Company fleet were the most important persons after the captain. They were responsible in managing the inventory on board, selling at the ports of call, buying and receiving the merchandise on their return voyage.
5. Local Revenues, Hong Kong Blue Book, 1870–1940, Hong Kong Government Reports [online]. Accessed 29. September 2023. https://sunzi.lib.hku.hk/hkgro/browse.jsp.
6. The Merck's family apothecary business dates back to the Engel-Apotheke or Angel Apothecary in Darmstadt, Germany when Jacob Frederick Merck purchased the town's second pharmacy in 1868.
7. Aspirin's anti-platelet function of aspirin was first discovered in the early 1950s by Lawrence L. Craven with substantial clinical studies verifyingits efficacy in the late 1980s. With extensive usage of Aspirin in patients with heart diseases since the 1990s, the Food and Drug Administration of the US issued its announcement that only selective patients under specialist care could benefit from daily aspirin therapy in its announcement of 7 December 2015. https://www.fda.gov/drugs/bioterrorism-and-drug-preparedness/daily-aspirin-therapy.
8. Streptomycin Treatment of Pulmonary Tuberculosis, *British Medical Journal,* no. 2 (1948):769–782. Accessed 29 September 2023. https://www.jameslindlibrary.org/medical-research-council-1948b/.
9. The first tea crop regulated the sailing times from England to Canton, which began in November. The trade season would last roughly until March of the following year, when the foreign community in Canton retired to Macao for the next six months. In 1686, Western men were allowed to reside within the trading zone during the trading seasons in the leased quarters built by authorized Chinese merchants, known as co-hong merchants, who were sponsors of their foreign partners.
10. The co-hong merchants were the local collaborators who were partners of the British tea and opium traders associated with the EIC to import legal and illegal opium in Guangzhou. The opium traders bypassed the Customs. Administration in Guangzhou to make substantial profits for each party.
11. East India Company and Raj 1785–1858, UK Parliament. Accessed 29 September 2023. https://www.parliament.uk/about/living-heritage/evolutionofparliament/legislativescrutiny/parliament-and-empire/parliament-and-the-american-colonies-before-1765/east-india-com pany-and-raj-1785-1858/.
12. Chawla, Sandeep et al. *A Century of International Drug Control*, (Vienna: United Nations Office on Drug and Crime Control, 2008), 23. Accessed 29 September 2023. https://www.unodc.org/documents/data-and-analysis/Studies/100_Years_of_Drug_Control.pdf.
13. Cassan, Benjamin, *William Jardine: Architect of the First Opium War*, Eastern Illinois University, Department of History, 2005 [online] 14, no. 1 (2005), 107–117. Accessed 29 September 2023. https://www.eiu.edu/historia/Cassan.pdf.
14. Tarantola, Arnaud, "Four Thousand Years of Concepts Relating to Rabies in Animals and Humans, Its Prevention and Its Cure". Tropical Medicine and Infectious Disease. 2, no. 2,

2017: 5. Accessed 29 September 2023. https://www.ncbi.nlm.nih.gov/pmc/articles/PMC608 2082/.

15. Based on modern immunity principles, using live rabies material is highly risky as the material has not been sterilized and could lead to serious repercussions including sepsis and cross contamination. It is therefore assumed that Ge Hong's reporting the use of rabies brain material was not based on his clinical experience and most likely from a secondary source.

16. Leung, AK, The business of vaccination in nineteenth-century Canton. *Late Imperial China*, Society for Qing Studies and The John Hopkins University Press, 29, No. 1 (2008): 7–39. https://www.hkihss.hku.hk/filemanager/content/others/angela-ki-che-leung/pdf/articles/2008_business.pdf.

17. Chang, C, The Localization of the Cowpox Vaccination in Early Nineteenth-Century China, Bulletin of Institute of History and Philology,78, no.4 (2007), 755–812, esp.757–761. https://www2.ihp.sinica.edu.tw/file/2902rSdirIK.pdf.

18. Belvins, S., Bronze, M., Robert Koch and the 'golden age' of bacteriology, *International Journal of Infectious Diseases*, 14 (2010), esp. 744–751.

19. Franc, A, Vetchy, D., and Fulopova, N., Commercially Available Enteric Empty Hard Capsules, Production. *Technology and Application,* Pharmaceuticals, MDPI, 2022, 15, 1398: 4. https://doi.org/10.3390/ph15111398.

20. In continental Europe, Marie Salomea Skłodowska Curie (1867–1934), a Polish born physicist and chemist, who together with her husband, Pierre Curie, and Henri Becquerel, in Paris, France received the Nobel Prize in Physics for their pioneering work in developing the "radioactivity" theory in 1905.

Chapter 3
Union Medical College and The "Cradle of Modern Medicine"

This chapter aims to shed light on the crucial role of British medical missionaries in China during the nineteenth century, focusing on the Union Medical College (协和医学堂, *Xihe Yixue Tang*, UMC), as a compelling case study. Examining the UMC's transformation from a charitable hospital to a privately funded university hospital between 1860 and 1949 reveals numerous opportunities and challenges.

China's first western hospital was the St. Raphael's Hospital (医人庙, *I Yan Miu*, or the Temple of Cures), opened by Bishop Belchior Carneiro in Macau in 1569. St. Raphael's Hospital pharmacy was officially opened with a full-time pharmacist in 1783 for the free supply of medicines to the poor. A century after, the Sisters of St. Paul de Chartres, a religious order originally hailing from France, expanded their Wanchai orphanage, known as Asile de la Sainte Enfance or "Asylum of the Holy Childhood." In 1898, recognizing the growing need for medical services among the underprivileged, they transformed the orphanage into a hospital which was renamed as the St. Paul's Hospital (圣保禄医院) in 1918. The Protestants also played an active role with Dr. William Lockhart (雒魏林, 1881–1896) of the London Missionary Society (LMS), built the Peking Hospital, locally known as the Free Healing Hospital (施医院, *Shiyiyuan*), in 1861 (Fig. 3.1).[1,2,3] Unfortunately, supporters of the Boxers Movement burnt down the Peking Hospital in the summer of 1900. Dr. Thomas Cochrane (1886–1953) arrived in Beijing to resume LMS's medical activities in the spring of 1902. With the help of his assistant, Li Xiaochun (李小川, Li Hsiao Chuan), Dr. Cochrane established China's first western medical College, UMC, with seed funding from the Empress Dowager Cixi (慈禧太后, the "Old Buddha") in 1903.

The UMC Hospital was formed after the Free Healing Hospital amalgamation with other medical institutions under the direction of the LMS, with a new purpose-built medical school and a 30-bed hospital in 1906 (Fig. 3.2). The American "Oil King" John Rockefeller (1839–1937), through his eponymous Rockefeller Foundation and its wholly owned subsidiary CMB, decided to acquire the UMC for the price of US $200,000 in 1915.[4] A prefix "Peking" was added to

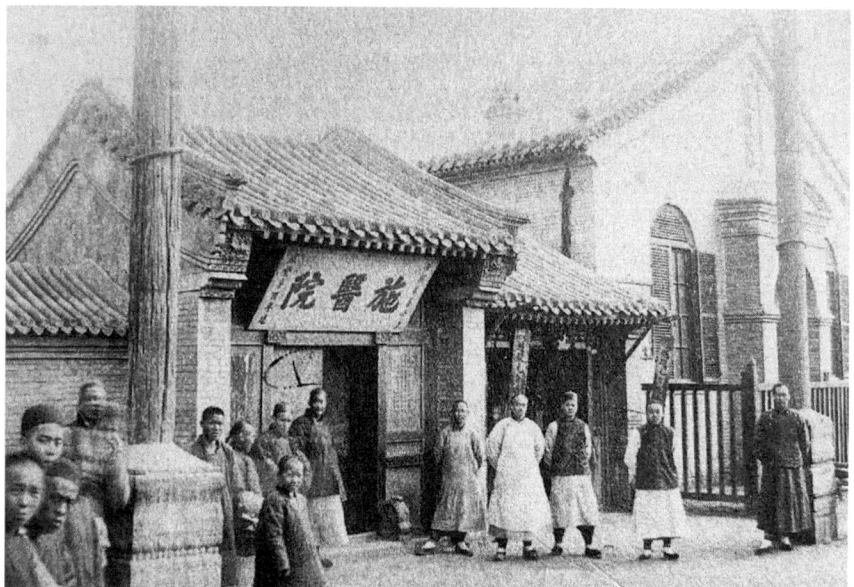

Fig. 3.1 Free Healing Hospital (施医院, *Shi Yi Yuan*), also called Two Flagstaffs Hospital (双旗竿医院, *Shuang Gigan Yiyua*n) by locals @ 1890s. *Credit* Dr. Thomas Cochrane III

the original name of UMC to become the Peking Union Medical College (PUMC). A total of US $7.6 million was spent on the project, which was many times over the original budget, due to lack of management control, the inadequate construction experience of the CMB, and high shipping costs during the First World War. A completely new PUMC Hospital was built in 1921, and is one of China's oldest Western hospitals, celebrating its 100th anniversary in 2021. PUMC Hospital continuously ranked as China's top general hospital for the thirteenth year in 2022.[5] Together with its affiliated medical institute, the UMC has been generally regarded as the "Cradle of Modern Medicine" since the 1920s. Frank McLean (1888–1968), a young professor of pharmacology and therapeutics at the Rockefeller Institute for Medical Research, became the PUMC's founding director. It was financed entirely by the CMB with a first-rate teaching faculty composed of researchers and clinicians.[6] From 1910 and 1941, PUMC Hospital's western-trained pharmacists established it as a model of hospital pharmacy. Zhu Zhu, said:

> Western pharmacists serving as lecturers in materia medica to medical and nursing students at the PUMC not only played a crucial role in educating students but also served as "gatekeepers" in the safe and cost-effective distribution of drugs and narcotics within the Hospital. The PUMC's pharmacy technician programme trained several hundred dispensing assistants, meeting half of China's needs in the 1910–1949 period. An unparalleled achievement in the history of pharmacy in China.[7]

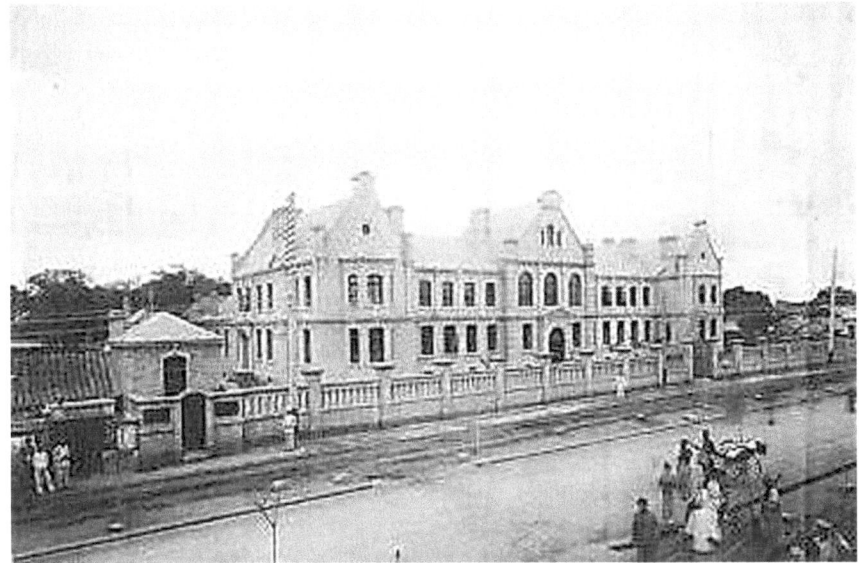

Fig. 3.2 The Union Medical College, Hataman Boulevard, Peking (now Chongwenmen Street, Beijing) @ 1906. *Credit* Dr. Thomas Cochrane III

Dr. Thomas Cochrane, The "Old Buddha" and The "Oil King"

Dr. William Lockhart (1811–1896) was instrumental in the opening up of four western hospitals in Chusan (Zhoushan, 1841), Hong Kong (1842), Shanghai (1844), and Beijing (1861) on the China coast. The PUMC could trace its humble beginnings to September 1861 when Dr. Lockhart moved to Beijing and became a senior physician to the British Legation. A month later, he helped the LMS to open the Peking Hospital. In the first year, he treated 22,144 patients, or more than 60 a day. Dr. Lockhart made significant contributions to medical services and the cause of evangelism in China during the late Manchu Qing dynasty. In 1864, Dr. John Dudgeon (德貞, 1837–1901) succeeded Dr. Lockhart as the head of LMS in Beijing.

   Dr. Dudgeon was born on 7 April, 1837 in Galston, Aryshire, Scotland. He graduated with a degree in Doctor of Medicine, and a Master of Surgery at the University of Glasgow in 1862. After joining LMS the following year, Dr. Dudgeon left Glasgow with his new wife on 21 July and arrived in Shanghai in December. In March 1864, he arrived in Beijing and immediately took over the position of Dr. Lockhart.[8] Dr. Dudgeon served as a physician to the British Legation in Beijing from 1864 to 1868. In 1865, he acquired a Buddhist temple with two flagstaffs at Chongwenmen Street (Hatamen Boulevard) and expanded the Peking Hospital (the "Hospital") at this new venue. The locals commonly called the hospital by two interchangeable names: the Free Healing Hospital and the Two Flagstaffs Hospital.

Dr. John Dudgeon was appointed Professor of Anatomy and Physiology at the Imperial College (同文馆, *Tongwen Guan*) of the Manchu Qing Government during the 1870s and 1880s. Over 10 years, Dr. Dudgeon translated Gray's Anatomy and Holden's Osteology into an 18-volume Chinese edition published in 1884. He was a champion of the anti-opium crusade in the 1870s. Dr. Dudgeon even opposed morphine as a substitute for opium when its habit-forming effects became known to be even worse than opium. However, after repeated conflicts with the LMS over prioritising evangelical over medical work, Dr. Dudgeon resigned in 1884. After that, he continued in private practice in Beijing until his death in February 1901.[9]

Dr. Thomas Cochrane (科龄, 1866–1953), a Scotsman who had studied medicine in Glasgow, served in Chaoyang, Manchuria, from 19 May 1887 to the spring of 1900.[10] In the middle of the Boxers Movement, the Free Healing Hospital was burnt down. The militant Boxers, organized by some court officials, created a violent uprising in 1899, finally crushed by the Eight-Nation Alliance in 1900. A year later, Cochrane returned to China from Britain and arrived Beijing in March 1902.[11] He had a competent auxiliary, Li Xiaochun to help out with the clinic (Fig. 3.3). Cochrane's dream was to build a medical college that could train practitioners of modern medicine in China (Fig. 3.4). Dr. Cochrane had treated many VIP patients of the Imperial Court. Then, one winter evening in 1903, he received an extraordinary patient, Li Lianying (李莲英, 1848–1911), the Chief Eunuch of the Manchu Qing Court, who was the personal attendant of the "Old Buddha". Dr. Cochrane fostered a friendship with Chief Eunuch Li Lianying when he performed a urological procedure to relieve excruciating pain from a swollen bladder which he suffered due to a castration completed before his admission into the court as a eunuch.[12] During Chief Eunuch Li's second visit, Dr. Cochrane expressed his wish to build a medical college and hospital to train physicians in China. His departing remarks were:

> Dr. Cochrane, please petition Empress Dowager as soon as possible. I will recommend your proposal strongly. However, I cannot guarantee the results, but I will make every endeavour to realize your wish.[13]

Shortly after, Dr. Cochrane visited his friend and a patient, Grand Councillor Natong (那桐, 1857–1925). Unfortunately, when they met, his mother was critically ill. Dr. Cochrane diagnosed her condition as pneumonia. She recovered quickly, thanks to Dr. Cochrane. As a gesture of gratitude, on behalf of Dr. Cochrane, Grand Councillor Natong petitioned the "Old Buddha" to build a medical college. Other foreign dignitaries also supported Dr. Cochrane behind the scenes. They included the British Resident Minister in Beijing, Sir Ernest Satow, British Legation Medical Officer Dr. Douglas Gray, and Sir Robert Hart, the Inspector-General of China's Imperial Maritime Custom Service.[14] After months of intensive lobbying, the "Old Buddha" approved a seed fund of £1400 sterling pounds (equivalent to 10,000 taels of silver) to build the medical college and a thirty-bed hospital on 26th May 1903. Senior officials of the imperial court further contributed another £1600. Emperor Guangxu (1871–1908) also granted land next to Dr. Cochrane's site for building the UMC and hospital.

Fig. 3.3 Dr. Thomas
Cochrane (1866–1953).
Founder of Union Medical
College, 1906. *Credit* Dr.
Thomas Cochrane III

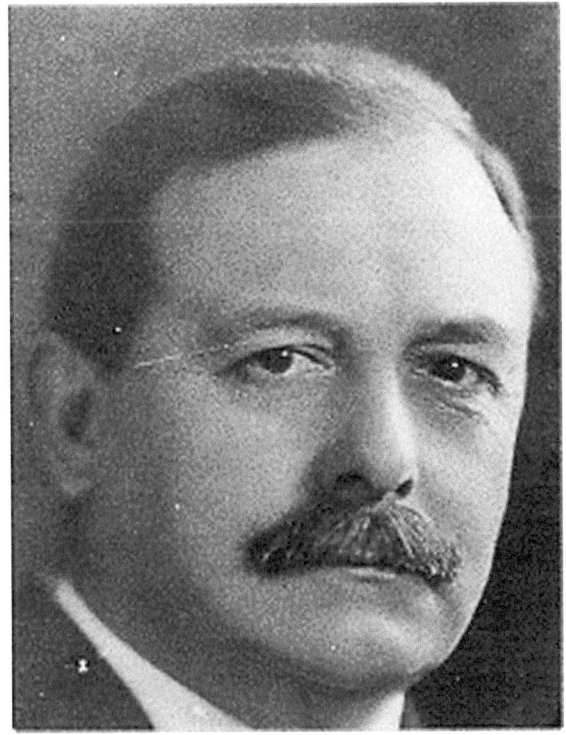

Donations continued to come from provincial governors, wealthy Chinese and foreign traders, entrepreneurs and individuals. The Arthington Trust also contributed to the LMS to build a new medical college and a thirty-bed teaching hospital with a consolidated total of £8680 (equivalent to 62,000 tales of silver).[15] The project was completed in 1906 and signalled the rebirth with a new Union Medical College name. (Image 4) The academic building was named Lockhart Hall, commemorating the founder of the Free Healing Hospital in 1861. The Grand Councillor Natong officiated at the opening ceremony on an auspicious day, the twentieth day of the first month in the lunar new year of the horse, on 13th February 1906, with 350 people in attendance. Two imperial princes, dukes, and representatives from the Great Powers and diplomatic corps participated in the inauguration.[16] "Great Powers" referred to as the Eight-Nation Alliance, included the original members of the Congress of Vienna of 1805; the Austrian Empire, France, Prussia, Russia and Great Britain with Italy, Japan, and the United States added a century later. The UMC was the only medical school recognized by the Board of Education of the Manchu Qing Government. Grand Councillor Natong said in the inauguration speech of the UMC:

> Dr. Thomas Cochrane is a gentleman eminent in his profession who spares no pains in carrying his project to a successful issue. One day, the College will become an instrument of incalculable benefit. Its fame will spread throughout the Chinese Empire.[17]

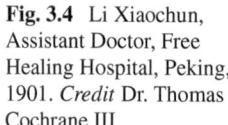

Fig. 3.4 Li Xiaochun,
Assistant Doctor, Free
Healing Hospital, Peking,
1901. *Credit* Dr. Thomas
Cochrane III

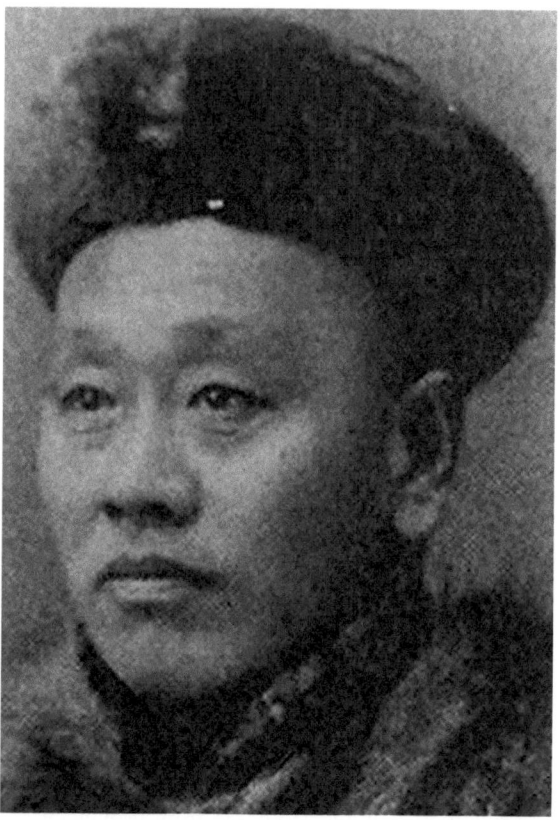

Sir Robert Hart (1863–1911), who was the most influential westerner at the Manchu Qing court, and Cockrane's patron, said in his speech:

> The students at the UMC will make scientific discoveries of worldwide importance. No country values education more than China, and it is only a matter of time before the College receives regular government support.[18]

In the same year, forty students were enrolled at the UMC to study medicine with a 5-year curriculum. Like other missionary medical colleges in China, the teaching medium was Chinese, but students also learned English. By then, quite the linguist, Dr. Cochrane was a fluent Mandarin speaker and had translated and published two textbooks: "Heath's Anatomy" in 1909 and "Heath's Osteology" in 1910. In those days, infectious diseases such as syphilis, hookworm, and tuberculosis were the most severe problems. By then, the UMC's staff consisted of 13 foreign doctors and one pharmacist for 95 medical students and 43 students in a preparatory department with a 1-year programme (Fig. 3.5).[19]

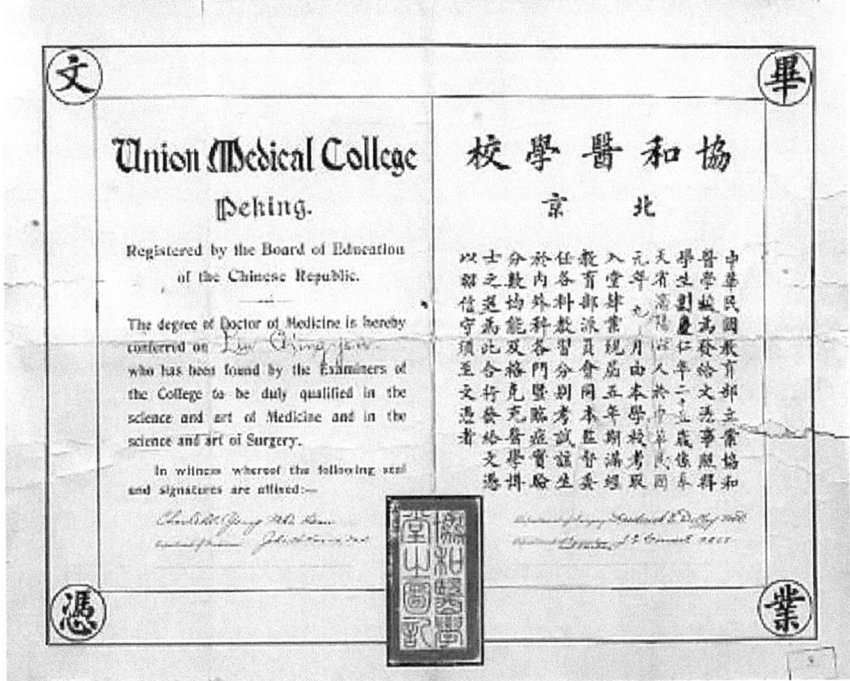

Fig. 3.5 Graduate Diploma of Union Medical College @ 1912. *Credit* Dr. Thomas Cochrane III

The pharmacist, Bernard Emms Read (1887–1949), a devout Christian and a pharmacist, was recruited by Dr. Cochrane as a lecturer in chemistry and pharmacy at the UMC and the pharmacy supervisor at the UMC Hospital in 1910.[20] Read was responsible for teaching pharmacy, pharmaceutics, dispensing, and practicum to second and third-year students, with many becoming hospital doctors after graduation. On 7th April 1911, Dr. Cochrane witnessed the graduation of 16 medical students after 5 years of studying at the UMC with a diploma issued by the Manchu Qing government's Ministry of Education (the Ministry) (Fig. 3.6). Thus, Dr. Cochrane's dream came true within 8 years of first communicating the idea to Chief Eunuch Li in 1903.

The Rockefeller Foundation was established in 1913 by the "Oil King", to bring western medicine to developing countries, including China. The first China Medical Commission (the Commission) organized by the Rockefeller Foundation arrived in Beijing on 18th April 1914, four months before World War I started in Europe. In 1914, 244 missionary hospitals and 446 western doctors served China's 400 million population.[21] The Commission representatives cited seventeen medical schools that were representative of the state of medical education in China. Amongst the sixteen other medical schools reviewed by the Commission, the UMC was the one that stood out as the most eligible candidate for Rockefeller Foundation investment. The Foundation set up the CMB on 30th November 1914 to implement the Commission's recommendations to build an influential medical school with a lasting impact in

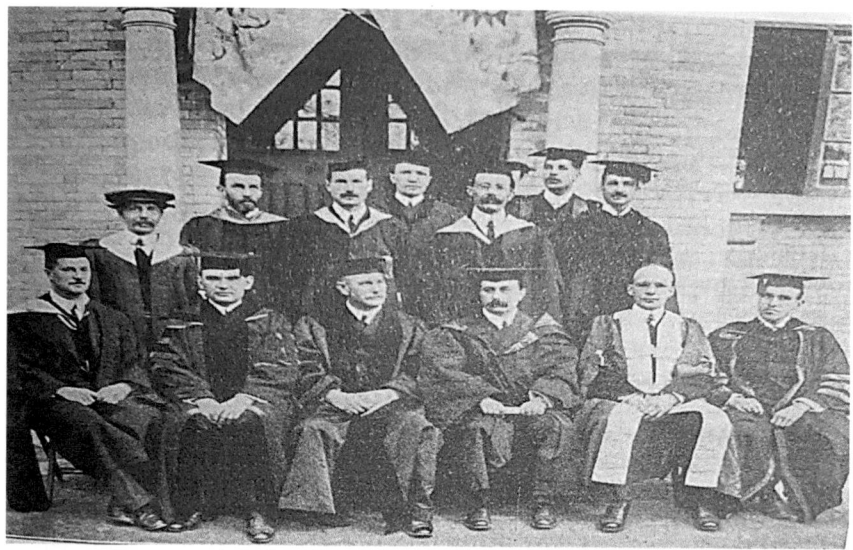

Fig. 3.6 In 1911, the UMC 15 professors including 14 medical doctors and 1 pharmacist. Front row, third person on the right, Dr Thomas Cochrane, second row, 1st person on the right, Bernard Read. *Credit* Dr Andy Adam.

China.[22] The logo of CMB is composed of a dragon representing China and a rod that is similar to the Rod of Asclepius representing medicine (Fig. 3.7). Wallace Buttrick, the first director of CMB, visited the missionary societies in England in April 1915 to enlist their support and established the terms for the final purchase of the UMC from the LMS. Following this, Dr. Cochrane, the medical director of the LMS, supported the sale of the assets of the UMC to CMB. Two months later, a memorandum was signed on 2nd June 1915 between the CMB and the LMS to acquire its properties for US$200,000.[23]

Dr. Cochrane's original intention was for the new medical school to continue to be taught in Chinese as more students could become medical doctors than a privileged few.[24] Buttrick led a second Commission to China in September and October 1915 to strategise on future public health and medical education investments. With the intensification of WWI, UMC faculty's 14 foreign medical personnel were reduced to just three. The majority returned to the frontlines of combat in Europe as field physicians. Buttrick submitted the trip report to the CMB and recommended focusing on medical education. To support the UMC in providing proper teaching and hospital services, the Rockefeller Foundation approved an additional US$1 million in funding for land, buildings and equipment in April 1916. In the same year, Bernard Read was awarded a CMB scholarship to study biochemistry and pharmacology at Yale University where he graduated in 1918 (Fig. 3.8).

Fig. 3.7 China Medical Board logo with Dragon and the rod of Asclepius symbolizing China and medicine. *Credit* China Medical Board

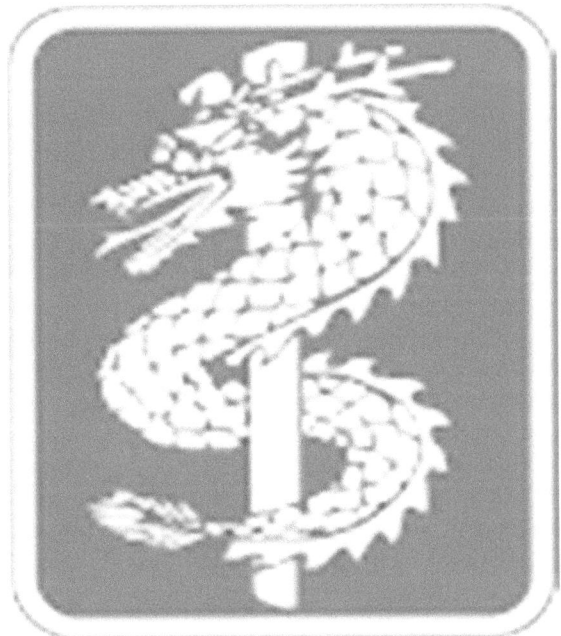

Fig. 3.8 Bernard Emms Read (1887–1949) Professor in Pharmacology, PUMC. *Credit* China Medical Board

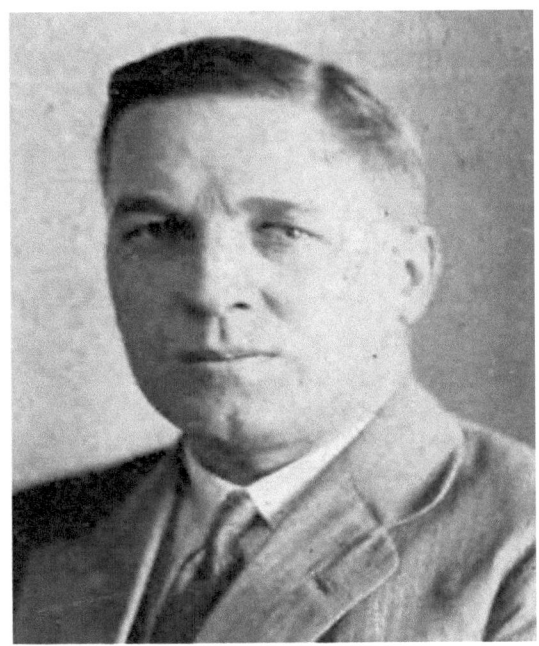

The decision of the CMB for the new medical school to be in Beijing was due to these critical factors: the city was the capital of three consecutive dynasties and would highly likely continue to be one; the national education centre with students from all corners of the country was there; Mandarin had become the official language of the ruling monarchs in the past several centuries; Its superior location with several buildings that CMB could put the new medical College into good use for some years to come; and it gave creditability to the UMC as the only government-recognized medical College.

The UMC was the best investment among the 16 missionary medical colleges and four private medical schools in China. The German Medical School for Chinese (德文医学堂, Deutsche Medizinschule für Chinesen, *Dewen Xixue Tang*) founded by a German physician Erich H. Paulun in 1907, had a better curriculum than the Harvard Medical School of China and was located in Shanghai. However, its teaching medium was German and not English.[25,26] The acquisition of the UMC by the Rockefeller Foundation transformed it from a charity organization to an upmarket, private medical college and hospital. The teaching medium of the first intake of the new medical faculty also changed from Chinese to English to attract a first-rate medical faculty from the US. The cornerstone of the newly renamed Peking Union Medical College (PUMC) was laid on 11th September 1917, when the first batch of eight students enrolled at its pre-medical school.[27]

The inauguration ceremony of the PUMC and the newly built 250-bed hospital started with an academic procession at 4.00 pm on 19th September 1921. CMB has now become the board governing the strategic direction of the PUMC When the Nationalist government relocated the capital from Beijing to Nanjing in 1928, the PUMC was again renamed as Peiping Union Medical College. The word *king*, as in Pe*king* in Chinese, referred to the capital city changed its name to *ping*, as in Pei*ping*—a peaceful city. The same year, CMB became an independent entity of the Rockefeller Foundation as the unexpectedly heavy demands of the PUMC placed a strain on the foundation's financial resources.[28] In the prime years from 1921 to 1942, the year the Japanese Imperial Army completely took over PUMC, it was the leading teaching hospital with a first-rate clinical research programme in Chinese medicine. (Chap. 8) At the end of the Second Sino-Japanese War in 1945, the CMB invested 10 million dollars to reopen the PUMC and its hospital. As a result, the PUMC Hospital reopened in 1948 for 2 years. In 1950, CMB exited the Mainland after the Communists founded the People's Republic of China on 1st October 1949. The PUMC Hospital changed its name to China Union Medical College Hospital as a teaching hospital.

British Pharmacists and the UMC

In the late nineteenth and early twentieth century, covering the late Manchu Qing dynasty and the early Nationalist Era in China, qualified pharmacists were trained professionally in retail chemists and druggists and hospital dispensaries in the UK and the US. Some of these young pharmacists had a pioneering spirit to make a difference in their missionary work in China. Bernard Read (伊博恩, 1887–1949) was the first British pharmacist to join the UMC He was a devout Christian from Brighton, England.[29] Read graduated with a Diploma from the Pharmaceutical Society of Great Britain (PSGB)'s School of Pharmacy in 1908 and registered as a pharmaceutical chemist in April 1909.[30] From 1909 to 1915, Read was an instructor in chemistry and pharmacy for pre-medical year students who initially enrolled at the UMC[31] Concurrently, Read was also the pharmacy supervisor of the UMC's hospital. After the CMB acquired the UMC, Read was groomed to be a pharmacology professor with scholarships to pursue advanced studies and research in the US. (See the section on *State and Private Research Institutes,* Chap. 7).

The second pharmacist, a former manager of A.S. Watson's Tianjin (Tisentsin) Branch, Alfred John Skinn (史京), was a natural successor of Read when he went on an MSc. Degree scholarship at Yale University in 1906–1908. Skinn was born in Bourne, Lincolnshire, England, in 1882. He qualified as a chemist and druggist with the PSGB in July 1910 and soon moved to Tianjin, a port city 66 miles (107 km) from Beijing.[32,33] Before joining the PUMC, Skinn had gained ample experience controlling drug costs as a dispensing and manufacturing chemist supplying to retail chemists and western hospitals and clinics in North China. Skinn served as the PUMC's hospital pharmacist from 1916 to 1917 while Read was away in the United States. When CMB acquired the PUMC in 1915, its hospital operations changed. It was no longer a charity but a privately funded hospital with most patients paying consulting fees. Hence, every department's financial management, particularly the pharmacy department where the supervisor booked daily transactions, had balancing costs and profitability as a top priority. The Hospital management recognized Skinn's business skills in controlling the costs of the Hospital pharmacy. In addition, when George Wilson, the PUMC's treasurer, was on leave for WWI service in Europe, Skinn served as the acting treasurer from 1917 until 1919. In Beijing, Skinn was also a junior warden of the freemasons of the China District of the International Chapter of the Grand Lodge of Massachusetts.[34] Skinn returned to Edinburgh, Scotland, in the early 1920s to study medicine and received his qualification as MB, ChB in July 1925 at 43. He later went to Hong Kong and entered private practice in 1930. Following the end of the Second World War, Skinn settled in Queensland, Australia and passed away in 1970 at 88.

The third pharmacist, Arthur John Daniel Britland (布兰德), succeeded Skinn in 1917. He was born on 13th August 1878.[35] He passed the minor examination, became a member of the PSGB and registered as a pharmaceutical chemist on 9th January 1902.[36] At thirty-eight, Britland joined the Anglican Mission to work as a pharmaceutical missionary in Beijing. Britland worked as the pharmacist at the PUMC

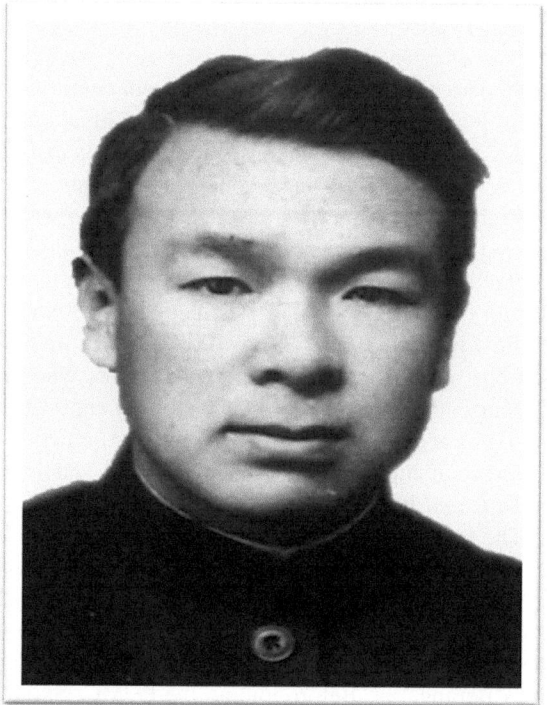

Hospital between 1917 and 1919. He supervised Moody Meng, who worked between 1917 and 1919. He supervised Moody Meng, who worked as a dispensary assistant there from 1916–1919. Britland sponsored Moody Meng's sea passage to study at the School of Pharmacy of London University in 1919.[37] After leaving the PUMC in 1920, Britland continued to live in Beijing and worked for the Church of England Peking Mission. While on leave in London, Britland interviewed Moody Meng on behalf of the PUMC for an assistant pharmacist position in mid-1924 (Fig. 3.9). Meng was offered the assistant pharmacist position to commence in January 1925, succeeding Yin-dah Hsu, who resigned in December 1924.[38] Britland was interned during the Japanese occupation in Weixian (Weihsien) in Shandong from 1943 until 1945. He returned to the United Kingdom after WWII and passed away on 21st November 1966.[39]

The fourth pharmacist, Xu Yinda (徐英达, Yin-Dah Hsu), was one of just two graduates from Yale College in China in 1916. Hsu received a 2-year CMB scholarship and graduated as a pharmaceutical chemist at the University of Maryland in the US in 1918. Hsu joined the PUMC's Hospital soon after graduation and worked as an assistant pharmacist until 1924. The fifth pharmacist, John Cameron (康约翰, 1891–1964), was born in Scotland in 1891 (Figs. 3.10 and 3.11). He received his MPS qualification in 1920 and moved to Beijing soon afterwards. He witnessed the opening of the enlarged PUMC upon its completion in 1921. In 1929, Cameron,

Moody Meng and an in-house trained assistant pharmacist, Tu Wan-Heng (杜万亨, Du Wanxiang), set up a pharmacy technician school in collaboration with the North China Pharmaceutical Society. When Cameron was away on his furlough in 1926 and 1931, Meng served as the acting pharmacy supervisor (Fig. 3.12). While still employed by the PUMC in 1939, Cameron was seconded to work in war service in Britain during WWII (1939–1945). He resigned from the PUMC the following year to take up a full-time position as Director, Medical Supplies, Middle East Section when he was with the Scottish Department of Health. During his 20 years as a lecturer in the PUMC and the Hospital pharmacy supervisor, Cameron was a leader who championed best-practice pharmacy management.

For example, Cameron was responsible for publishing four out of the six hospital formularies to promote the rational use of drugs, manufacturing of pharmaceuticals, quality, safe storage and distribution of narcotic medicines and poisons. Cameron was an Honorary Fellow of the American Pharmaceutical Association, the PSGB, the Chemical Society, the Royal Geological Society and the Royal Society of Edinburgh. He passed away in Vancouver, Canada, in 1964 at 73.[40]

The sixth pharmacist, Moody Meng (孟目的, 1897–1983), was born in October 1897 to a Protestant family in Baoding County, Hebei Province, about ninety-three miles or one-hundred-and-fifty kilometres southwest of Bejing. His father was a

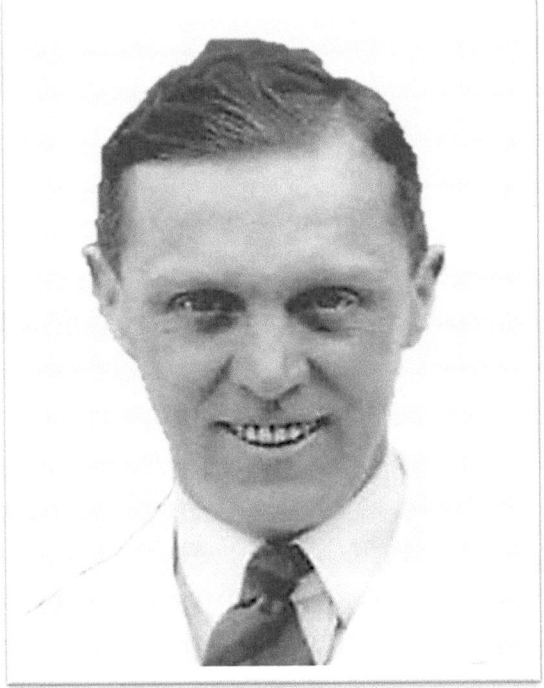

Fig. 3.10 John Cameron in laboratory coat @1925. *Credit* Meng Zhaoyi and Meng Xianwei

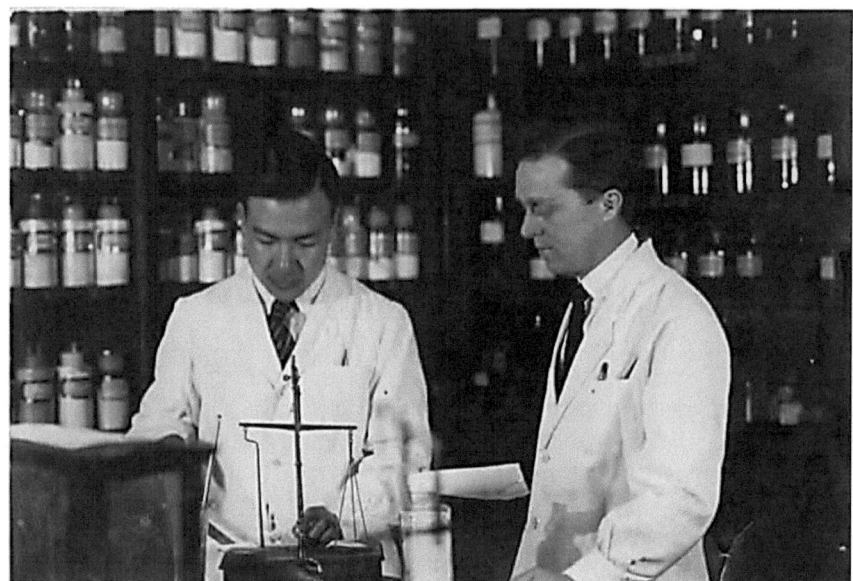

Fig. 3.11 Moody Meng (left) and John Cameron (right) in Dispensing Room of PUMC Hospital @1925. *Credit* Meng Zhaoyi and Meng Xianwei

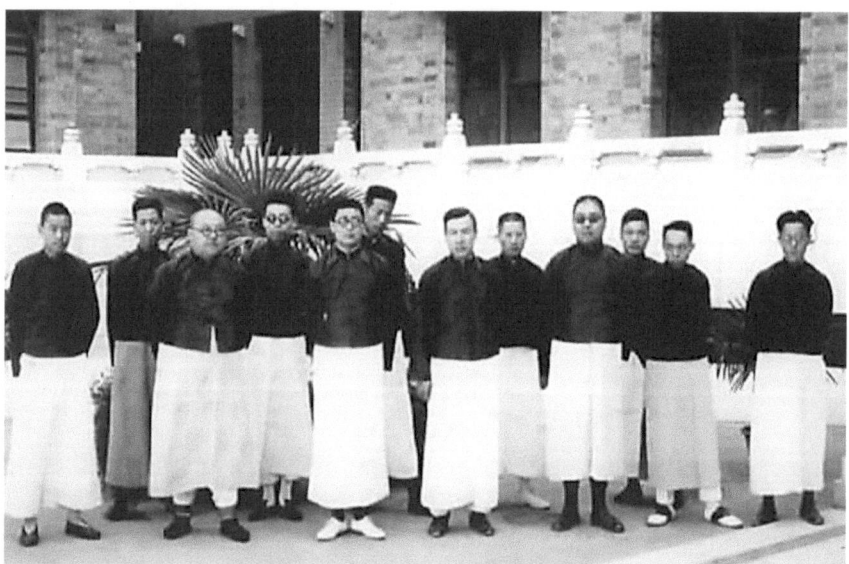

Fig. 3.12 Moody Meng (right, 4th from front row), acting pharmacy supervisor, and Tu Wan-Heng, assistant pharmacist, (left, 3rd from front row) and the pharmacy staff of the PUMC College in June 1926. *Credit* Meng Zhaoyi and Meng Xianwei

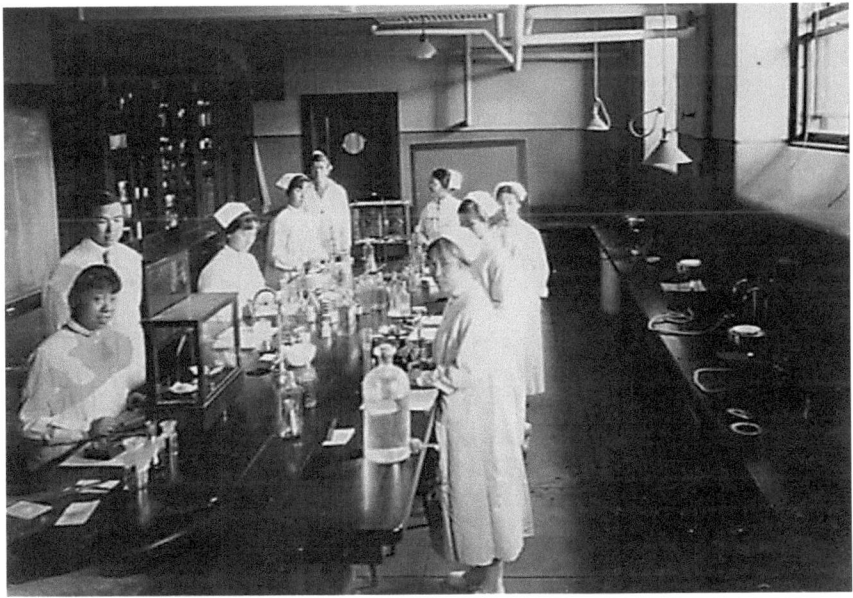

Fig. 3.13 Moody Meng, (standing with tie and laboratory coat, second from left) and student nurses attending a dispensing class. @1926. *Credit* Meng Zhaoyi and Meng Xianwei

pastor of an independent church.[41] After attending high school, Meng was recommended by his cousin, Major K.J. Meng, to work at the pharmacy department of the PUMC Hospital as a dispensary assistant in 1916 while attending courses under Britland there.[42] With financial help reportedly from Britland for the passage to London, England in 1919, Meng went to work at Allen and Hanbury in 1920 to save up the tuition fees needed to attend the Diploma Course at the School of Pharmacy, the University of London in 1921. Meng graduated in 1923 and qualified as a pharmaceutical chemist with the PSGB on 23 April 1924.[43]

In addition to his pharmacy duties, Meng also conducted practicums in dispensing for nurses (Fig. 3.13). Then in January 1929, Dr Heng J. Liu (刘瑞恒, Liu Ruiheng), the newly appointed Vice Minister at the Ministry of Health (MoH), invited Meng to take leave from PUMC Hospital to undertake the editorial work on the first edition of the Chinese Pharmacopoeia (中华药典第一版) (See the section on *The 1930 Chinese Pharmacopoeia*, Chap. 8)[44]. Meng's secondment was initially for six months but was subsequently extended to over a year. He returned to PUMC Hospital in May 1930 to be the acting supervisor of the pharmacy department when Cameron was on a year-long leave between 1st July 1930 and 31st July 1931 (Figs. 3.14 and 3.15). Meng edited two publications: the *Pharmaceutical Journal of the North China Pharmaceutical Society* in 1930 and a booklet entitled *Posology-Percentage-Poisons* published in 1931. Upon Cameron's return to work in August 1931, Meng's relationship with Cameron deteriorated, purportedly due to Meng not having obtained the prior approval of PUMC for the two publications.[45] As a result, Meng discussed

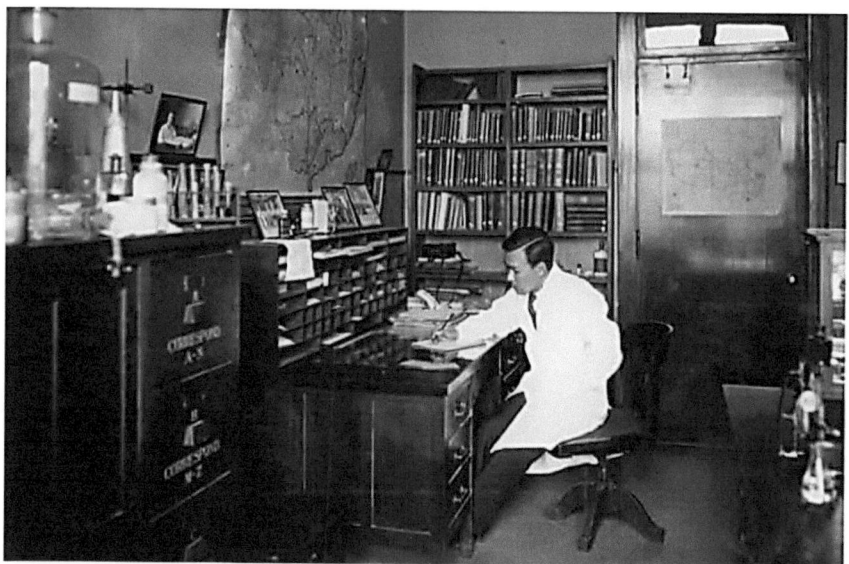

Fig. 3.14 Moody Meng as acting pharmacy supervisor when Cameron was on furlough in 1930. *Credit* Meng Zhaoyi and Meng Xianwei

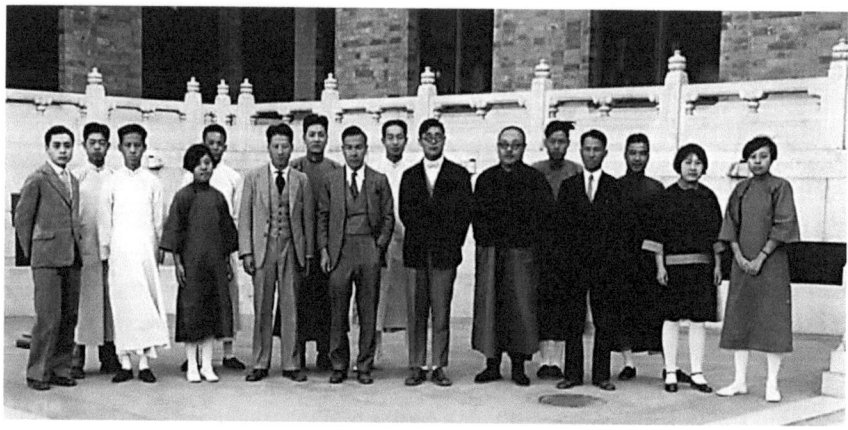

Fig. 3.15 Moody Meng (right, 6th from front row), acting pharmacy supervisor, and Du Wanxiang, assistant pharmacist, (left, 5th from front row) and the pharmacy staff of the PUMC in traditional robes in September 1930. *Credit* Meng Zhaoyi and Meng Xianwei

this with Dr. Heng J. Liu and was offered a temporary assignment to work in the National Flood Relief Project under the now-renamed National Health Administration (NHA) on 1st September 1931. Whilst on assignment there, Meng was offered a full-time position by Dr. Heng J. Liu to head the Central Field Station of the NHA to control the supply of drugs and oversee the practice of pharmacists. Meng resigned from PUMC in January 1932 to take up this new full-time position. He subsequently founded the National College of Pharmacy in Nanjing in 1936 with funding from the Ministry of Education.[46]

The seventh and last western trained pharmacist was (叶青桐, Arthur Tye, Ye Qingtung, Wide-Gile prounication Yeh Ching-Tung). He was of Chinese descent and was born as a British subject in Rutherglen, Victoria, Australia, in 1909. Tye received his pharmaceutical chemist qualification at the Melbourne College of Pharmacy in 1930 and joined the staff of PUMC as an assistant pharmacist on 1st April 1932, succeeding Meng. Tye also served as a lecturer in pharmacology at the PUMC When Cameron returned to the United Kingdom and joined the War Office in 1939, Tye became the acting supervisor of the pharmacy department until December 1941, when the United States declared war on Japan, which had already occupied Peiping since 1937.[47]

Hospital Formularies and Rational Use of *Xiyao*

In a tradition of leading western hospitals such as Guy's Hospital of London, Johns Hopkins Hospital of Baltimore and others in the late nineteenth and early twentieth centuries, hospital formularies were developed as a guidebook for the rational use of drugs by young doctors and nurses. By 1910, the UMC had become a medical institution with a regular intake of medical students and a busy 30-bed teaching hospital serving mostly poor patients. Therefore, it was time for the UMC to develop a hospital formulary (the Formulary) to serve as a teaching aid and a guidebook for medical interns, students, and nurses. Soon after Read's arrival, he published the "First Edition of the Union Medical College Hospital Pharmacopoeia" (an interchangeable word for "Formulary" in the early twentieth century) in 1910. From 1922 to 1942, five more editions of the Formulary were published by the UMC and PUMC Among the *Xiyao* (western drugs and formulations) listed in UMC's 1910 Pharmacopoeia, the pharmacy department manufactured forty-seven commonly dispensed formulations and purchased seven branded pharmacopoeia drugs, including aspirin, from importers and suppliers. British and US physicians prescribed these *Xiyao* in their clinical work. Meanwhile, PUMC's outpatient clinics and operating theatres stocked vaccines, sera, and anaesthetics for routine use. However, these biological medicines would most likely be under the responsibility of the bacteriological and surgical departments.

After changing hands from LMS to CMB in 1915, a new 250-bed hospital named PUMC Hospital with a large medical faculty with many academic staff and senior physicians opened in 1921. The 1922 PUMC Hospital's Formulary included a statement that the Formulary was to be used in conjunction with the "Useful Drugs", published by the *Journal of the American Medical Association* in 1921. Cameron's arrival as the pharmacy supervisor in 1921 was timely in coordinating the Second Edition of the 1922 Formulary. The number of drugs increased from seven in 1910 to 189 in 1922, representing a 27-fold increase. This was due to a fully-fledged medical

Table 3.1 A selective list of publications of John Cameron, supervisor of pharmacy, PUMC Hospital, 1924–1927

#	Month/Year	Paper	*Journal*	Country
1	August 1924	The Chemical purity of chemical tetrachloride	*China Medical Journal*	China
2	April 1925	Observations on hydrogen peroxide		
3	May 1925	Eradication of cockroach		
4	June 6, 1925	The old and the new in pharmacy in China	*Pharmaceutical Journal*	UK
5	August 1926	Some observations on pharmacy in Great Britain		
6	December 1926	The danger of purchasing anywhere	*China Medical Journal*	China
7	March 1927	Pharmacy in China 1927	*American Druggist*	US
8	March 1927	A pharmaceutical aspect of China in 1927	*American Journal of Pharmacy*	US
9	April 1927	Adulterations	*China Medical Journal*	China
10	April 1927	Pharmaceutical sterilization		
11	May, June and July 1927	A few practical suggestions for hospital pharmacies in China		

Source Authors Compilation

faculty with many sub-specialties in internal medicine, a much larger fee-paying outpatient clinic, and many US physicians with a different prescribing and dispensing habit than their British missionary counterparts. Free treatments in the fiscal year ending 30th June 1922 accounted for 12% of prescriptions (3355 of 27,976) or 18% of out-patient treatments (13,615 of 74,763). These numbers were far fewer than the UMC Hospital, which provided free dispensed medicines to the public.[48] Given the large expenditure budget of the PUMC and Hospital, cost control of every department, particularly the pharmacy department, would be a top priority. The objectives of the 1922 Formulary, as stated in its Foreword, were:

> First, to promote the teaching of rational drug therapy within the institution, and second, to secure the greatest degree of economy compatible with the welfare of patients of the Hospital. The Hospital Committee also agreed to a special list of drugs in the experimental stage which might at some future date be included in the Formulary. Additions and deletions from this list were to be made from time to time by the Hospital Committee, on the recommendation of the head of a clinical department.[49]

Cameron was a prolific writer and published many originally researched papers on pharmacy practice in Chinese and Western pharmaceutical Journals (Table 3.1)

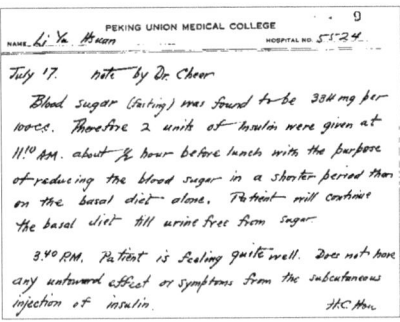

Fig. 3.16 China's First Insulin patient discharge and in-patient records—Li Yu Hsun, September 13, 1923. *Credit* Peking Union Medical College Hospital

He shared his views in the 1927 Formulary with readers in an article published in the National Medical Journal. It read in part:

> In the Peking Union Medical College for many years, we have had a Formulary of all the drugs and pharmaceutical chemicals used in the Hospital. We have recently published our third edition (October 1927), and it occurred to the writer that it might serve a very useful purpose in China if this publication were printed in Chinese. We have suggested to the Committee on the Hospital that such a publication would be great in many of the smaller hospitals in China. Their decision in the matter will be awaited with interest.[50]

Generic or pharmacopoeia drugs had replaced almost all patented medicines in PUMC's 1927 Formulary. Although the number of prescriptions dispensed increased to 36,250 for out-patients, the total number of dispensed items dropped to 70,000, or 94% of the 1922 level. The Formulary also included four antisera that met Non-official Remedies standards (1927 NNR Standards), four antitoxins, of which two met U.S.P. specifications (diphtheria antitoxin and tetanus antitoxin), two met NNR standards, and four vaccines.[51,52,53] Exceptionally, breakthrough drugs such as insulin were prescribed on a needed basis. Insulin was imported 5 months after its launch in North America, and a PUMC Hospital discharge record on 19 September 1923 showed China's first insulin case was a diabetic patient named Li Yu Hsuan. He was admitted for foot gangrene due to perforated foot and thumb ulcers in July 1923 (Fig. 3.16).

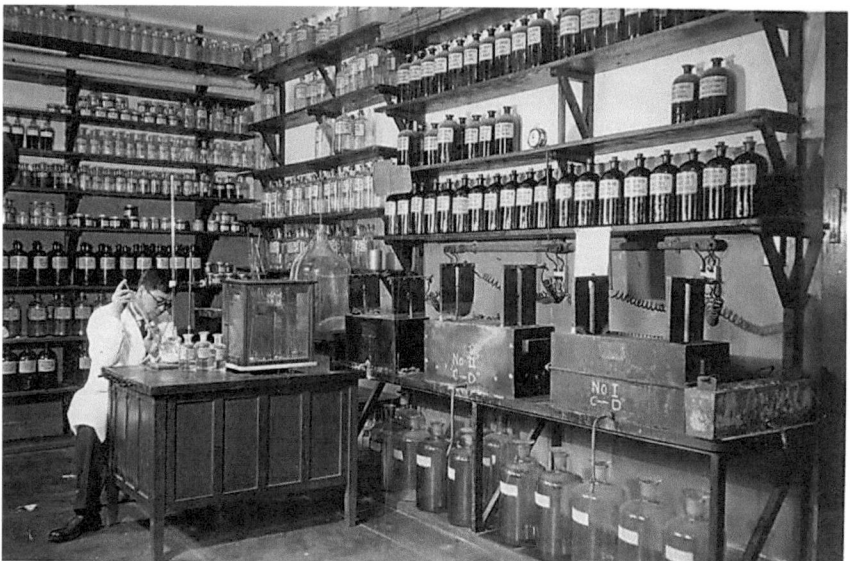

Fig. 3.17 Tu Wen-Heng, senior assistant pharmacist, PUMC pharmacy laboratory @ 1930. *Credit* Meng Zhaoyi and Meng Xianwei

The Formulary had a significant revision that the supply of standardized generic drugs by PUMC Hospital's pharmacy department met the British or the United States Pharmacopoeia specifications. In addition, for cost saving purposes, the pharmacy department had installed manufacturing facilities such as a distillation plant, tabletting machine, ampoule filling and sealing equipment, mixers and grinders within the Hospital compound, which was a norm of British or US hospitals at the time.[54]

Adulterated or sub-standard drugs of dubious origin supplied by pharmaceutical traders were tested routinely for incoming raw materials, purified water for oral mixtures, liquids and injectables, and finished products for a host of own manufactured pharmaceuticals.[55] Therefore, a laboratory was purposefully built with equipment to test its manufactured products routinely. An example was the making of Hydrogen Peroxide 10% Solution, which rapidly decreased within a few days after bottling. This also involved the determination of refractive index saponification value, halogenation reaction of chlorine, or iodine etc. Tu Wen-Heng, a senior assistant pharmacist, was in charge of the pharmaceutical laboratory (Fig. 3.17). An interesting category of the 1927 Formulary was the in-house toiletries that the pharmacy department produced for in-patients, such as toothpaste and powder. Each soap, talcum powder and skin whitening emulsion made by PUMC Hospital had 10 and 50% strengths. Among the OTC drugs and toiletries, these commodities were popular

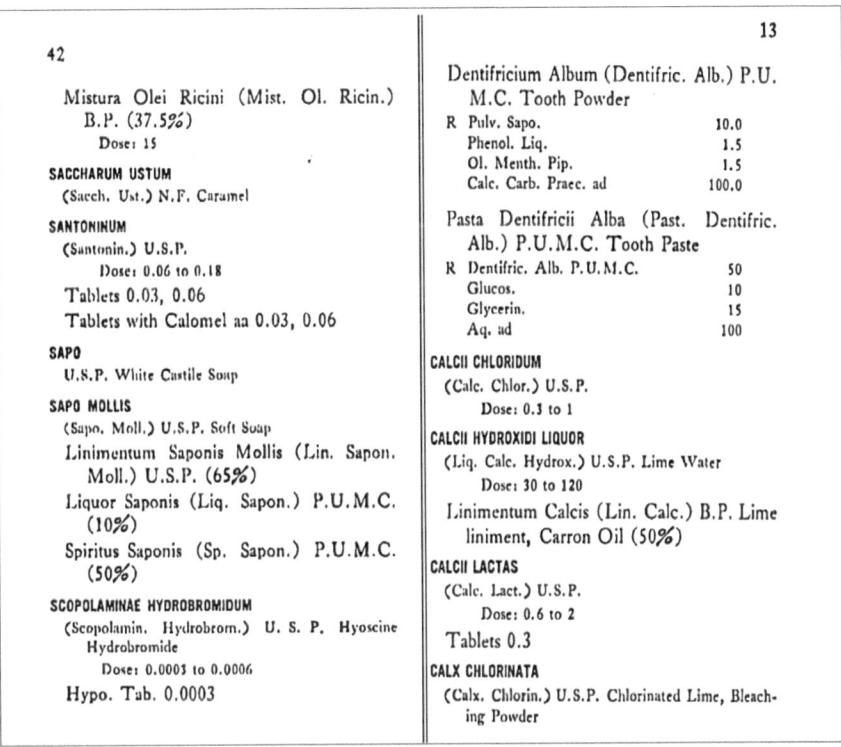

Fig. 3.18 1927 Formulary, medicines and toiletries manufactured by PUMC Hospital Pharmacy staff. *Credit* Peking Union Medical College, China Medical Board

items sold to the public in the dispensary shop (Fig. 3.18).[56] Between 1922 and 1932, the annual compound growth rate (CAGR) in the number of finished drugs only increased by 2.4% per annum, and the number of formulations remained stable in the range of 46–54.

The Great Depression and subsequent years showed an even smaller growth of pharmacopoeia drugs from 240 to 293 or 1.47% per annum from 1932 to 1942. From 1910 to 1941, the Hospital committee published six formularies with the pharmacy department as the coordinator and "gatekeeper" in the rational use of drugs. Merely fifty-four medicines and pharmaceutical preparations were listed in the 1910 Pharmacopoeia, which jumped to 354 in 1942, representing 6.3 multiples or a 6% annual compound increase over 32 years.

Knowledge Dissemination, Basic Research and Development

John Bowers, the author of Western Medicine in a Chinese Palace, viewed PUMC's research work after the CMB's acquisition of the UMC in China could be summarized as:

> The scientific contributions of the research programmes at PUMC between 1919 and 1941 were outstanding, especially for their attacks on health problems of China such as communicable diseases and parasitology and nutritional deficiencies. The introduction of ephedrine stands as the greatest contributions to modern medicine from that of an indigenous system of medicine. In its relatively brief lifespan, PUMC soon became the leadimg medical centre in Asia, its influence extending throughout that vast region.[57]

Another observation of Bowers could be more thought-provoking and partially explains the smooth transition in the public health arena and the continuation of the macro policy despite the change of governments from the Nationalist to the Communist on 1st October 1949:

> That PUMC was strikingly successful in training the leaders of medicine for China is attested by the fact that when it closed in December 1941, fewer than ten of its (hundreds) graduates were in private practice. Virtually all of the alumni were teaching medicine, leading hospital medical services, or in government positions in public health. A survey shortly before the nationalization of the school showed that six of the national medical schools of China were under the leadership of PUMC graduates and that six others were headed by individuals who had received part of their training at PUMC.[58]

Internally, besides the Hospital formularies, they also conducted lectures and prepared newsletters. The PUMC published several books on pharmacy practice and collaborated with the North China Pharmaceutical Society to train pharmacy technicians en masse in 1929. (See the section on *State Investments in Capacity Building* in Chap. 6) In the case of PUMC's training program for pharmacy technicians, the training materials were all in English, as the trainers set the examination questions. The PUMC's British pharmacists played an exemplary role in the knowledge dissemination of pharmacy practice management inside the Hospital to medical interns, students, nurses, and pharmacy technicians. Externally, they published their practice learning, project outcomes, and professional reports to counterparts in professional journals in China and the western world in leading medical and pharmaceutical journals. Cameron joined the PUMC after he qualified as a pharmaceutical chemist in the UK in 1920. After years of working as an apprentice in a dispensing chemist, he was eager to come to Beijing to share best practice pharmacy management with his colleagues at the PUMC and fellow pharmacists in Beijing and around China.

Seven western-trained pharmacists worked at the PUMC in the 32 years from 1909 to 1941. Together, they left a legacy as the "champions of modern pharmaceutical management" in China. The successive pharmacy supervisors of Li Qinghua and Chen Lanying, who served the PUMC Hospital from 1947–1948, and 1948–1988 were pharmacy graduates of local universities. The CMB's acquisition of UMC in 1915 remains a controversial subject in modern China. On the one hand, PUMC was regarded by the medical profession as the "Cradle of Medicine" and trained many talents like Read, Meng, and Zhao who made advances in their respective fields; on the other hand, it's Hospital served a much small number of poor patients than when it was set up as the Free Healing Hospital 55 years earlier!

The academic faculty of the PUMC conducted active research programmes in pharmacognosy, beginning in the early 1920s. Chaulmoogra oil and ephedrine were two of several natural drugs the PUMC's scientists researched and supplied, gaining global recognition in that decade.[59] Like many other university medical colleges or hospitals in the UK or the US, PUMC actively produced essential drugs not commonly available or at high prices in-house in the first half of the twentieth century. Dr. Ralph Seem, medical superintendent of the PUMC Hospital, reported on the work of chaulmoogra oil in his annual report ending 30th June 1922:

> At a conference on leprosy held at the PUMC during the opening exercises in September 1921, it was agreed that the Peking Union Medical College could contribute a service to China and Korea by undertaking the production of the ethyl esters of chaulmoogra oil. At that time, ethyl esters were very difficult to obtain in the market and very expensive. They were being quoted by one manufacturer at about $300 per liter. The production of these esters by the Dean's method was undertaken in the Chemical Laboratory with the aid of Miss Ruth A. Wood, formerly of Dr. Dean's laboratory at the University of Hawaii.
>
> They are now being produced in quantity. The price at which the product is distributed depends on the cost of production and hence on demand. Up to the present date at that time, June 30, 1922, about 60,000 c.c. (60 L) had been distributed in China and Korea. It had first been priced at $30 per litre before reducing to $25 per litre. From 1st July 1922, the production of the ethyl esters was placed under the direction of Mr B.E. Read, of the Department of Pharmacology, and any inquiries or orders for the product may be addressed to him.[60]

Later in the year, Read was awarded a second fellowship for his PhD in the drug metabolism of chaulmoogra oil at Yale University, which he completed in 1924. During Read's study leave, Carl Frederic Schmidt (1893–1988) joined as an associate professor of the Department of Pharmacology, Physiology, and Physiological Chemistry of the PUMC in 1922. His 2-year assignment at the College was to develop an educational pharmacology programme and identify Chinese materia medica with therapeutic values. After a disappointing first year in the research of Chinese materia medica, Schmidt had an assistant, K.K. Chen, a pharmacist with a PhD in biochemistry and physiology at the University of Wisconsin, in the second year. Together they reviewed the commonly used Chinese materia medica and pursued detailed pharmacological studies in *Ephedra sinica* (Chinese name, *Mahuang*) (Fig. 3.19).[61] Chen

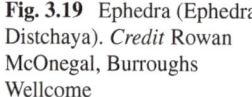

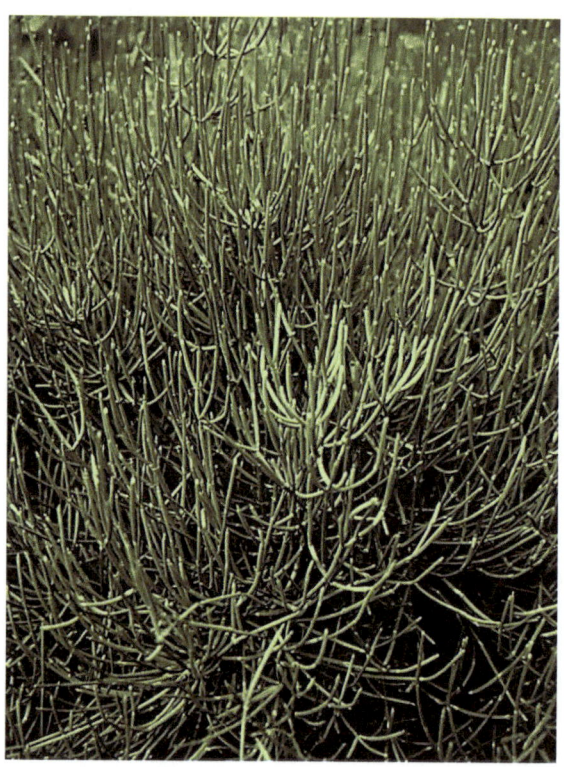

Fig. 3.19 Ephedra (Ephedra Distchaya). *Credit* Rowan McOnegal, Burroughs Wellcome

and Schmidt jointly conducted a thorough investigation of ephedrine, which eventually showed it to be an effective chemical structure similar to adrenaline (called epinephrine in the US).[62]

Upon completing his 2-year stint at the PUMC in 1924, Chen returned to the University of Wisconsin as a research associate and continued his clinical research in ephedrine while working on his medical doctor degree there. With help from Bernard Read and Zhao Chenggu (赵承嘏, T. Q. Chou, 1885–1966) in China, Chen subsequently joined Lilly as the Director of Pharmacologic Research in 1929 (Fig. 3.20).[63] He eventually produced an oral, long-acting ephedrine drug for children's allergic diseases, including bronchial asthma and hay fever (Fig. 3.21).[64]

Fig. 3.20 Ko Kuei Chen (1989–1988). Courtesy of Meng Zhaoyi and Meng Xianwei

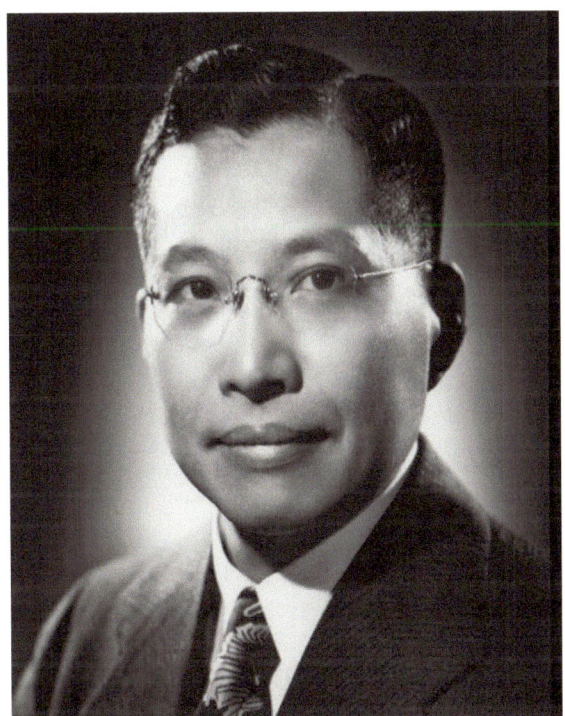

Fig. 3.21 Ephedrine products, (Ephedra Ma-huang), 1930. *Credit* Wikipedia

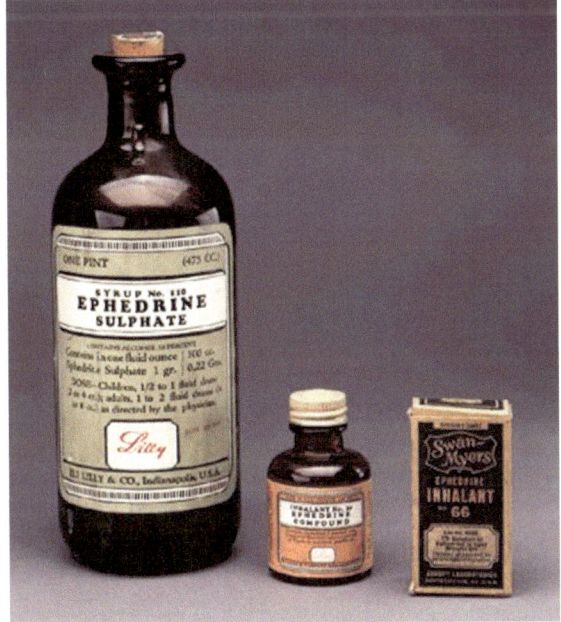

Notes and References

1. The London Missionary Society had been founded in England in 1795 by evangelical Angli-
    cans and various non-conformist groups. Congregational missions were established in Oceania
    and Africa, but Presbyterian missionaries were also particularly active in China.
2. Goodall, N. *History of the London Missionary Society 1895–1945* (London: Oxford University
    Press 1954).
3. Hughes, A, *Biographical History of William Lockhart,* School of Oriental and African Studies,
    University of London. Accessed 29 September 2023. http://archiveshub.ac.uk/data/gb102-ms3
    80645.
4. Bowers, JZ, *Western Medicine in a Chinese Palace. Peking Union Medical College, 1917–1951*
    (New York, USA: The Josiah Macy Jr Foundation, 1972), 43.
5. *Beijing Hospitals Top Annual Comprehensive Rankings of Chinese Hospitals*, English, The
    People's Government of Beijing Municipality, 30 November 2022. Accessed 18 April 2023.
    www.English.beiing.gov.cn.
6. Ferguson, ME, *China Medical Board and Peking Union Medical College Hospital: A Chronicle
    of Fruitful Collaboration (1914–1951)*. (New York: China Medical Board, 1970), 30–34.
7. Personal interview of Zhu Zhu, research fellow of PUMC Hospital Pharmacy Department,
    April 19, 2023.
8. Gao, X.高晞," De zhen chuan—yige yingguo chuanjiao shì yu zhongguo yixue xiandai-
    hua", 德贞传——一个英 国传教士与中国医学现代化, [*A Biography of John Dundgeon, A
    British Missionary and Modernization of Medical Education in the Late Qing Period*. Fudan]
    (Shanghai: Fudan University Press, 2009), pp. 300–301.
9. Bowers, *Western Medicine in a Chinese Palace*, 6.
10. Adam, A, *Thomas Cochrane and the Dragon Throne* (London, SPCK 2018), 84.
11. Adams, *Thomas Cochrane*, 99.
12. Adams, *Thomas Cochrane*, 135.
13. Adams, *Thomas Cochrane*, 139.
14. Adams, *Thomas Cochrane*, 141.
15. Adams, *Thomas Cochrane*, 141.
16. Adams, *Thomas Cochrane*, 151.
17. Adams, *Thomas Cochrane*, 151.
18. Adams, *Thomas Cochrane*, 151.
19. Adams, *Thomas Cochrane*, 37–38.
20. Bowers, *Western Medicine*, 223.
21. Bowers, *Western Medicine*, 38.
22. Bowers, *Western Medicine*, 38.
23. Bowers, *Western Medicine*, 43.
24. *Medicine in China, Education*, China Medical Board of the Rockefeller Foundation, (Chicago,
    The University of Chicago Press, 1914). Accessed 29 September 2023. https://centennial.chi
    namedicalboard.org/sites/chinamedicalboard.org.100/files/Medicine_in_China.pdf.
25. Bowers, *Western Medicine*, 51.
26. Apparently, the Paulun Medical College was not deemed to be an acquisition candidate of the
    China Medical Board as the German curriculum was focused on laboratory medicine rather
    than clinical medicine, as was practiced in the UK and the US in the early 1900s.
27. Bowers, *Western Medicine*, 65.
28. Ninkovich, Frank, "The Rockefeller Foundation, China, and Cultural Change", *The Journal
    of American History,* 70, No. 4 (1984): 799–820. Accessed 29 September 2023. http://www3.
    nccu.edu.tw/~lorenzo/Ninkovich%20Rockefeller%20Foundation.pdf.
29. Schwartz, KL, *"Bernard Emms Read: 17 May 1887 to 13 June 1949"*. J. Hist Med Allied Sci
    1950; V (Spring), pp. 216–217.
30. Annual Register of Pharmaceutical Chemists and Chemists and Druggist. (London: Pharma-
    ceutical Society of Great Britain 1919), 264.

31. Bernard Emms Read Employment Record, (PUMC Archive in Beijing), Accessed December 19, 2022.
32. Annual Register, 1919: 294.
33. The Pharmaceutical Society of Great Britain Calendar 1912 (London: The Pharmaceutical Society of Great Britain, 1912). Accessed September 5, 2022.
34. Abbott, LM and Hamilton, FW. *Proceedings of the Most Worshipful Grand Lodge of Ancient Free and Accepted Masons of the Commonwealth of Massachusetts for The Year 1917* (Cambridge, Mass: Caustic-Claflin Company, 1918), lxiv.
35. The Complete List of Weihsen Inmates, Weihsien Picture Gallery. Accessed 29 September 2023. http://www.weihsien-paintings.org/RonBridge/habitants/weihsien02.pdf.
36. Annual Register, 1919: 62.
37. Chiu, Patrick, "British Pharmacists and the Peking Union Medical College Hospital, 1910–1941", *Pharmaceutical Historian* 47, no. 3 (2017), 57–65, esp. 62. Accessed 29 September 2023. https://www.ingentaconnect.com/content/bshp/ph/2017/00000047/00000003/art00002?crawler=truee.
38. PUMC Internal memorandum of December 31,1924 from John Cameron, Pharmacist to Ms. Alberta Worthington, Assistant Secretary of CMB in Beijing (PUMC Internal Archive), Accessed December 19, 2022.
39. Announcement, The Chemist and Druggist 186, 1966: 582.
40. Biographical Index of Former Fellows of the Royal Society of Edinburgh 1783–2002, Part 1. Edinburgh: The Royal Society of Edinburgh, 1966: 154.
41. China Medical Board internal memorandum between L. Carrington Goodrich, Assistant Director of the CMB to Henry Houghton, Director of the CMB of June 11, 1924 (PUMC Archive). Accessed December 19, 2022.
42. Personal correspondence between Roger S. Greene, Director of CMB and Major K.J. Meng, Moody Meng'scousin, regarding Moody's employment at the PUMC Pharmacy, of July 5, 1916 (PUMC Archive). Accessed December 19, 2022.
43. UMC Internal memorandum of December 31, 1924, from John Cameron, Pharmacist to Ms. Alberta Worthington, Assistant Secretary of CMB in Beijing (PUMC Archive). Accessed December 19, 2022.
44. Chiu, *British Pharmacists*, 63.
45. Confidential correspondence between Roger S. Greene, Director of PUMC and Dr J.B. Grant regarding Moody's relationship with John Cameron of 9 November 1931. (PUMC Archive). Accessed, December 16, 2022.
46. Chiu, *British Pharmacists*, 63.
47. Arthur Tye emigrated to the United States in 1947, entered the Ohio State University College of Pharmacy and Completed a PhD degree on the quantitation of analgesic actions of opiates in 1950. He was appointed as an assistant professor in 1950 and subsequently served as assistant dean and professor of pharmacy until his retirement in 1970. Tye passed away in Santa Rosa, Sonoma County, California, in 1987 at the age of 78.
48. Report of the Out-Patient Department, Fourteenth Annual Report of the Medical Superintendent, Peking Union Medical PUMCH. Peking, China. Year Ending 20 June 1922, 21. Accessed 29 September 2023. https://findit.library.yale.edu/?f%5Byale_genre_sim%5D%5B%5D=Books%2C+Journals+%26+Pamphlets&q=Bdx+P39h&search_field=Call+number&sort=date_dtsi+asc%2C+sort_ssi+asc&utf8=%E2%9C%93.
49. Formulary, Peking Union Medical College, PUMC Press, June 1922, 1.
50. Cameron, John, "A Chinese Pharmacopoeia"—When? *The National Medical Journal* 13, no.6 (1927), 449–453.
51. During the 1926/27 fiscal year, the number of out-patient items dispensed jumped from 36,250 to 70,000, or an average of 200 prescriptions a day. Prescriptions filled for inpatients and staff members, including repeats, amounted to 21,300. The total number of prescriptions filled by the pharmacy during the year was 91,300, an average of over 300 per working day.

52. Zhu Zhu and Zhang Bo, "The 1927 Formulary of Peking's First Western Teaching Hospital", *Pharmaceutical Historian* 51, no. 2 (2021), 33–40.esp. 35. Accessed 29 September 2023. https://docserver.ingentaconnect.com/deliver/connect/bshp/00791393/v51n2/s1.pdf?exp ires=1683457769&id=0000&titleid=72010666&checksum=699A1151C8730B1E85D6A 751870532DB&host=https://www.ingentaconnect.com.
53. Zhu Zhu, The 1927 Formulary, 37–38.
54. Zhu Zhu, The 1927 Formulary, 38.
55. Zhu Zhu, The 1927 Formulary, 39.
56. Zhu Zhu, The 1927 Formulary, 38.
57. Bowers, *Western Medicine,* 223.
58. Bowers, *Western Medicine*, 223.
59. Leprosy was a severe and chronic illness but not a fatal one. In the early 1920s, China had 1.5 million lepers. Therefore, the only effective drug treatment was by chaulmoogra oil. Prior to the discovery of the prodrug. Promin, a precursor of dapsone, by Parke Davis in 1941, the ethyl esters of chaulmoogra oil was used initially in India in the late 1910s and later to the rest of the world. The use of chaulmoogra oil (also called *Hydnocarpus* oil) for treatment of leprosy in India can be traced back to as early as 600 BC in *Sushruta Samhita.*
60. Fourteenth Annual Report of the Medical Superintendent, Peking Union Medical College Hospital, 1922: 24–25.
61. The Japanese scientist Nagajosi Nagai first studied Mahuang in 1887, isolating its active principle called ephedrine, with limited if any pharmacological studies.
62. Koelle, G, *A Biographical Memoir of Carl Frederic Schmidt, 1893–1988* (Washington D.C., National Academies Press, 1995), 273–289, esp. 276–278. http://www.nasonline.org/public ations/biographical-memoirs/memoir-pdfs/schmidt-carl.pdf.
63. Chen, KK, "Two Pharmacological Traditions: Notes from Experience". The *Annual Review of Pharmacology and Toxicology* 21, (1981), 1–6. Accessed 29 September 2023. https://www. annualreviews.org/doi/pdf/10.1146/annurev.pa.21.040181.000245.
64. Ephedrine was the first drug available as an oral dosage form for children asthma.

Chapter 4
The Rise of Western Chemists

This chapter delves into the intriguing story of how three expatriate retailers initiated and flourished their businesses in the vibrant cities of Hong Kong and Shanghai in the latter half of the nineteenth century. The rise of Ningbo entrepreneurs, some were dispensing assistants at these western chemists, established superior nationwide distribution channels, who ultimately reshaped the business landscape across the eighty treaty ports by the 1930s.

China lost the First Opium War (1839–1842) which led to the subsequent signing of the Treaty of Nanking (the Treaty) with the United Kingdom in 1842. As a result, five treaty ports along the eastern coast were opened for foreign traders, including western retail pharmacies, known as chemists and druggists (or simply as chemists). The emergence of western chemists was first reported in an advertisement placed by Drs Alexander Anderson and Peter Young on 1 January 1843 (Fig. 4.1). Among the colonies of the Western powers in Asia, Macau had an early start in hospital services. Historical records revealed Dr. T B Watson's clinic, the only British medical practitioner in Macau had an onsite dispenser and two chemists and druggists opened for business in 1848: De Freitas Dispensary in Praya Manduco and De Seabra's Dispensary in Praya Grande.[1] In the same year, Hong Kong had eighteen Chinese medicine herbalists and six chemists and druggists in the newly founded British Colony (Table 4.1).[2]

Located south of the mouth of the Yangtze River, which originates in the Qinghai-Tibetan plateau and runs through nine provinces, Shanghai became the natural commercial hub and the most vibrant entrepot for the domestic and overseas markets for a century from 1844 to 1943. By 1880, China had 30–40 million opium smokers out of an estimated population of 450 million. Initially imported but later mass produced "opium cures", narcotic substitutes of opium, were marketed by western chemists: the British Dispensary (operated by McTavish and Lehmann), Hong Kong Dispensary (A.S. Watson), Laou Teh Kee (Shanghai Medical Store operated by J. Llewellyn) and others in China. Their brands of "opium cures" became the suppliers of the hotly sought after over-the-counter medicines by habitual narcotic users.

© The Author(s), under exclusive license to Springer Nature Singapore Pte Ltd. 2023   67
P. Chiu, *A History of Western Pharmacy in China*,
https://doi.org/10.1007/978-981-99-8635-4_4

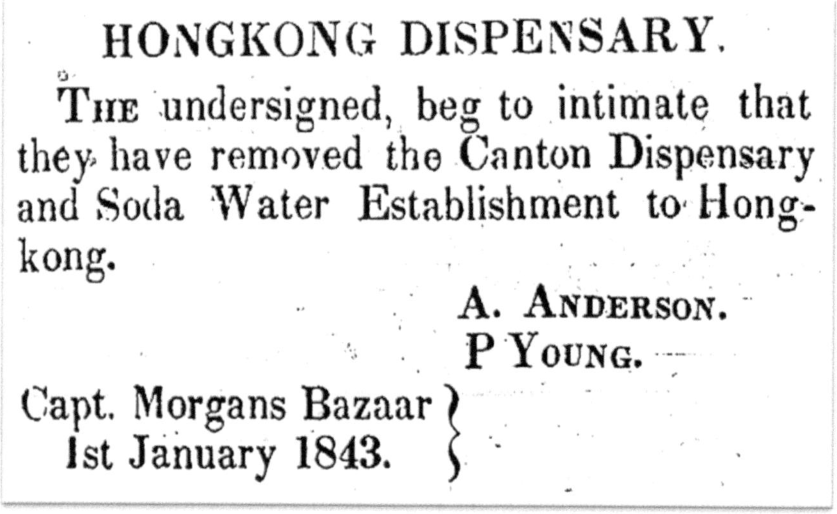

> # HONGKONG DISPENSARY.
>
> THE undersigned, beg to intimate that they have removed the Canton Dispensary and Soda Water Establishment to Hongkong.
>
> A. ANDERSON.
> P YOUNG.
>
> Capt. Morgans Bazaar }
> 1st January 1843.   }

Fig. 4.1 Hong Kong Dispensary opening advertisement, Capt. Morgan Bazaar. *Credit* Friend of China and Hong Kong Gazette, Thursday, 5 January 1843

Table 4.1 List of Hong Kong chemists and druggists in 1848

Chemists and druggists	Location	Manager/proprietor
Hong Kong Dispensary	Queen's Road	James Hume Young
Victoria Dispensary	Pottinger Street	Thomas Hunter and George K Barton
Medical Hall	Queen's Road	Alexander S Taylor
Stocker's & Co.'s Dispensary	Queen's Road	Charles Stocker
Farriers	Queen's Road East	George Frazer
Castles & Co	Stanley Street	Not known

Credit Hong Kong Almanck 1848

Western owned retail and wholesale chemists in Shanghai had a near monopoly of imported medicines until the first Chinese owned Great China Dispensary, founded by former employees of the British Dispensary (previously called the British Hospital), in 1888. Great China and other local entrepreneur owned pharmacies competed directly with their former employers for the lucrative "opium cures" market in Shanghai and the rest of China. Although Macau had retail drug stores much earlier, its first retail chemist with a qualified pharmacist came in much later than Hong Kong or Shanghai. Pedro Nolasco da Silva founded the Farmacie Popular (Bianmin Yaofang) in 1895. Pedro Nolasco's third son, *Henrique Maria* (1884–1969), graduated in pharmacy and law at the Goa Medical School and moved Fharmacia Popular to larger premises at number 95 on the same avenue in 1907. Farmacie Popular then

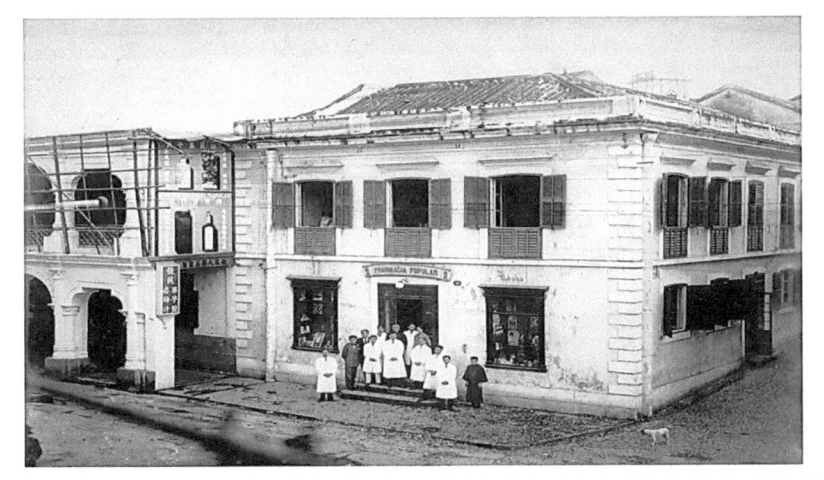

Fig. 4.2 Farmacie Popular, to 16 Largo do Senado, Macau. c.1916. *Credit* Farmacie Popular, Macau

moved to 16 Largo do Senado, a building owned by the Fraternity of the Macau Holy House of Mercy in 1916 and remained there until now (Figs. 4.2 and 4.3).

The Boxers Movement (1900–1901) also burnt down foreign owned businesses, including the A.S. Watson's store in Qianmen (Chien Men, "Gate of the Zenith Sun"), Beijing in the summer of 1900, driving both Chinese and expatriate entrepreneurs to Shanghai for good. A series of natural, financial and political disasters occurred in the following decade were to lead to the collapse of the Manchu Qing Empire in 1911.

Treaty of Nanking, Hong Kong and Shanghai

Commodore Gordon Bremer, commander-in-chief of British forces in China, landed at Possession Point, Hong Kong, on 25th January 1841. However, military conflicts between the British and Chinese continued for another one-and-a-half years. The Treaty of Nanking was finally signed between the Manchu Qing and British officials on 29 August 1842, aboard the HMS *Cornwallis* anchored in Nanjing.[3] Hong Kong Island was ceded to Britain in perpetuity, with five coastal ports in Eastern and Southern China opened to foreign traders and missionaries. Among the six cities, Hong Kong had a head start as a trade hub in taking over Canton in serving the southern provinces. However, disputes arose from the Treaty with Article II, which documented the opening of the five treaty ports with conditions of trade published in the *London Gazette* on 7 November 1843:

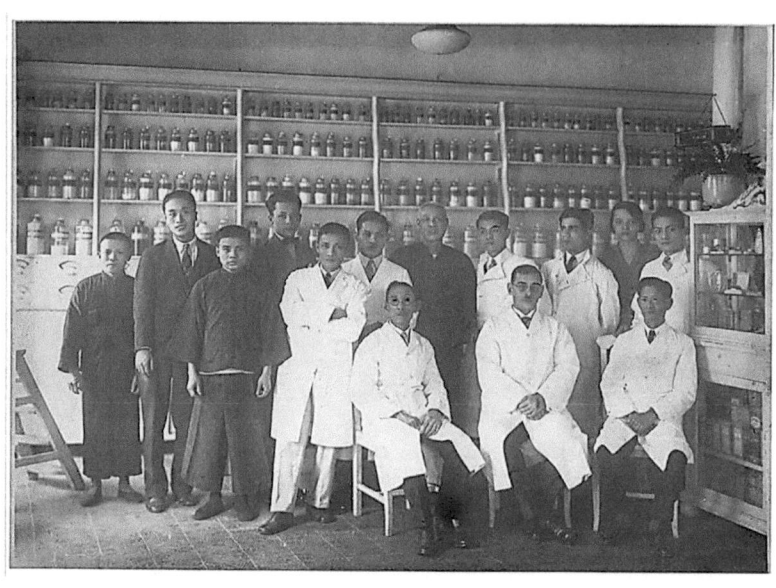

Fig. 4.3 Henrique Maria (1884–1969, front low, middle seat), pharmacist, and staff. *Credit* Pharmacie Popular, Macau

> His Majesty, the Emperor of China, agree's that British subjects, with their families and establishments, shall be allowed to reside, for the purpose of carrying on their mercantile pursuits, without molestation or restraint, at the cities and towns of Canton, Amoy, Foochow foo, Ningpo, and Shanghai; and Her Majesty the Queen of Great Britain, will appoint Superintendents, or Consular Officers, to reside at each of the above-named cities or towns.[4,5]

The Chinese version of the Treaty used the words "ports for British Superintendents, or Consular Officers, to reside at the five cities and townships". It omitted the words "British subjects, with their families". Strict implementation of the Treaty was carried out by a Manchu official, Aisin-Gioro Kiying (Keying, or previously Chi-Ying in Chinese), Viceroy of Guangdong (Kwangtung) and Guangxi (Kwangsi) Provinces, from 1844 to 1848, and Ye Mingchen (Yeh Ming-Cheng) from 1852 to 1858. As a result, the British and other western traders shifted their trading activities from Canton to Hong Kong and Shanghai. Since Hong Kong became a crown colony of the United Kingdom, the burgeoning economy was primarily due to its unique strategic location as an entrepot for trade between China and the rest of the world. Its institutional and legal systems familiar to the western world are also advantages.

Shanghai became a treaty port on 17 November 1843. By 1844, JM & Co. the opium trader that drove the First Opium War between China and Britain, and ten other foreign businesses opened their branches in Shanghai. [6] The International Settlement and the French Concession in Shanghai elected their nationals as representatives to manage the "business districts" like small expatriate colonies with by-laws, regulations and, most importantly, extra-territorial rights. The Treaty provided the United States and France with the same terms and conditions. Both countries signed their respective treaties with the Manchu Qing government for trade privileges and extraterritorial rights on the 3rd of July and 24th of October of 1844.

Shanghai was ready to take off with the International Settlements and the French Concession rapid growth which soon surpassed Hong Kong and the other treaty ports in the following decades (Fig. 4.4). The influx of Indian Parsi, Iraqi Jews, and Western entrepreneurs from 1860 to 1900 made Shanghai a global city like London, New York, or Paris. A sevenfold increase in trade value was recorded from 57.2 million taels in 1859 to 392.7 million taels of white silver in 1905.[7]

The success of turning Shanghai into China's de facto international trade and opium centre was due to several reasons:

Gong Mujiu, the Shanghai Daotai ("Taotai", modern-day mayor) and Maritime Customs Superintendent, co-operated fully upon request by Captain George Balfour, the deputy British Superintendent of Trade. The timely opening of a separate customs house dedicated to foreign ships near the settlement of the British traders in 1845 uplifted the image of Shanghai from a sleepy fishing town to a regional maritime trade hub.

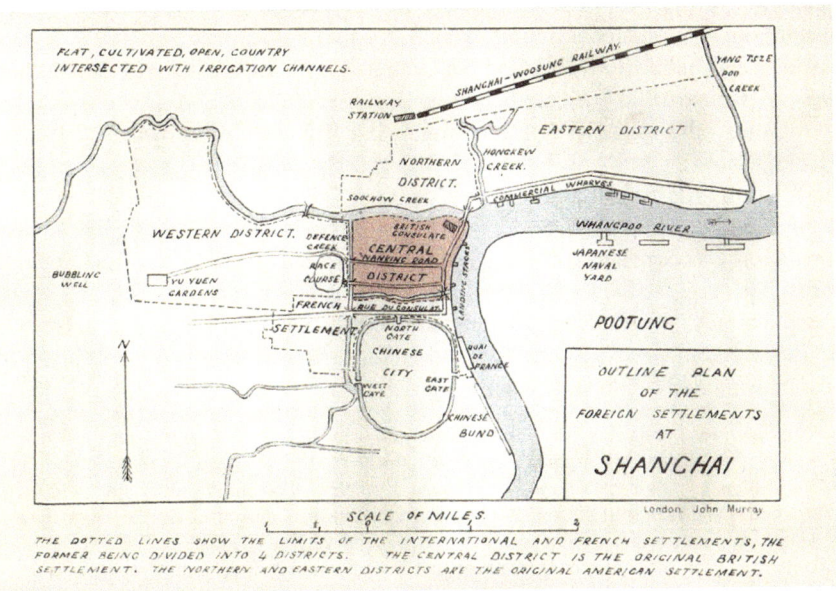

Fig. 4.4 1845–1863. The Shanghai International Settlements and the French Concession 1907. *Credit* The University Libraries, The University of Texas at Austin

Hundreds of thousands of refugees from the nearby eastern provinces of Shanghai fled the social disturbances caused by the "Small Swords Society" in the 1840s. Even more refugees fled from the rebellion of the self-proclaimed "Christian converts" of the "Taiping Heavenly Kingdom" from 1850 to 1864 which brought in abundant labour to support increasing harbour activities and the local economy.

The Shanghai Municipal Council (SMC), established in 1854 by a group of foreign land lessees, was set up to allow the business to be conducted in a *laissez-faire* and safe environment. British, French and US expatriate business leaders of Shanghai-based trading companies provided "extraterritorial" town management and public security services to the residents in the International Settlement in 1854. The SMC laid down by-laws and held the monopoly on essential utilities, including electricity, water and gas, public transportation, revenue collection, control of opium sales and public security. Regulations relating to police, fire, port, prostitution, and waste collection, were strictly implemented to provide a safe business environment within its assigned territory. Despite the vast contribution of SMC to Shanghai's growth as a modern city was close to a century from 1854 to 1943, however, its direct involvement in opium is a blemish on its history.[8] In 1862, the French Concession opted out of the arrangement and formed its municipal council. The following year, the British and US merged their concessions to form the Shanghai International Settlement and continued the management of the SMC until August 1942.[9]

Shanghai's growth was further boosted when the Boxers Movement turned violent in 1900. The Boxers drove away many businesses to Shanghai when churches and commercial properties were burnt and looted in Beijing and Tianjin in June 1900. In addition, A.S. Watson's Beijing branch was burnt down in a big explosion of its warehouse's chemical inventory in the Qianmen area, opposite the Legation Quarters, on 16 June 1900.[10] The other treaty ports served as regional bespoke centres by reaching out to nearby cities and towns like Tianjin for Northern and Hankou (Hankow, now a district of Wuhan) for Central. But they were far less vibrant than Shanghai. By the end of the nineteenth century, Shanghai had earned its reputation as the "Pearl of the Orient". As a result of its thriving economy, Shanghai's general population exceeded that of Hong Kong with 241,000 in 1895, and its expatriate population surpassed that of Hong Kong with 13,700 ten years later in 1905 giving rise to a vibrant western chemist and narcotic drug business (Chart 4.1, Table 4.2). Dr. Zhaong Yongan, an authority on modern China's narcotics history, had his views on the Shanghai Municipal Council:

> The SMC was the most senior administrative power in the international settlement, whose role was to manage and promote the development of the settlement. Within China, the International Settlement also was considered a model settlement. Their exclusive rights to control and license the legal sale and consumption of opium made opium a powerful factor within the semi-colonial power struggles in the settlement, situating the SMC in the centre between the influence of Chinese and British authorities as well as of missionary associations.[11]

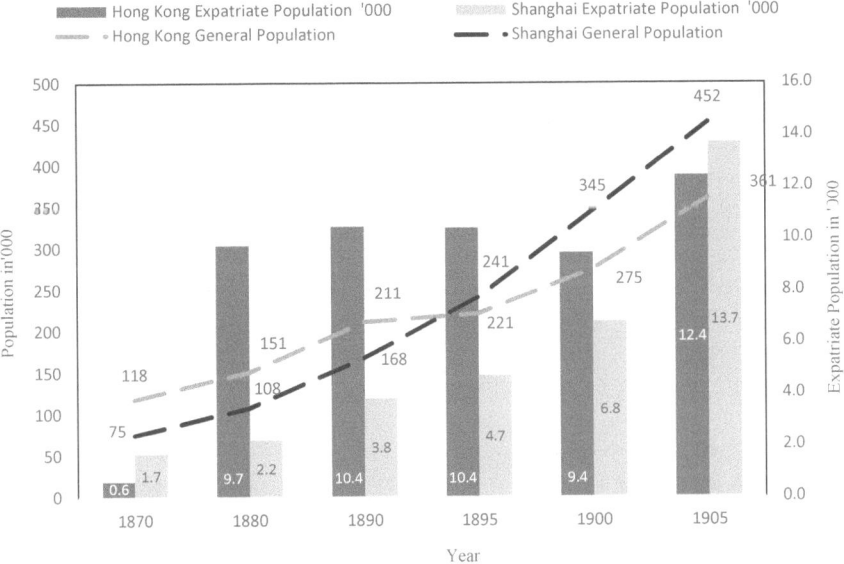

Chart 4.1 1870–1907 General and expatriate population in colonial Hong Kong and Shanghai international settlements. *Credit* Hong Kong Blue Book, Twentieth Century Impressions of Hong Kong, Shanghai, and Other Treaty Ports of China

China's First Retail and Manufacturing Chemist: Hong Kong Dispensary

Dr. Thomas Boswell (T. B., 1815–1860) sold his medical practice in Macau and moved to Hong Kong when taking over the shares of Dr. Alexander Anderson's Hong Kong Dispensary in 1856. Before T. B. joined the business, his predecessor, John Preston, appointed J. Llewellyn as the partner of the Shanghai branch of the Hong Kong Dispensary in 1853. Watson's health deteriorated, and his nephew, Alexander Skirving (AS), joined as the manager of the Dispensary in 1858. But AS was neither a trained medical doctor nor a chemist and soon changed the Dispensary's direction to that of a marine supplier. However, his strategy was delayed for a year due to a fire at the Dispensary in 1859 when it was rebuilt with larger premises at 16 Queen's Road Central (now New World Tower). The Dispensary became the leading chemist supplying laudanum (10% opium or 1% powdered morphine) tincture, proprietary medicines, toiletries, and sundries to the freighters, which would stock up for sailors who felt ill or became injured without a ship surgeon on board and required immediate pain relief. With the departure of Llewellyn from Shanghai for Ningbo in 1860, AS formed a partnership with S.W. Cleave to set up Watson, Cleave & Co., Pharmaceutical Chemists (Fig. 4.5). After building the marine supplier business consecutively

Table 4.2 Western and Japanese chemists in the late Qing and early Republican period (1850–1910)

#	Year	Chemist and druggist	Country of origin	Responsible person	Location
1	1850	British Hospital	UK	M.G. de Souza	1 The Bund (Nanjing Road/ Szechuan Road), name changed to British Dispensary in 1880
2	1850	Shanghai Dispensary	UK	J.P. Lock	Location not known
3	1853	Hong Kong Dispensary	UK	J. Llewellyn (1860), S.W. Cleave	1 Park Lane, (See Shanghai Medical Hall). Moved to 16 Nanjing Road East in 1860
4	1860	Shanghai Medical Hall (J.Llewellyn)	UK	E.C. Kirby	1 Park Lane (Traded as J.Llewellyn/ Lauo The Kee)
5	1866	Pharmacie de L'Union	Germany	T. Koffer	Corner of Kwuangtung Road and Jiangsu Road
6	1878	Rakuzendo	Japan	Kishida Ginko	32 Broadway
7	1887	Pharmacie Francaise	France	S. Soubellat	Corner of Hankow road and Honan road
8	1893	Pharmacie Central	France	Ernest E. Berthel	325 Broadway

Credit The Hongkong Almanack and Directory for the year of the Lord 1850, Noronha's Office, Hong Kong. https://archive.org/details/hongkongalmanack1850/mode/2up

over seven years in Hong Kong, AS's health deteriorated suddenly. Soon after celebrating the silver anniversary, AS sold the business to W.M. Bell, returned to the UK in 1865, and passed away the following year (Chart 4.2).

John David Humphreys (1837–1897, JDH), a "back-packer" in today's terms, travelled from London, England, to Calcutta (Kolkata), India, in the late 1840s and learnt business skills there. After spending 15 years in Calcutta, JDH married Jesse Lambert in 1864, and the couple immediately joined the "gold rush" in New South Wales, Australia. After a couple of years there without luck, JDH tried his last gambit in Hong Kong in 1866. He joined the Dispensary as the bookkeeper. Six years later, Arthur Hunt, another employee of the Dispensary, and JDH acquired Bell's shares and began to trade as A.S. Watson in 1872. With continuing booming business as a marine supplier, JDH acquired Hunt's shares and became A.S. Watson's sole proprietor in 1874. JDH's friendship with the bankers and opium traders allowed him to expand into the hotel and property development business in the mid-1870s. He also saw the

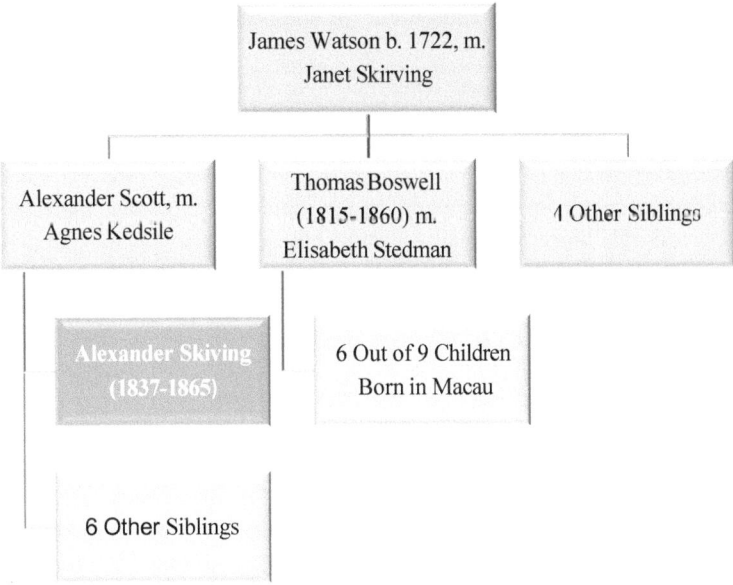

Chart 4.2 Family tree of A. S. Watson. *Credit* Hong Kong Society for the History of Pharmacy

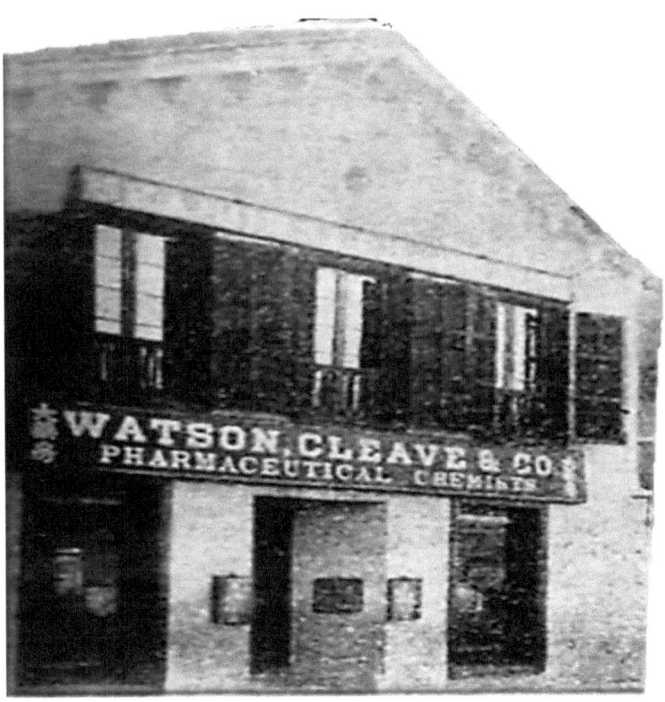

Fig. 4.5 Watson, Cleave & Co., pharmaceutical chemists, Shanghai, @1860s. *Credit* Hong Kong Society for the History of Pharmacy

market for local production of soda water for hotels and restaurants in Hong Kong and the transiting freighters.

A.S. Watson soon expanded its manufacturing capacity by opening a new workshop at 1–3 Stanley Street, Central (now Hing Wai Building with entry at 36 Queen's Road Central) in 1875. Six flavours of soda water and proprietary medicines, such as "Watson's Worm Cakes" (santonin containing anthelmintics), were produced and distributed throughout the treaty ports on the mainland. However, the top-selling and most profitable Watson's brand was none other than the laudanum and "opium cures" produced locally as substitutes for opium smokers in Hong Kong. A.S. Watson expanded beyond China; its first overseas branch opened in Manila, the Philippines, in 1883. At the same time, A.S. Watson was preparing to grow on the mainland and went for an initial public offering. As a result, it became Hong Kong's number 15 limited liability company in 1882. JDH' eldest son, Henry, was born in Hong Kong in 1867 and went to boarding school in the South Sea in England. He qualified as a pharmaceutical chemist of the Pharmaceutical Society for Great Britain in 1888 and returned to Hong Kong as A.S. Watson's pharmacy manager the following year. In addition to the highly profitable "opium cures", he soon consolidated the family retail and manufacturing chemist business by focusing on soda water, and proprietary medicines with Watson's brand (Figs. 4.6, 4.7, 4.8 and 4.9).

In the following decade, Henry grew the business in China and the Philippines and succeeded his father as the chairman of A.S. Watson in 1897. Violence suddenly erupted during the Boxers Movement in Northern China in 1900. A.S. Watson withdrew from the Beijing market soon after its store at Qianmen was burnt down in the summer of 1900 and reprioritized its mainland business with a focus on Shanghai to serve both the eastern and central regions. By 1908, A.S. Watson had gained its flagship store's reputation as Asia's only modern retail pharmacy (Fig. 4.10). Its Alexander Building store in Hong Kong was the talk of the town from the Straits Settlements in Southeast Asia to Shanghai on the East China Coast in 1908, and Kelly and Walsh's book had the following description:

> The ground and first floors of that magnificent and imposing block known as Alexandra Buildings are occupied by the Hong Kong Dispensary, otherwise the well-known firm of A.S. Watson & Co. Ltd., Chemists, Druggists, Soda Water Manufacturers, etc. Travellers passing through Hong Kong should pay a visit to the Hong Kong Dispensary, where they may obtain every requisite for their voyage, including toilet articles, medicines, perfumery, tobacco, cigars and wines of the very finest quality, at prices that will compare favourably with those ruling at home or any place along the route.[12]

The following year, A.S. Watson acquired the two chemist shops, including the Hongkew Medical Hall of the British Dispensary, operated by McTavish and Lehman, in Shanghai. Donald Mennie's responsibilities increased, and he became the managing director of A.S. Watson North China. The most significant impact on China's economy in the 1910s came from the flooding in the Yangtze River (1909–1910), the collapse of the rubber commodity market in the Shanghai Stock Exchange (1910), and the Manchurian Plague (1910–1911). The final straw was the Wuhan revolution of 1911, overthrowing the dynasty. These cumulatively led to a sharp depreciation of the Chinese silver dollar by fifty per cent in 1912 with

Fig. 4.6 A. S. Watson's
Soda Water in
Torpedo-shaped glass bottle.
@1870. *Credit* Hong Kong
Society for the History of
Pharmacy

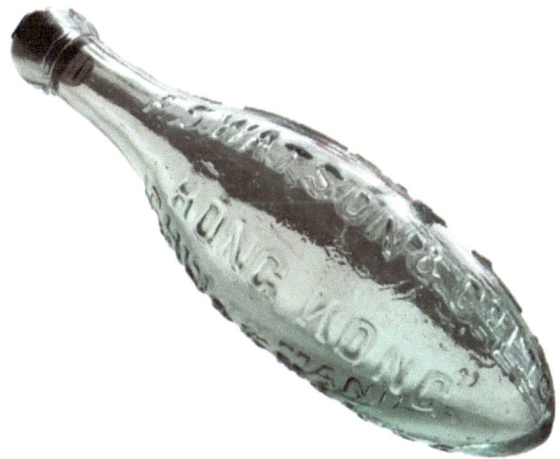

Fig. 4.7 A. S. Watson's
Ginger Beer in ceramic jar.
@1870s. *Credit* Hong Kong
Society for the History of
Pharmacy

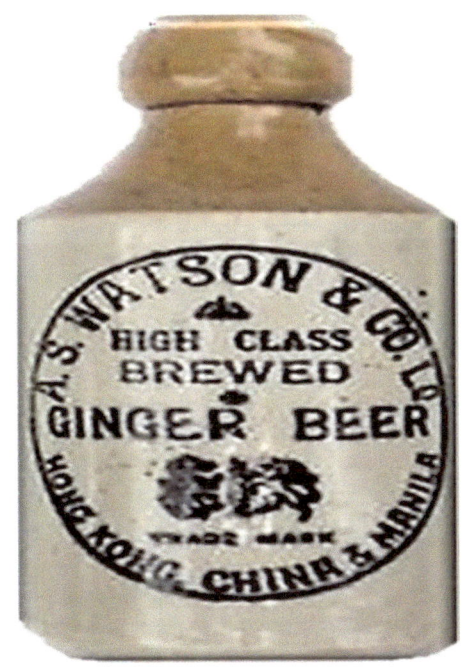

massive bankruptcies and closures of Shanghai's British or European-owned retail pharmacies. Due to heavy bad debts in the marketplace, A.S. Watson sold off its retail pharmacy and soda water business in the Philippines to improve its cash flow in 1912. The majority shareholding of Watson's 60-year-old Shanghai business, including the

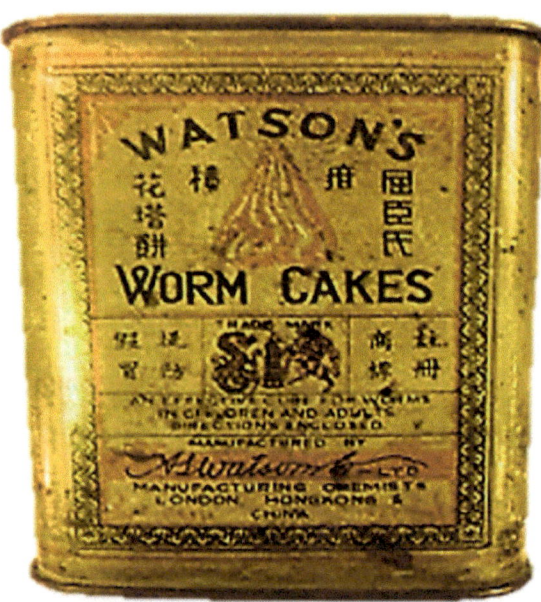

Fig. 4.8 Watson's Santonin Bonbons @1930. *Credit* Hong Kong Society for the History of Pharmacy

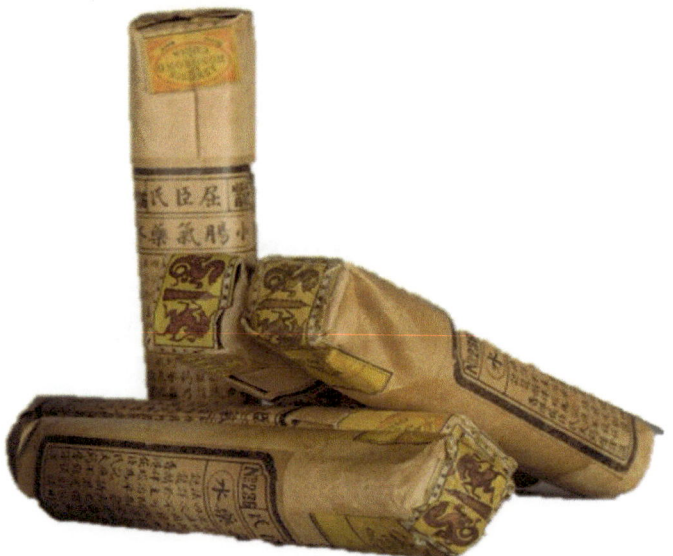

Fig. 4.9 Watson's Inguinal Hernia Medicine. *Credit* Courtesy of Burnaby Village Museum

Fig. 4.10 Alexandra
Building, Central, Hong
Kong @1920. The Alexandra
building in Gloucester road,
Central, Hong Kong, was the
"talk of the town" from the
straits settlements to
Shanghai when built in 1908.
Credit Hong Kong Society
for the History of Pharmacy

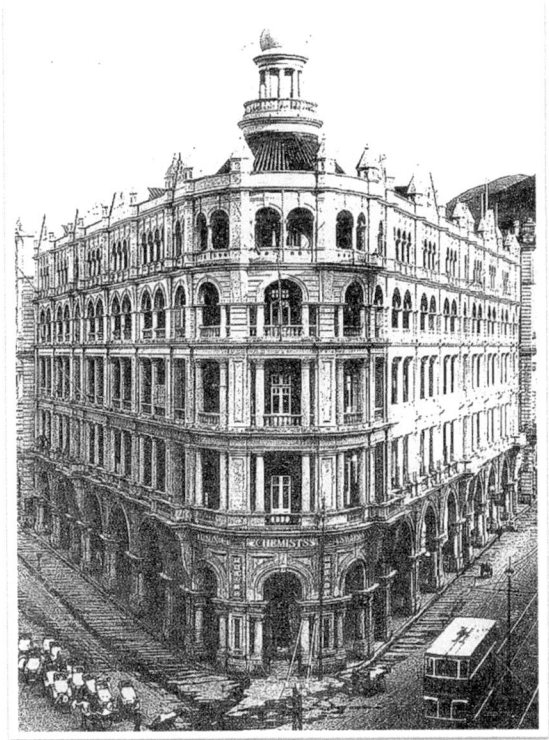

retail chemist shops and soda water manufacturing facilities, was sold to its manager, Donald Mennie, at a fraction of its original investments, in 1917.[13]

A.S. Watson survived these tumultuous periods and WWI because it was the market leader in the "opium cures" until the 1920s when Chinese manufacturing chemists and Japanese narcotic drug dealers took over the mainland market.[14] As a result, A.S. Watson took the initiative to expand its proprietary medicines portfolio and the distributor business in Taiwan during this period. (See the sections on *Narcotic Substitutes and Western Chemists* in Chap. 5).[15] During the heydays of A.S. Watson in the early 1920s, its annual calendar posters displaying a portfolio of its best-selling soda water and proprietary medicines were a hotly sought-after collector item by drug store customers in China and Southeast Asia (Fig. 4.11). Global recession (1929–1932) hurt A.S. Watson's business as hundreds of thousands of Chinese labourers, habitual users of "opium cures" who worked in the mines and plantations in Southeast Asia, were repatriated back to Mainland. In the following years, there was little or no demand for tin and rubber commodities for industrialized markets in Europe and the US. Prior to his departure for retirement in Canada, Henry Humphreys held the 48th annual general meeting of A.S. Watson on 21 March 1933. Excerpts of his last report as the chairman of the board of directors give insight:

I regret that I now come before you with an account that, compared with the previous year's report, must be considered disappointing; I feel this especially as this is the last occasion that I shall preside at the Company's annual meeting. Profits have generally responded to our activities, but unfortunately, the prevailing world-wide business and financial depression have adversely affected the Company's business, especially in its more profitable departments. This factor is responsible in a great measure for the poor results shown. In regard to this Company's business, this will be more readily understood when the fact is appreciated that on account of the lack of business during the past year or so, hundreds of thousands of Chinese who had for years been a source of considerable revenue and profit to the Company have been expatriated from Indochina, Straits Settlements, FMS and the Dutch Indies.[16]

Finally, A.S. Watson exited the mainland market in 1950 after the 1946–1949 Chinese civil war. However, it marched on as a British colonial chemist in Hong Kong until it was completely taken over by Li Ka-Shing's Cheung Kong Holdings Group Ltd. in 1981. [17] A.S. Watson re-entered the mainland market in 1984 which then transformed into a 3780 health and beauty retail outlets in China by mid-2023 alone making its original dream come true.

Fig. 4.11 Watson The Chemist, 1921 calendar poster. The Chinese character "*Zhen*" meaning "*Auspicious*" with beverages, proprietary medicines and toiletries (without the opium cures) shown at the bottom of the poster. *Credit* Roy Delbyck

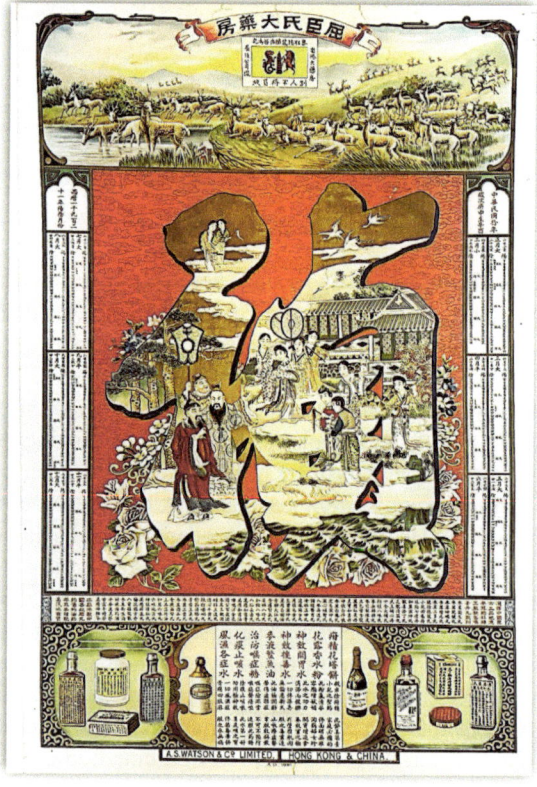

Shanghai's First Western Retail Pharmacy: British Dispensary

The British Hospital was opened for business serving the expatriate resident population and seamen in 1850 by a Macanese, M.G. de Souza, in the Bund area of Shanghai.[18,19] Souza was a former dispenser at the Dispensary in Hong Kong, and he replicated his employer's business practice to serve as a marine supplier to the transiting freighters. In the early 1870s, C.S. Churton became the British Hospital's new owner. While keeping its marine supplier wholesale business in the Bund, he opened a branch on Nanjing East Road in Shanghai in 1873 and a retail outlet in Hankow. The British Hospital soon began its journey as a wholesale and manufacturing chemist. The most popular items were the "opium cures" with different formulations of morphine, codeine and dionin in powder, lozenges, and pill forms for habitual opium smokers (See Chap. 5). Churton transferred the shareholding of the British Hospital to James McTavish and Paul Lehmann in 1880, who dropped the name "Hospital" and replaced it with "Dispensary" to trade as the British Dispensary.

McTavish and Lehman registered the business as a limited liability company in Hong Kong. The British Dispensary was actively engaged in the distribution business. It also became the agency of Allen and Hanburys, Wyeth and Brothers, Valentines Meat Juice, and Dr. Jayne's Family Medicine. In 1884, MacTavish and Lehman opened the Hongkew (Hongqiao) Medical Hall branch at No. 1 Suzhou River (Fig. 4.12). Stewart McLeish became the store manager, and Paul O'Brien Twigg joined as an assistant of the British Dispenasry. Four years later, the Dispensary opened another branch in Tianjin and stepped up its media advertising campaign (Fig. 4.13). In the same year, three experienced Chinese dispensers, including the manager Gu Songquan opened Shanghai's first Chinese-owned western chemist— Great China Dispensary. Other Chinese dispensers working for expatriate owned chemists soon followed their move.

After being trained at the Dispensary for 15 years, Twigg returned to the UK, took the Chemist and Druggist examination with the PSGB and became a qualified pharmacist in 1899. The Boxers Movement was causing havoc in Beijing with the burning down of western businesses. Donald Mennie (1875–1944), a chemist with the Beijing branch of the British Dispensary, exited from Beijing to join the Hongqiao Branch operated by the MacTavish & Lehman Ltd. in Shanghai.[20] As a safe haven, Shanghai's economy grew and Twigg's connections with the heads of pharmacies in Shanghai's western hospitals motivated him to return and open his retail pharmacy, P O'Brien Twigg Dispensary (Twigg's Dispensary), in late 1900. With increasing competition from local players, the MacTavish and Lehman's retail pharmacy business continued with growing difficulties. Its two retail outlets were acquired by A.S. Watson in 1909. A.S. Watson's North China business was subsequently acquired by Donald Mennie, who became the owner-manager of A.S. Watson of North China in 1917 which caused some relief.[21]

Fig. 4.12 MaTavish &
Lehmann Ltd. Hongkou
Branch @1908. *Credit* Hong
Kong Society for the History
of Pharmacy

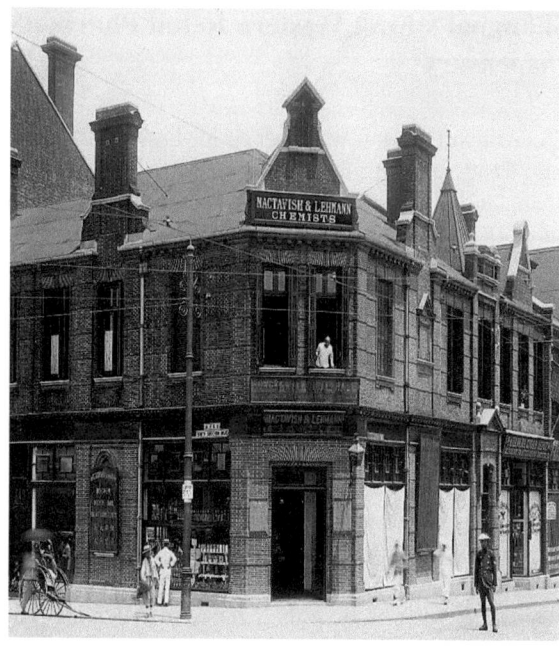

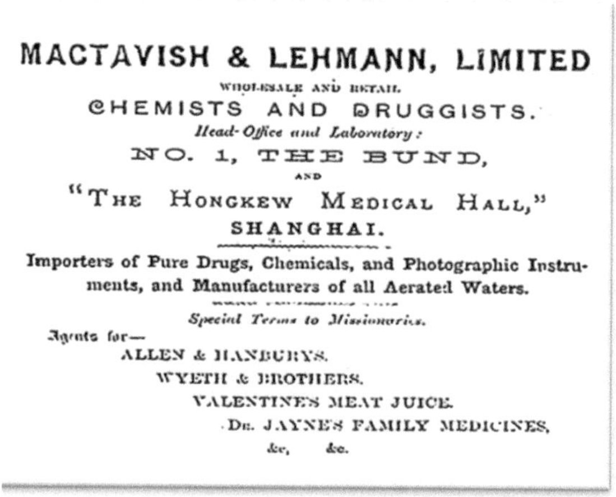

Fig. 4.13 Inside front cover
advertisement of
MacTavish & Lehmann,
Limited, Shanghai in Shun
Pao, 2, June 1894. *Credit*
The China Medical Journal

MACTAVISH & LEHMANN, LIMITED

WHOLESALE AND RETAIL.

CHEMISTS AND DRUGGISTS.

Head-Office and Laboratory:

NO. 1, THE BUND,

AND

"THE HONGKEW MEDICAL HALL,"

SHANGHAI.

Importers of Pure Drugs, Chemicals, and Photographic Instruments, and Manufacturers of all Aerated Waters.

Special Terms to Missionaries.

Agents for—

ALLEN & HANBURYS.

WYETH & BROTHERS.

VALENTINE'S MEAT JUICE.

Dr. JAYNE'S FAMILY MEDICINES,

&c,   &c.

The stock market crash in the Wall Street of New York occurred on 29 October 1929, resulting in the global recession and badly hitting Shanghai's retail market. In addition, the military clashes between the Japanese and the Nationalist armies in the suburbs of Shanghai in 1932 led to worsening financial situation. A year later, the Twigg's Dispensary was sold to a former Chinese employee who owned the Puji Dispensary. This signalled the beginning of the end of expatriate owned pharmacies in Shanghai.

The supply of "opium cures" by Chinse entrepreneurs and Japanese pharmaceutical companies replaced their western industry players in the 1910s until the 1940s. The Nationalist Government could not tackle the social ills effectively until the arrival of the Chinese Communists in 1949.

Leading Marketer of Toiletries—Shanghai Medical Hall

In 1860, Llewellyn decided to leave the partnership with the Dispensary operated by A.S. Watson in Shanghai and moved to Ningbo to start a new chemist business. Llewellyn sold his share of the business to E.C. Kirby, who opted to part ways with A.S. Watson.[22] Kirby registered a new trade name Shanghai Medical Hall (SMH), operated by Messrs. J. Llewellyn & Co. (Llewellyn) The latter registered the Chinese name Laou Teh Kee with the Shanghai Municipal Council in 1861 and it became the first Shanghai registered Chemist and Druggist. A.S. Watson acted promptly and partnered with S W Cleave to continue the Dispensary's business at 16 Nanjing Road, across the road. In 1867, J. Bradfield became the proprietor of SMH.[23]

In the next couple of decades, SMH focused on its private label personal care and drug products. These included thirteen toiletries, four health supplements, four "opium cures", four children's syrups, and eight oral internal and external use preparations. Exports of SMH's products under the Laou Tch Kee brand went as far as Japan and India. Laou Teh Kee was one of the earlier importers of "opium cures" which had a wide range of dosage forms such as lozenges, powders, and syrup, to fit the different needs of the habitual users. SMH became Kodak's distributor of photographic supplies in 1892.[24] In addition, Llewellyn's Laou Teh Kee brand of toiletries enjoyed recognition as a leading brand in Japan in 1878 (Fig. 4.14). In 1882, telephones were installed in Shanghai with 100 subscribers. Laou Teh Kee was one of the earliest customers with a number 72. It expanded with a branch opened at the corner of Fuzhou (Foochow) Road and Shaanix (Shensi) Road in February 1884. Four years later, Bradfield grew Laou Teh Kee's business by leaps and bounds with its flagship store at the Bund in Shanghai (Fig. 4.15), and seventeen branches including the co-branded Laou Teh Kee Chemist with local partners in Beijing, Suzhou, Hangzhou, Yangzhou, Yantai, Hankou and other locations.

In 1888, Bradfield had a dispute with the local employees leading to the departure of Zhuang Lingchen, an experienced and well-connected Chinese comprador, and two other dispensers of SMH left later in the year. [25] Like Gu of the Shanghai Dispensary, Zhuang and two other colleagues started up their own chemist, Great China Dispensary (中西药房 "Zhongxi Yaofang") and competed directly with Laou Teh Kee on the same range of imported and locally produced "opium cures". The departure of Zhuang and others dealt a big blow to Laou Teh Kee's "opium cures" business. G. A. Watkins, a long time employee of Laou Teh Kee acquired the business from Bradfield's and rebuilt the retail and manufacturing business in 1889.[26] Under Watkins leadership, a new soda water plant was soon installed and business entered into a new phase with the soda water contributing a significant portion of its business

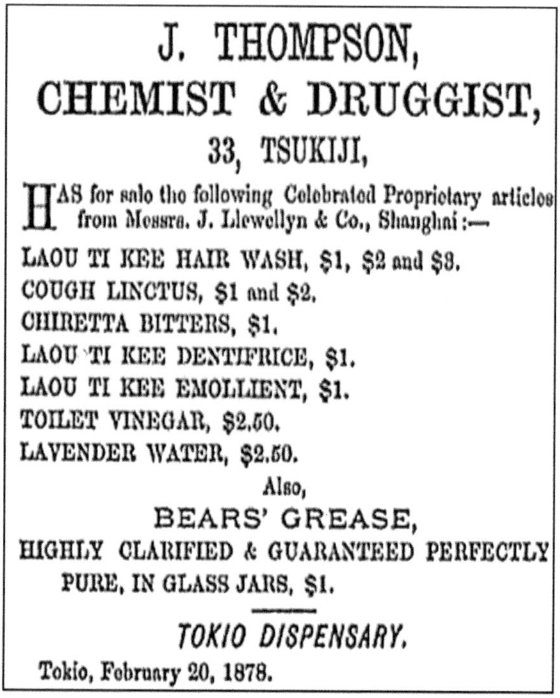

Fig. 4.14 Classified advertisement of J. Llewellyn & Co. brand of personal care products placed by J. Thompson Chemist and Druggist on 20 February 1878 for the edition of 23 March 1878. *Credit* Tokiyo Times

J. THOMPSON,

CHEMIST & DRUGGIST,

33, TSUKIJI,

HAS for sale the following Celebrated Proprietary articles from Messrs. J. Llewellyn & Co., Shanghai:—

LAOU TI KEE HAIR WASH, $1, $2 and $3.

COUGH LINCTUS, $1 and $2.

CHIRETTA BITTERS, $1.

LAOU TI KEE DENTIFRICE, $1.

LAOU TI KEE EMOLLIENT, $1.

TOILET VINEGAR, $2.50.

LAVENDER WATER, $2.50.

Also,

BEARS' GREASE,

HIGHLY CLARIFIED & GUARANTEED PERFECTLY PURE, IN GLASS JARS, $1.

TOKIO DISPENSARY.

Tokio, February 20, 1878.

in the next couple of decades. At the 25th general meeting of Messrs. J. Llewellyn and Co. Ltd. held at Shanghai on April 30, 1914, Mr. C.W. Wrightson, chairman of the board of directors, said:

> Your Directors, recognizing the advantages to be gained by an extension of the aerated water branch of your business, decided to install an entirely new and up to date plant, and I am pleased to inform you that the new factory, situated on the North Szechuen Road, commenced business on the first of this month and though we have only the results of a month's working, our expectations have so far been fully realized, the quality of our waters subjected to the new electric process of sterilization proving highly satisfactory; and your Directors have every confidence in the future of this branch of the business.[27]

Shanghai's four largest western chemists, British Dispensary, Koeffer Dispensary, Laou Teh Kee, and A.S. Watson, collectively served as pioneers of western retail, wholesale, and manufacturing chemists in China (See the section on *Research of Ethical Pharmaceuticals* in Chap. 7). They produced quality branded *Xiyao*, "opium cures", proprietary medicines, and health supplements for the local and overseas markets. Their Chinese employees eventually succeeded as prominent retail and manufacturing chemists in the first half of the twentieth century. The rise of the western chemists in China was led by the dozens of expatriate owned dispensaries operating in the colonies of Hong Kong, Macau, and the treaty ports of Shanghai and others in the second half of the nineteenth century. They became the driving force behind the transformation of Chinese medicine pharmacy, which also stocked

Fig. 4.15 Laou Teh Kee
Dispensary. Operated by J
Llewellyn & Co., Shanghai.
c. 1910. *Credit* Hong Kong
Society for the History of
Pharmacy

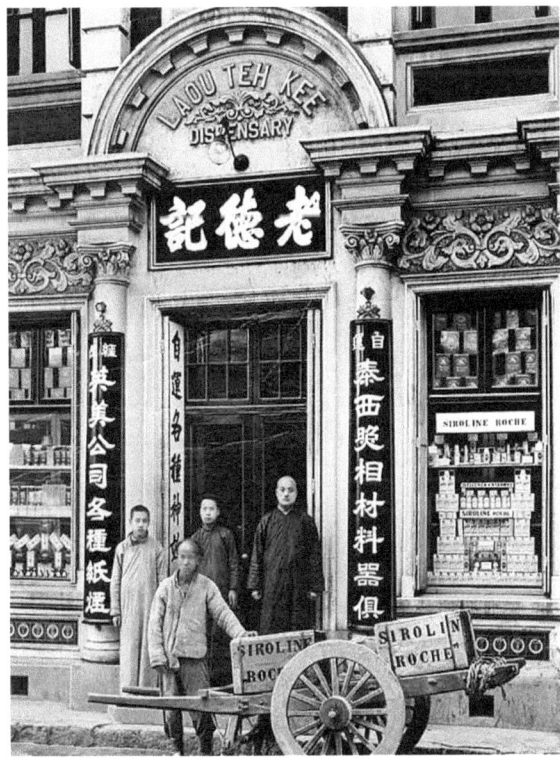

up "opium cures" and novel proprietary medicines containing herbal ingredients
in the first half of the twentieth. By the mid-1910s, Chinese chemists had gained
their economy of scale in establishing their private label brands of "opium cures"
and proprietary medicines with local production facilities. As a result, they enjoyed
far higher profit margins than imported brands from Japan, Europe, the UK or the
US. Besides, Chinese chemists worked "round the clock all year round", and few
independent expatriate chemists worked such hours.

During the Second Sino-Japanese War of 1937–1945, all western pharmacies,
including those in Hong Kong were closed. Finally, the foundation of the People's
Republic of China in October 1949 reset the pace of development in the private sector.
The state was again responsible for planning, supplying and distributing medicines
to the mass market like the Song emperors a millennium ago. The growth of western
retail chemists in modern China is another controversial subject. Western chemists
offered a new retail and consumer marketing concept of private label proprietary
medicines, toiletries, soda water, and photographic supplies like any reputable British
or US high street chemist. At the same time, these western and their Chinese counterparts also supplied "opium cures", which were social ills well worth in-depth
study!

This chapter documents the success of entrepreneurs who adeptly aligned with local customary practices and flourished in free market economies with their "opium cures", anti-wormer bonbons, soda water, photographic supplies in the second half of the nineteenth century. Shanghai surpassed Colonial Hong Kong as a prominent trading hub, as the latter was burdened with increasing laws and regulations when the Opium Ordinance came into effect in 1893. The natural disasters, political and economic turmoil occurred in the late 1900s, drove the Ningbo entrepreneurs operating in Shanghai, to acquire their western counterparts, who were facing financial difficulties, and ultimately reshaped the business landscape across the eighty treaty ports by the 1930s.

Notes and References

1. Tarrant, William, *The Hong Kong Almanck and Directory for the Year 1848*, (Hong Kong, Noronya 1848), 74–75. Accessed 12 March 2023. https://archive.org/details/1848hongkong almanachdirectory/page/n71/mode/2up.
2. Chiu, Patrick, "The First Hundred Years of Western Pharmacy in Colonial Hong Kong (1841–1940)", *Pharmaceutical Historian 46*, no. 3 (2016): 42–49, esp. 43. Accessed 29 September 2023. https://leopard.tu-braunschweig.de/rsc/viewer/dbbs_derivate_00044174/Pharmaceutical-Historian-2016-3.pdf?page=5.
3. The original text of the Treaty of Nanking has been archived by the Ministry of Foreign Affairs, Republic of China at the National Palace Museum, Taipei, Taiwan since 1949. Accessed 29 September 2023. https://web.archive.org/web/20140514235850/http://libdb1.npm.gov.tw/tts cgi/capimg2.exe?1%3A121345731%3A910000108001-0-0.pdf.
4. Articles II and III, Treaty between HER MAJESTY and the EMPEROR of CHINA, *The London Gazette,* no. (1843):3597–3603. Accessed 29 September 2023. https://www.thegaz ette.co.uk/London/issue/20276/page/3597/.
5. The Treaty of Nanking of 1842 had two official versions: some parts of the Chinese version differed which restricted the entry of foreign traders and missionaries into Guangzhou for temporary residency. The English version simply left out such conditions of stay.
6. By 1848, 28 commercial companies and 86 foreigners were stationed in Shanghai of whom 21 or 75% were British companies followed by 7 American business organizations, and one company each of British India and France. There were also 63 of 73% of British nationals, including businessmen and missionaries, 17 or 20% of US citizens and 6 or 7% of French and Indian nationals.
7. Wright A. Ed., "Shanghai Shipping, Commerce and Customs", *Twentieth Century Impressions of Shanghai, and Other Treaty Ports of China: Their History, People, Commerce and Resources,* (London, Lloyd's Greater Britain Publishing Co. Ltd. 1908), 1–848, esp. 454.
8. Zhang, Y, Du, Y, 'Lessons in ambivalence: The Shanghai Municipal Council's Opium Policies, 1906–1917', *International Journal of Drug Policy* 37, 2016, 136–142, esp. 137. Accessed 29 September 2023. https://www.researchgate.net/publication/309381993_Lessons_in_ambival ence_The_Shanghai_Municipal_Council's_opium_policies_1906-1917.
9. The Shanghai British Concession was formally established on November 20, 1846, the US Concession two years later in 1848 and the French Concession in 1849. To effectively implement the extra-territorial jurisdiction, the British and United States governments merged their two respective concessions into the Shanghai International Settlement on September 21, 1863. The International Settlement ended in December 1941 when the Japanese military declared war on the US and abolished the duties of the SMC.

10. "Peking: Report of Captain John T. Myers", *Siege of Peking, May to August 1900, United States Naval Hospital, Tientsin, China*, September 26, 1900. Accessed 29 September 2023. https://www.history.navy.mil/research/library/online-reading-room/title-list-alphabetically/b/boxer-rebellion-usnavy-1900-1901/selected-documents-boxer-rebellion/siege-peking-may-august-1900/peking-report-of-captain-john-t-myers.html.

11. Zhang, *Lessons in ambivalence,* 138.

12. "Hong Kong, The World's Shop Window", *Handbook to Hong Kong*, (Hong Kong, Kelly and Walsh, 1908), 106–112.

13. Chiu, *Transformation from Colonial Chemists,* 29.

14. Chiu, *Transformation from Colonial Chemist,* 38–39.

15. Chiu, *Transformation from Colonial Chemist,* 36–38, 65.

16. "Messrs. A.S. Watson & Co. Ltd., Disappointing Year Revealed at Annual Meeting, Hong Kong". Hong Kong. Daily News, March 22, 1933: 6. https://mmis.hkpl.gov.hk/old-hk-collection.

17. Chiu, *Transformation from Colonial Chemist*, 54.

18. The word *"Hospital"* as in the case of British Hospital was misleading in today's understanding. The first western hospital in Shanghai in the mid-nineteenth century is widely accepted as the Chinese Hospital founded by Dr. William Lockhart (1811–1896) of the London Missionary Society, an evangelical missionary society, in 1844. The British Hospital might have a few beds on site for sick seamen who stayed there more as a convalescent home than a medical institution.

19. Macanese are those of Portuguese ancestry who have settled down in Macau for several generations since the early seventeenth century. Many came from Goa, India, and some from Brazil and Lusophone Africa.

20. Chiu, *Transformation from Colonial Chemist,* 25.

21. Chiu, *Transformation from Colonial Chemist,* 29–30.

22. Chiu, *Transformation from Colonial Chemist,* 6–7.

23. *China Directory for 1867* (Hong Kong: A. Shortrede & Co., 1867), J9. Accessed 29 September 2023. https://www.chinafamilies.net/wp-content/uploads/2018/07/1867-China-Directory-v6ptsp.pdf.

24. List of Principal Kodak Dealers, The Kodak Manual, June 1892: 39. Accessed 29 September 2023. https://www.pacificrimcamera.com/rl/02391/02391.pdf.

25. "Shanghai Jindai Xiyao Hangye Shi" 上海近代西药行业史, [Shanghai's Modern Pharmaceutical Industry], "Shanghai Shehui Kexueyuan Chuban She" 上海社会科学院出版社 [Shanghai Academy of Social Sciences Press, 1988], 233.

26. *The Chronicle and Directory for China, Corea, Japan, The Philippines, Cochin-China, Annam, Tonquin, Siam, Borneo, Straits Settlements, Malay Sates, etc. for the Year 1889*, (Hong Kong, Daily Press 1889): 446. Accessed 29 September 2023. https://wellcomecollection.org/works/uf8r7ew3/items.

27. J. Llewellyn & Co., Hong Kong Telegraph, 5 May 1914: 8. Accessed 29 September 2023. https://mmis.hkpl.gov.hk/web/guest/old-hk-collection?from_menu=Y&dummy=.

Chapter 5
"Opium Cures", Proprietary Medicines and Soda Water

This chapter examines the dramatic surge of "opium cures", fueled by their novelty appeal and newspaper advertisements, in substituting opium smoking. The considerable profitability of the "opium cures" and its user-friendly forms of pills, powders, tablets and injections motivated numerous small-scale traders to establish retail outlets across the country, ultimately resulting in a pervasive epidemic of narcotic addiction in the 1890s. Paradoxically, leading western retailers and wholesalers expanded into proprietary medicines and soda water, laying the foundation for China's burgeoning pharmaceutical industry in the early twentieth century.

From the Divine Farmer's Classic of Materia Medica, complied by apothecary scholars in the Eastern Han dynasty (25–220), to Li Shizhen's "*Compendium of Materia Medica*" released in 1596 (the 21st year of the reign of Emperor Shenzhong, r. 1573–1620) in the Ming dynasty, Chinese medicine men had accumulated ample knowledge and expertise in the formulation and research for the most suitable herbal medicines to treat its people. The nineteenth century saw a sea change in the breakthroughs of pharmacy with the extraction and isolation of alkaloids, synthesis of drugs for surgical anaesthesia, and discovery of potent narcotic medicines for cough and pain suppression. In the first half of the twentieth century, advances in chemistry, microbiology, pharmaceutics, manufacturing technology and sterilization techniques further drove eastern traditional and western pharmacy practices apart. Naturally, potent cough suppressants and pain killing drugs with increasing potency, such as laudanum, cocaine, morphine, and heroin, used as medicines, also have equally and increasingly habit-forming effects. These mass-produced narcotic drugs yielded substantial profits to the manufacturing chemists in Europe and the UK in the nineteenth century.[1] However, rapid business growth stalled when the restriction on the sales of heroin and other narcotic drugs was imposed in Europe, the UK and the US in the early 1910s. In China, western chemists began advertising imported and soon locally produced laudanum or "opium cures" in Shun Pao (申报, *Shenbao*, Shanghai News) when launched in 1872. With opium smokers reaching a staggering thirty million as ready consumers of "opium cures" in the 1880s, Chinese-owned western chemists began to sprout up and engaged in the lucrative retailing

© The Author(s), under exclusive license to Springer Nature Singapore Pte Ltd. 2023   89
P. Chiu, *A History of Western Pharmacy in China*,
https://doi.org/10.1007/978-981-99-8635-4_5

and wholesaling of "opium cures" in Shanghai once dominated by their British and European employers.

In the late 1880s, local Shanghaiese chemists began a twenty-year journey of gradually taking over the domestic "opium cures" market.[2] By the 1900s, exports of "opium cures" to Taiwan and Southeast Asian markets rose due to the demand of hundreds of thousands of Chinese migrant workers and bonded labourers from the southern provinces of China working in the rubber plantations and tine mines in these countries. Chinese chemists followed in the footsteps of their western counterparts as distributors of imported "opium cures", proprietary medicines and toiletries. They soon marketed their private-label brands of laudanum mixed with herbal medicines containing grounded opium powders for all common illnesses, offering cough, diarrhoea, or pain relief. An explosive growth of "opium cures" and imported proprietary medicines was recorded in the 1900s, and such drugs flooded the market from Harbin to Hainan a decade later. China's first soda fountain set was installed at the Canton Dispensary in 1832. With the operation of Albany Pumping Station for freshwater supply from the Pokfulam Reservoir to the Central District of Hong Kong and a new ice factory in Hong Kong in 1874, A. S. Watson began to produce a range of flavoured soda water in its new plant in 1876. Other local dispensaries, such as Dakin Dispensary, Koeffer Dispensary and a couple of local businesses soon followed suit.[3]

Narcotic Substitutes and Western Chemists

Friedrich Sertürner (1783–1841) was a German pharmacist who pioneered modern pharmacy and had a lasting impact in transforming the pharmacy profession from a state of apothecary to a scientific discipline. His biggest achievement was the discovery of the colourless crystals of pure morphine by precipitation, published in 1817.[4] Mass production of morphine was, however, successfully carried out by Emmanuel Merk, who turned the family's retail pharmacy in Darmstadt in 1827, making the business the largest chemical and pharmaceutical manufacturer in Germany and the world in the nineteenth century.[5] Today, discussing opium and "opium cures" sales might show indifference to the morale scourge this was on Chinese society. However, a different perspective was provided by Ellen Castlelow in her article "Opium in Victorian Britain":

> Opium and other narcotic drugs played an important part in Victorian life. Shocking though it might be to us in the twenty-first century, in Victorian times, it was possible to walk into a chemist and buy, without prescription, laudanum, cocaine and even arsenic. The most popular preparation was laudanum, an alcoholic herbal mixture containing 10% opium. Called the 'aspirin of the nineteenth century,' laudanum was a popular painkiller and relaxant, recommended for all sorts of ailments including coughs, rheumatism, 'women's troubles' and also, perhaps most disturbingly, as a soporific for babies and young children. And as twenty or twenty-five drops of laudanum could be bought for just a penny, it was also affordable. The 1868 Pharmacy Act attempted to control the sale and supply of opium-based preparations by ensuring that they could only be sold by registered chemists. However, this was largely ineffective, as there was no limit on the amount the chemist could sell to the public.[6]

After the Second Opium War ended in 1860 with the opening of more treaty ports and unrestricted and duty-free import of opium into China, opium smoking became a national "leisure drug" across all walks of life. According to the Chinese delegation to the International Opium Commission of Shanghai (1909) the number of addicts increased to between 21.5 and 25 million (or 5.4–6.3% of the total population) by 1906.[7] The opium pipe was a status symbol of the wealthy smokers at home and in the opium dens, as in the case of Hong Kong in the nineteenth century (Fig. 5.1). Domestic farming of opium poppy also rapidly escalated after 1860, and exports to the rest of the world grew and exceeded imports in 1880. Laou Teh Kee was an early western chemist to advertise imported brands of laudanum as "opium cures" in Shun Pao in Shanghai in 1874 (Fig. 5.2).[8] Laou Teh Kee's goal was for these apothecaries to stock up on western opium substitutes for consumption by local opium smokers. JDH, the sole owner of A. S. Watson since 1874, saw the growth of the opium-smoking phenomenon tied in with Shanghai's unique location at the mouth of the Yangtze River, which was evolving as the nationwide logistic centre. In 1882, he entrusted John Davey as the Shanghai Dispensary manager and James Jones as the assistant to prepare for the roll-out of A. S. Watson's brand of "opium cures".[9] Sales of imported "opium cures" were initially slow due to their high price, as labourers could not afford to pay for these narcotic substitutes, however, the consumption of "opium cures" as opium substitutes increased with rapid growth in opium cultivation surpassing imported opium at 6500 MTs in 1880.[10]

To finance Humphrey's first stage of A. S. Watson's strategic plan to become China's leading retail and manufacturing chemist, 200,000 silver dollars were raised as additional capital from its shareholders.[11]

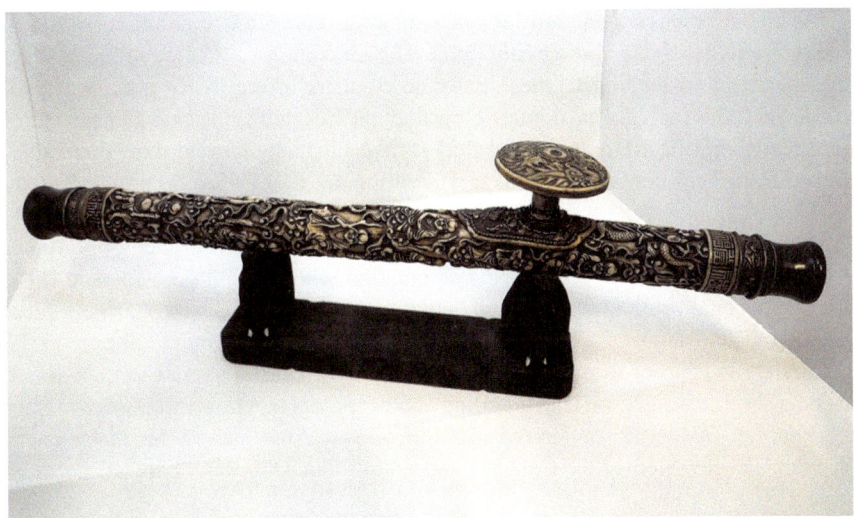

Fig. 5.1 Cloisonne opium pipe @nineteenth century. Engraved on the pipe-bow are the two five-talon dragons, representing the imperial status of the Qing dynasty. *Credit* Hong Kong Police Museum

Fig. 5.2 "Opium
cures"—Laudanum (opium
tincture). 1880–1940. *Credit
Science Museum, Wellcome
Foundation*

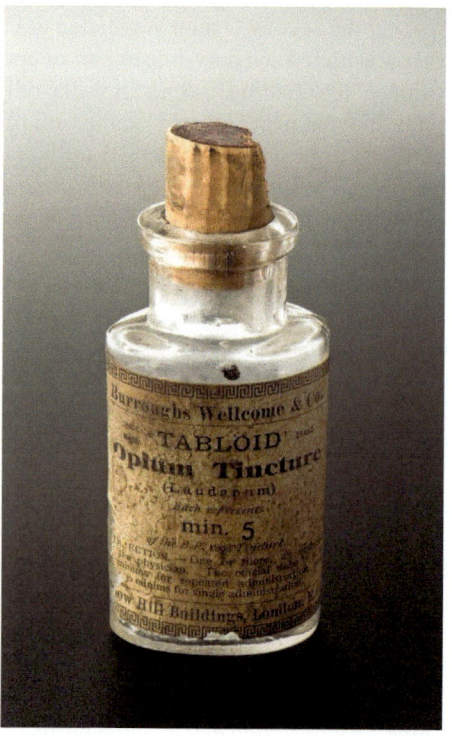

The objective was to generate demand for "opium cures" and to improve inventory holding by its stockists in the treaty ports. The marketing campaign with classified advertisements in leading Chinese daily newspapers in the treaty ports was well timed. With the increase in domestic production of opium, the prevalence rate of opium consumption in China skyrocketed. As a result, the opium smoking population jumped from 3 million in the 1830s to 15 million, or 3% of the total population, by 1890.[12],[13]

A study of A. S. Watson's business history revealed that its golden opportunity arrived in early 1893. A. S. Watson's association with "opium cures" made it the largest retail chain with over a hundred outlets and the most advanced pharmaceutical and soda water manufacturer at the turn of the twentieth century.[14] Other than the soda water, and earlier forms of "opium cures", A. S. Watson's retail and wholesale business showed a quantum leap in selling another potent narcotic, morphine, directly to the public. This trend accelerated after followers of American medical missionary Dr. John Glasgow Kerr of the Canton Hospital introduced morphine injections as an "opium cure" for menial workers.

These habitual narcotic users found they could save more than 80% on "highs" by injecting morphine under the skin. Moreover, the hypodermic morphine injections were much cheaper than purchasing dross or residual opium scraps collected from smoked opium pipes. In the second quarter of 1893, 1000 people took two shots daily. Drug users who opted for morphine injection to opium smoking without supervision quickly suffered many casualties with overdosing and from infection when sharing needles to save costs. Even adding up the charges for the morphine injections administered by the medical doctor, it was still much cheaper than smoking low quality opium dross.[15] (See the section on *Localization of Western Retail and Manufacturing Chemists* in Chap. 9) All western chemists, including A. S. Watson, had long queues outside each morning for morphine supplies. The impact on business at the time was such that Hau Fook Hong, the official 'opium farmer' representing the licensed opium dens, sent a formal letter requesting the then Colonial Treasurer on 24 May 1893 to address the loss of opium revenues due to the intensifying competition from morphine injections (Fig. 5.3).[16] The term "opium farmer" referred to a master franchise holder of opium supply, granted the franchise for a given period by the colonial Government in the nineteenth and early twentieth centuries. The master franchise holder operated as an agent who supplied the prepared opium to the licensed opium dens and was not a de facto farmer who cultivated opium by profession. Because of this, the Morphine Ordinance 1893 was promulgated on 23 September by the Hong Kong government, prohibiting the unauthorized use of morphine injections without medical supervision or a prescription issued by a medical practitioner. However, while the move temporarily halted the use of morphine injection locally, it had little or no impact on the mainland, where there were no laws governing the sales of "opium cures".

A. S. Watson mitigated its loss of the morphine injection market in Hong Kong by expanding its distribution channels on the mainland and exporting its branded "opium cures" to Taiwan and Southeast Asia.[17] At the turn of the twentieth century, A. S. Watson became a leading "opium cures" brand in Taiwan (Figs. 5.4 and 5.5). Chinse entrepreneurs and Japanese pharmaceutical companies stepped up their efforts in producing "opium cures" in 1910s and they continued to supply the China and Southeast Asian markets until the 1940s. Taiwan was used by Japanese pharmaceutical companies as a base for cultivating coca trees for cocaine production in Japan.[18] "Opium cures", the highly habit-forming narcotic drugs essentially had a major share of the opium addiction market. As a result, the narcotic addiction peril persisted for another eight decades from the 1870s to 1940 in China. Neither the Manchu Qing nor the Nationalist Government could tackle the social ills effectively.

"Secret Remedies" and Proprietary Medicines

In the Anglophone world of the UK and its colonies and the US in the nineteenth century, proprietary medicines, backed with heavy advertising in newspapers, billboards and other marketing channels, were sold as "secret remedies" to treat a host of minor illnesses and discomforts. Dr. Michael Jepson, a British pharmaceutical historian, wrote:

> Many "secret remedies" contained little more than a few vegetable extracts, but others did contain active constituents that might include opium, or heavy metals such as mercury, antimony, lead or arsenic, which were variously used for treating coughs, colds, consumption

Sirs,

The Prepared Opium Ordinance of 1891, section 10, provides for the preparation and sale of prepared opium, and the word "preparation" by the interpretation clause in the Ordinance is stated thus: the subjecting of opium of any kind to any degree of artificial heat, for any purpose whatever shall be taken to be the preparing of such opium. In the latter part of section 10 it is provided "that no medical practitioner, chemist or druggist, not being a Chinese, or being such and having a European or American diploma, shall be prevented from preparing or selling opium bona fide for medical purpose".

Within the last few months a number of establishments have been opened in Hongkong, to which those who have acquired the habit of opium-smoking have been induced to resort for the purpose of having a preparation of opium administered by means of subcutaneous injections. As the charge made for each injection is very small, large number of Chinese have been induced to frequent these houses, and, we believe, that a considerable diminution in the receipts of the Farm arising from the sale of prepared opium for local consumption has been working to this cause. Under these circumstances we would ask you to be good enough to suggest to the Government either some modifications to the law with reference to the sale of preparations of opium, or else that a law might be passed making the subcutaneous injection of drugs, except under certain restrictions and by a duly qualified medical men, a punishable offence.

We are informed that a large number of persons have been seriously injured in their health by having recourse to places above mentioned, and as the practice is at the same time likely to affect permanently the revenue of the Colony as well as the present Opium Farmers, we feel justified in urging you to bring the matter to the serious attention of the Colonial Government.

We have the honour to be,

Sir,

Your most obedient Servants,

HAU FOOK COMPANY
Opium Farmers.

Fig. 5.3 Letter from Hau Fook Company to the colonial secretary, 24th May, 1893. *Source* Hong Kong Government Gazette, 16 September 1893. 970–971

(wasting away of the body), venereal and skin diseases. Only the official name and concentrations of poisons included in the Pharmacy Act of 1868 were required to be declared on the label of medicines containing them. In Britain, full disclosure of all active ingredients of a substance recommended as medicine only became obligatory with the passage of the Medicines Act in 1941.[19]

Import and sales of western proprietary medicines in China can be dated back to early 1841 when Drs. Alexander Anderson and Peter Young opened their matshed

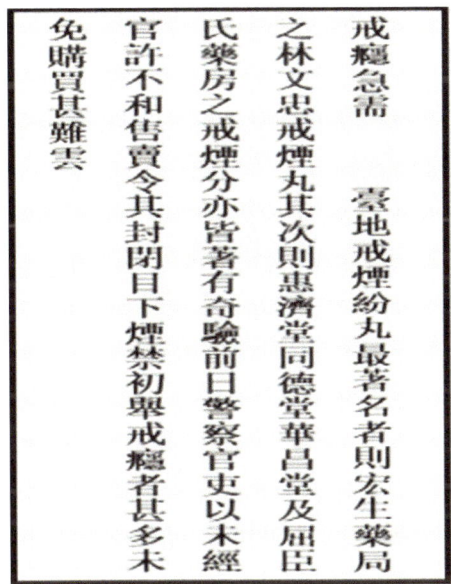

Fig. 5.4 News of *"Urgent needs for "opium cures" in Taiwan"*. Shortage of "opium cures" in Taiwan as police restricted trade, A. S. Watson among affected brand owners. *Credit* Taiwan Daily News, 3 April 1897

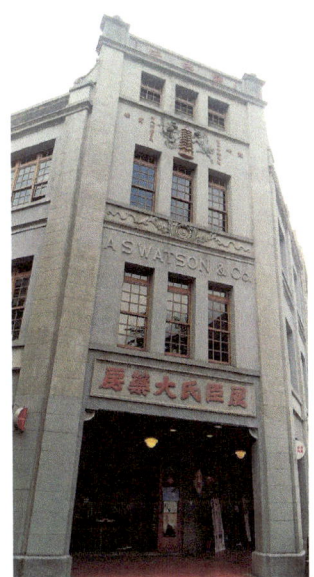

Fig. 5.5 A. S. Watson retail chemist façade, Taipei, Taiwan @1928. *Credit* Kalun Chiu

dispensary in Hong Kong. Advertisements for British and US brands of proprietary medicines started appearing in The North China Herald in 1851.[20] Hong Kong and Shanghai importers were invariably western and Japanese traders. Initially, their target consumers were Chinese residents living in the treaty ports of China and in Hong Kong. They soon reached out to those consumers living in the provinces. In the late nineteenth century, agents of American and British pharmaceutical houses advertised their proprietary medicines in newspapers to local consumers with highly exaggerated claims. The British, Japanese and US brands marketed included 'Moffat's Life Pills' and 'Phoenix Bitters', 'Holloway's Pills and Ointments', 'Scott's Cod Liver Oil', 'Haseline Snow Cream', and 'Eno Fruit Salts' were some of the popular proprietary medicines and toiletries imported for the China consumer market (Table 5.1).

In the second half of the nineteenth century, most proprietary medicines would seek trade mark registration but not patent protection since a registered patent medicine would need to reveal its list of active ingredients and the method of manufacture, which few manufacturers would do. Many manufacturing chemists also made exaggerated claims that such drugs could cure life threatening conditions. Hence, the term "quack medicine" was used to refer to ineffective and unsafe medicines. The British Medical Association published a booklet on "Secret remedies, what they cost and what they contain." in 1909. Excerpts given included:

> The wrapper around the jars of Burgess's Lion Ointment: was headed 'amputation avoided, the knife superseded', before stating that it had become the "most popular remedy for curing all diseases of the skin, ulcers, abscesses (including tuberculosis), piles, venereal sores, tumours, toothache, gatherings (pains) in the ear, deafness", and about thirty conditions. The label declared it to be a vegetable preparation, but on examination it was found to contain

Table 5.1 Key brands of imported or locally manufactured proprietary medicines, 1851–1911

#	Year	Brand	Original manufacturer	Country/ Territory origin	Agent, if any	Product range
1	1851	*Moffat*	John Maffat	US	Fogg and Co	*Moffat's Life Pills and Phoenix Bitters*
2	1855	*Holloway*	Prof. Holloway	UK	Hall and Holtz	*Holloway's pills and ointments*
3	1886	*A. S. Watson*	A. S. Watson Co. Ltd	British Hong Kong	Own brand and agents for others	Private label brand of baby food, "Opium Cures", proprietary medicines, soda water, toiletries, wines, spirits
4	1890	*Great Eastern*	Great Eastern Dispensary	China	Own brand	No.1 OTC/proprietary manufacturer with a range of *Dr T C Yale Stimulat Remedy (1905), Rentan (1910), Balingji (1923), Vinnin, Mytone* etc

(continued)

Table 5.1 (continued)

#	Year	Brand	Original manufacturer	Country/ Territory origin	Agent, if any	Product range
5	1900	*Scott's Emulsion*	Scott & Browne Ltd	US	Brunner Mond and Co. Ltd	*Scott's Cod Liver Oil* was the most popular fish oil in China in the early twentieth century
6		*Star*	Star laboratory	British Hong Kong	Own brand	*Shi Tak Chee Chi Chong Shui* —a morphine containing anti-diarrhoea tincture
7	1903	*Dr D Jayne*	Dr D Jayne & Sons Ltd	US	Own brand	*Jayne's expectorant, tonic vermufge,* and other drugs
8	1905	*Jintan*	Morishita Jintan Co., Ltd	Japan	Tao & Co	*Jintan* was the most popular OTC Japanese *Kampo* (TCMformula) in China
9	1907	*Sanatogen*	Bauer Chemical Co	Germany	Melchers and Co	*Santogen* bran tonic
10	1908	*William's*	Dr. William's Medicine Company	Canada	Own brand	Iron containing *Pink Pills for Pale People*—Tonic for Blood
11	1909	*Doans*	Doan's Pharmacy	Canada	Foster, McCllean & Co	*Doan's back ache kidney pills* etc. by Doan's pharmacy
12	1910	*Kepler*	Burroughs Wellcome	UK	Own brand	*Kepler Cod Liver Oil, Quinine Sugar Coated Tablets,* and *Haseline Snow* Cream etc. The latter was the most favourable facial cream of the female market in China
13	1911	*Eno's fruit salt*	JC Eno & Company	UK	H C Dickson & Co. Ltd	*Eno's* Fruit Salt

Credit Transformation from Colonial Chemist to Global Health and Beauty Retailer A. S. Watson, [Shanghai's Modern Pharmaceutical Industry] etc.

lead oleate, beeswax, resin, olive oil, water and lard. Beecham's Pills, on examination, was found to contain aloes, powdered ginger and powdered soap. The wrapper claimed that the pills were composed entirely of medicinal herbs' and cured well over 30 conditions, some of which came under inclusive headings such as 'all nervous affections, kidney and urinary disorders, flushings of heat and maladies of indiscretion', in addition to constipation, headache and bilious or liver complaints.[21]

    In China, western retail chemists were serving the needs of the expatriate popu-
lation. They were also the first to produce a dozen-bottle batch size of laudanum for
cough, cold, indigestion, and diarrhoea for the local consumer market. In addition,
marine suppliers had stocked up and advertised branded proprietary medicines, alco-
hols and spirits, beverages and food and sundry items for transiting freighters from
the early 1840s in Hong Kong and well into the first few decades of the twentieth
century in the treaty ports. It was not until the eldest son of JDH, Henry, qualified
as a pharmaceutical chemist, a senior rank of chemist and druggist, in the UK in
1888, that A. S. Watson was ready to achieve a second quantum leap in its retail
and manufacturing chemist business. Henry' returned to Hong Kong and joined the
family business as the pharmacist and manager of the retail and manufacturing operations in 1889. His first assignment was to develop a long-term strategic plan for A.
S. Watson. Henry achieved this within the first six months by registering the trade
marks of wines, spirits and soft drinks (items 1–47), opium smoker's cures (items
60–67 and 74–75), infant food (item 56), and toiletries (items 48–49, 57–73, and 78)
(Fig. 5.6).
    Henry's goal was to diversify A. S. Watson's portfolio of proprietary medicines
with an over emphasis on "opium cures" to that of proprietary medicines by
introducing a highly effective children's worm purgative, "Watson's Anthelmintic
Bonbons", in 1889 (Fig. 5.7). The first Watson's anti-wormer drug produced with
economy of scale was santonin (*Latin santoninum*). Santonin's commercial history
could be traced back to 1849 and an American pharmacist Charles Pfizer and his
cousin, Charles Erhardt, a candy maker from Germany. The two cousins established
Charles Pfizer and Company in Brooklyn, New York City. They produced an herbal
bonbon containing santonin, a highly effective therapeutic but equally toxic anti-
intestinal parasitic drug sourced from Siberia and Turkmenistan. The first edition of
the British Pharmacopoeia listed santonin as a standard drug in 1864.[22,23] Although
A. S. Watson was not the first producer of santonin anthelmintic, its brand of was
the most successful when launched soon after the colonial government of Hong
Kong approved A. S. Watson's trade mark registration in the summer of 1889. It was
rebranded as "Watson's Worm Cakes" in the 1930s with a longer shelf-life for the
hot and humid summer months in the southern provinces of the mainland, Taiwan,
and the Strait Settlements of Southeast Asia (Fig. 5.8).
    Star Talbot (施德芝, Sze Tak Chee, Shi Dezhi, 1861–1935), a Eurasian marine
supplier turned proprietary medicine maker from late 1890–1930, developed
Shanghai's first proprietary medicine around the 1900s (Fig. 5.9). He came from
a humble background; Talbot's British father was a sailor, and his mother was from
the treaty port of Ningbo. He grew up in Hong Kong and graduated from Queen's
College, attended mainly by Eurasians.[24] He went to Shanghai as a teenager and
worked for expatriate traders in the marine supply chain. In 1900, Talbot acquired
an opium smoking cessation formula from a Shanghai Chinese medicine dispensary and turned part of his photography studio, Sze Yuen Ming Photographer, into a
compounding room to produce Star Talbot's brand of *Sze Tak Chee Chi Chung Shui*
(General-Purpose Formulation for Illnesses)—a morphine containing tincture -into a
multifunctional medicine. He was the first to put his headshot onto the medicine box

THE HONGKONG GOVERNMENT GAZETTE, 11TH MAY, 1889. 427

GOVERNMENT NOTIFICATION.—No. 228.

Notice is hereby given that Messrs. A. S. WATSON & Co., LIMITED, of Victoria, Hongkong, have complied with the requirements of Ordinances 16 of 1873, and 8 of 1886, for the registration in this Colony of their Marks as applied to Wines, Spirits, Liquors, Medicines, Perfumes, Erated Waters, and other articles of a Dispensing Chemist and Druggist, as more particularly set forth in the following Schedule and that the same have been duly registered, viz.:—

SCHEDULE.

1. Watson's Vin de Quinquina.
2. Do. Prickly Heat Lotion.
3. Hongkong Tai Yeuk Fong Hair Wash (English and Spanish.)
4. Watson's Chiretta Bitters.
5. Do Tonic Bitters.
6. Watson's Finest Selected Old Scotch Malt Whiskey (Mellow Brand) " Glenorchy."
7. Watson's Finest Selected Old Scotch Malt Whiskey "Aberlour Glenlivet."
8. Old Irish Whiskey (A quality.)
9. John Jameson's Fine Old Irish Whiskey (B quality.)
10. Very fine Old Irish Whiskey (C quality.)
11. Watson's H.K.D. Blend of the Finest Scotch Malt Whiskies (D quality.)
12. Watson's very Old Liqueur Scotch Whiskey (E quality.)
13. Finest Old Jamaica Rum.
14. Superior very old Cognac Brandy (B quality.)
15. Very old Liqueur Cognac Brandy (C quality.)
16. Hennessy's Finest very old Liqueur Cognac Brandy 1872 Vintage (D quality.)
17. Sherry Pale Dry (Light Dinner Wine (A quality.)
18. Sherry Superior Pale Dry (good) Dinner Wine (B quality.)
19. Sherry Natural Manzanilla (superior quality) (C quality.)
20. Sherry superior Old Pale Dry (C C quality.)
21. Sherry very superior Old Pale Dry (D quality).
22. Sherry extra superior Old Pale Dry (E quality) very finest quality old bottled.
23. Genuine Breakfast Claret (A quality.)
24. St. Estephe (B quality.)
25. St. Julien (C quality.)
26. La Rose (D quality.)
27. Thorne's Blend Old Scotch Whiskey.
28. John Jameson's Old Irish Whiskey.
29. Fine Old Irish Whiskey.
30. Hennessy's Old Pale Brandy.
31. Finest Old Jamaica Rum.
32. Finest Old Genuine Bourbon Whiskey.
33. Finest Old Tom Gin.
34. Pale Dry Creaming Champagne (Brand G. R. S. & Co., Epernay.)
35. Pot Brand with Name, Address and Trade Mark printed on.
36. Watson's Phosphoric Champagne.
37. Lithia Water.
38. Effervescent Gingerade.
39. Sarsaparilla Water.
40. Sparkling Raspberryade.
41. Seltzer Water.
42. Ginger Ale.
43. Tonic Water.
44. Soda Water.
45. Lemonade.
46. Pure Supercarbonated Potash Water.
47. Watson's Mineral Tonic Water.
48. (Chinese) White Face Powder No. 140.
49. („) Rouge Powder No. 128.
50. Watson's Anthelmicetic Bon-Bons or Worm Tablets No. 132 (Label printed in English and Chinese) ......$1 size.
51. Do. do. 50 cts. „
52. Do. do. 25 „ „
53. Do. do. 10 „ „
54. Worm Bon-Bons (Chinese.)
55. Watson's Anthelmicetic Bon-Bons or Worm Tablets.
56. Watson's Infant's Food (Chinese.)
57. Envelope for Ching Fun (Chinese.)
58. Watson's Florida Water (Chinese) 30 cts. size.
59. Do. (Do.)10 „
60. Opium Smoker's Cure Pills No. 201 (Chinese) $1 size.
61. Do. Do. 50 cts. „
62. Do. Do. 25 „ „
63. Do. Do. 10 „ „
64. Opium Smoker's Cure Lozenges No. 202 (Chinese)......$1 size.
65. Do. Do. 50 cts. „
66. Do. Do. 25 „ „
67. Do. Do. 10 „ „
68. Red Face Powder No. 203 (Chinese.)
69. Hand-bill for Red Face Powder No. 203 (Chi.)
70. Do. Pink Colour do.
71. Do. Blue do. do.
72. Do. Wh. Face Powder No. 140 (Chi.)
73. Do. Rouge Powder No. 128 (Chi.)
74. Do. Opium Smoker's Cure Pills No. 201 (Chinese.)
75. Do. Opium Smoker's Cure Lozenges No. 202 (Chinese.)
76. Do. Bon-Bons No. 132 (Chinese) large size.
77. Do. Bon-Bons No. 132 (Chinese) small size.
78. Watson's Oriental Tooth Powder.

&c.. &c., &c.

By Command,

FREDERICK STEWART,
Colonial Secretary.

Colonial Secretary's Office, Hongkong, 7th May, 1889.

Fig. 5.6 Registered trade marks of A. S. Watson & Co. Ltd. 11th May 1889. *Credit* Hong Kong Government Gazette

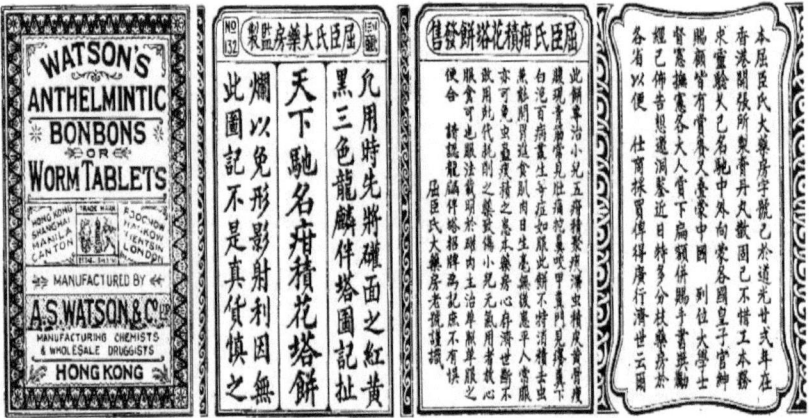

Fig. 5.7 A.S. Watson's Anthelmintic bonbons package label 1889. *Credit* Hong Kong Government Gazette

Fig. 5.8 A.S. Watson's Worm Tablets: 1930 label with cone shaped sugar candy as brand logo. *Credit* Hong Kong Government Gazette

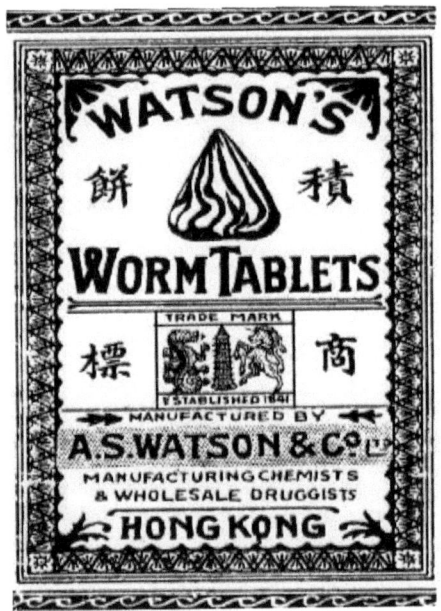

and package insert, which became a hallmark for all Chinese proprietary medicines (Fig. 5.10).

Although the Great Eastern Dispensary (中法药房, "*Zhong Fa Yaofang*") was not the first Chinese-owned chemist to open for business in the Shanghai International Settlements or the French Concession, it was indeed the most innovative marketer in modern China's health and beauty industry. With the explosive growth in trade

Fig. 5.9 Star Talbot (Sze
Tak Chee, *Sze Dezhi*) c. 1900
in Shanghai. *Credit* Hong
Kong Society for the History
of Pharmacy

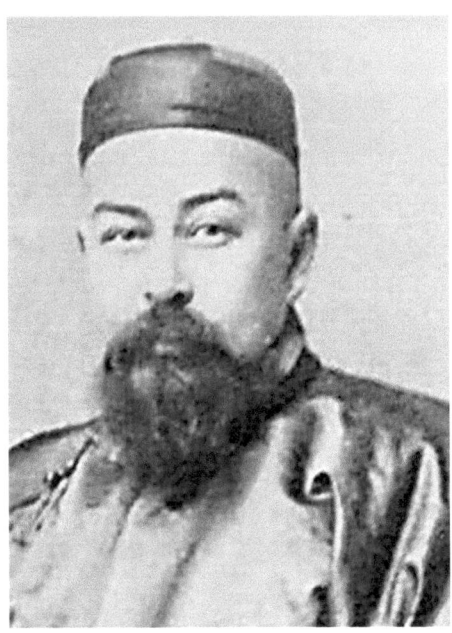

and the narcotic business in the 1880s, an influx of migrant workers from the eastern
provinces flocked into Shanghai's French Concession.

Huang Chujiu (黄楚九，Wong Tsu-Chiu, 1872-1931) of the Great Eastern
Dispensary marketed an imported brand of an ophthalmic drug in his Chinese
medicine apothecary in the French Concession in the 1890 (Fig. 5.11). The Great
Eastern Dispensary relocated again to larger retail premises in another part of the
French Concession—Foochow Road (Fuzhou Road, Si Malu) in 1904 Fig. 5.12). In
the meantime, local agents of American and British pharmaceutical houses advertised their proprietary medicines in local newspapers to consumers with highly
exaggerated claims.

In 1901, Great Eastern Dispensary, the most creative Ningboese owned dispensary
in Shanghai started to roll out its private-label brand of "opium cures". With his
first pot of gold from selling the "opium cures", the owner manager, Huang Chujiu
subsequently launched Dr. T. C. Yale's Brain Tonic, (艾罗补脑汁，"*Ailuo Bunao
Zhi*"), a brain tonic containing caffeine, herbal ingredients and multivitamins in
1905. By then, consumers in Shanghai embraced all things foreign. At the same
time, local entrepreneurs were dared to challenge the status quo of Chinese medicine
remedy by launching health supplements for the brain, heart and blood, and kidneys
with heavy advertising and marketing in local media. The word "*Yale*" in the Dr.
T. C. Yale's Brain Tonic was chosen to capitalize on the public's perception that
western medicine had faster onset than Chinese medicine, which would restore the
yin and yang balance. Incidentally, the transliteration of the word Yale had the same
meaning as the Shanghainese pronunciation of the surname "*Huang*" or "*Yellow*",

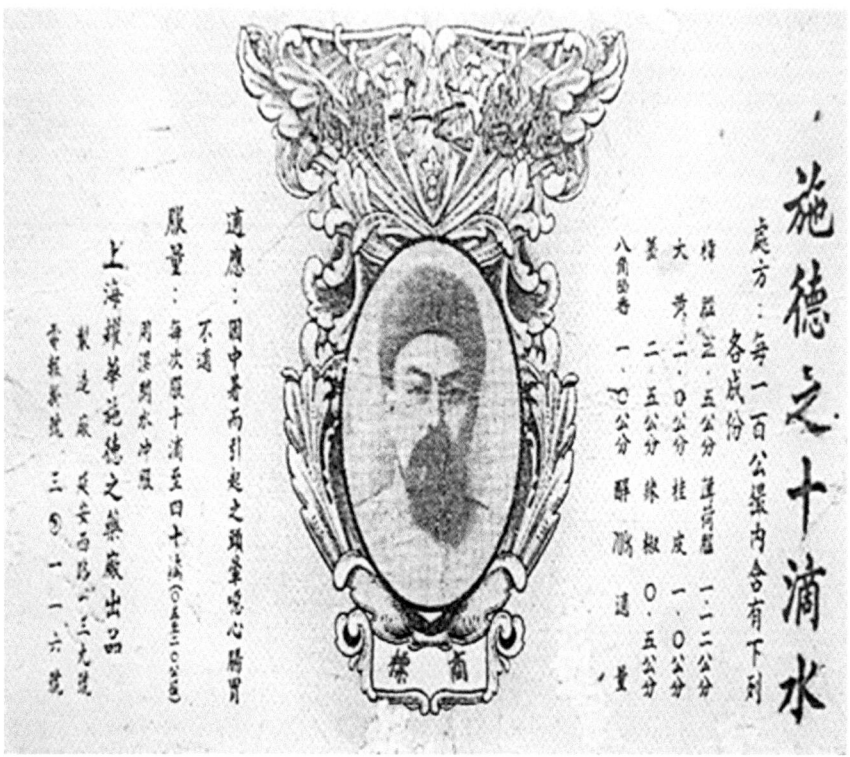

Fig. 5.10 Product insert of *Sze Tak Chee Ten-Drop Water* with Star Talbot's Headshot in the centre. c. 1910 in Shanghai. *Credit* Hong Kong Society for the History of Pharmacy

the owner of Great Eastern Dispensary. In addition, his initials of T C for Tsu-Chiu also corresponded to the brand's T C Yale.[25,26] Chang Ning articulated the success of Dr. T. C. Yale fit this trend and marketed the new concept of the "brain" in western medicine as.

> Of those changes, the most stunning was a new idea of the function of the brain. Rather insignificant in the past, the brain, along with the nervous system, replaced the heart as the centre of the body and thus as a volition, will and memory. Though medical historians have done much to illuminate the impact of this transformation on intellectuals and physicians, little research has traced its impact on Chinese culture and consumer life. By analyzing the surge of Ailuo Brain Tonic and other brain-related stimulants in the late Qing, I argue that the medicine men selling and promoting brain tonics played an essential role in the transformation. The drug stores sold not only drugs but also the new concept of the brain.[27]

The Great Eastern Dispensary continued to launch other proprietary medicines, including *Vinnin Stomach Remedy* and *Mytone Pain,* in the 1900s to the 1920s (Fig. 5.13). A subsidiary of the Great Eastern Dispensary, Longfu Drug Company, launched a proprietary medicine, *Rentan* (人丹), caught the Shanghai consumer

Fig. 5.11 Wong Tsu-Chu (1872–1931), owner of Great Eastern Dispensary, Shanghai. C. 1900. *Credit* Hong Kong Society for the History of Pharmacy

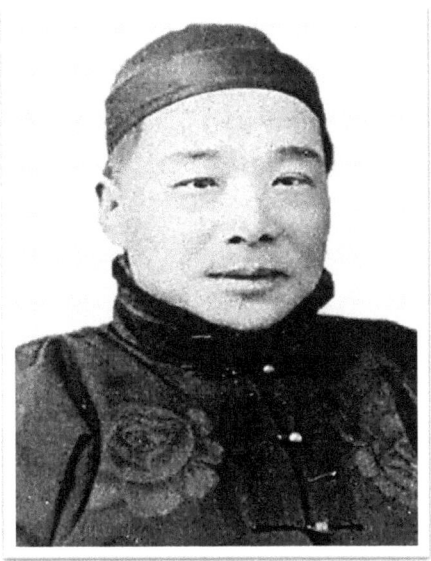

Fig. 5.12 Great Eastern Dispensary, flagship store at Foochow Road, Shanghai. C. 1904. *Credit* Hong Kong Society for the History of Pharmacy

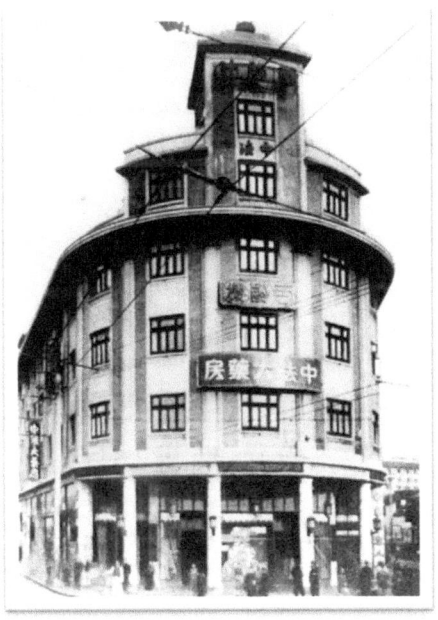

Fig. 5.13 Great Eastern
Dispensary's star products.
Top left: *Dr T C Yale Brain
Tonic.* @1905. Bottom left:
Vennin Stomch Remedy,
@1920, and bottom right,
Mytone Pain Killer. @1920.
Credit Hong Kong Society
for the History of Pharmacy

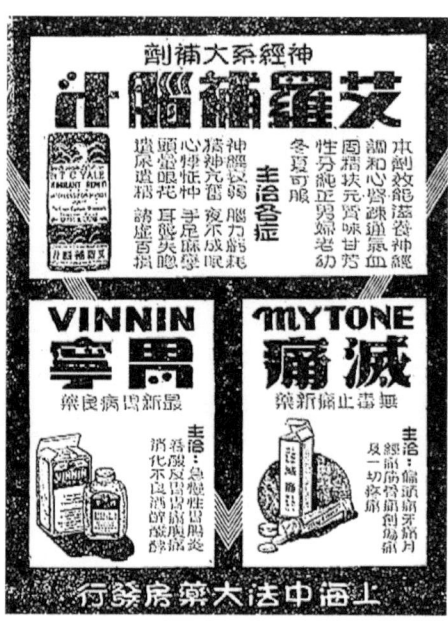

market by storm in 1910. Toa & Co. (东亚商社), the Shanghai agent of an all-purpose herbal remedy, Jitan (仁丹), manufactured by the Morishita family, claimed *Rentan* was a copy of the Jitan brand made by the Morishita family in Japan. The latter sued Great Eastern Dispensary's subsidiary, *Jiufu* Pharmaceutical Co. (九福制药公司), alleging its infringement of trade mark of Jitan which brought free publicity to Rendan, a consumer health herbal remedy. (See Chap. 8's Section on Intellectual Property Laws etc. In the early twentieth century, Great Eastern made a significant foray into the proprietary medicines market, drawing inspiration from the remarkable success of local brands such as "Liang Peiji Fever Pills" (梁培基发冷丸).[28] Foreign brands such as Doan's Ointment and Scott's Cod Liver Fish Oil demonstrated immense popularity and market traction, serving as catalysts for Great Eastern's venture into this industry (Figs. 5.14 and 5.15).

Holland Water and Flavoured Beverages

Soda water, mimicking natural sparking mineral water, had been bottled and served to patrons of spas in Europe and the US for the "health benefits" of such bubbling water since the early eighteenth century. In 1807, a patent based on the initial design of Joseph Priestly was granted to Henry Thompson in the production of carbonated water in the UK. After that, retail chemists on both sides of the Atlantic installed soda fountains for their patrons when shopping and waiting for their filled prescriptions. James Bradford, a port surgeon, reportedly installed Asia and China's first soda fountain in his Canton Dispensary to subsidize the funding of the free ophthalmic

Fig. 5.14 Calendar girl poster of *Doan's Ointment* by Foster McClellan Co. of London, UK. c. 1910. *Credit* Hong Kong Society for the History of Pharmacy

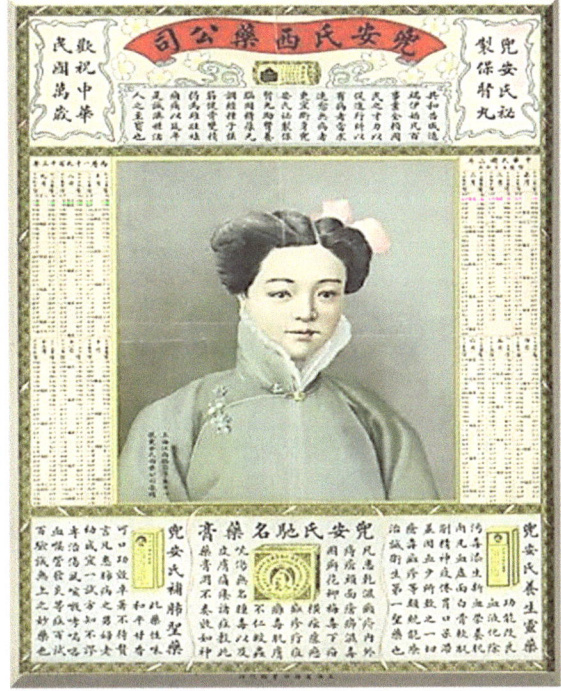

clinic, also known as the Canton Ophthalmic Hospital, in 1832. Shipments of bottled water became frequent in Hong Kong when ice was available to chill the bubbly drinks after the First Opium War. As the first freighters to ship soda water carried the Dutch EIC Company flag, locals called the bottled gas mineral water "Holland Water".

Soon after Hong Kong's first ice factory was built by two Scotsmen with steady supply of ice in 1874, A. S. Watson installed a distillation plant at its pharmaceutical workshop at 1–3 Stanley Street, Central, Hong Kong.[29] A. S. Watson launched its range of six-flavour Holland Water in 1876.[30] Ge Yuanxi (葛元熙), a travel writer based in Shanghai, reported the flavoured Holland Water in his *Huyouzaji* (沪游杂记) Shanghai Travel News guidebook:

> In summer, there is Holland Water and Lemonade, which are filled with carbonated water by machines. Be careful when opening the bottle, its plug bursts out like a bullet. Drinking it can dispel the summer heat.[31]

The launch of A. S. Watson's flavoured Holland Water in the City of Victoria was an instant hit, with the fizzy drinks contained in a torpedo-shaped green glass bottle. Both the soft drink and the glass bottle were new to the consumers.[32] Other than the local advertisements in the newspapers, the hand-drawn wooden carts transported

Fig. 5.15 Scott's Emulsion
of Cod Liver Oil,
advertisement. c. 1920.
Credit Hong Kong Society
for the History of Pharmacy

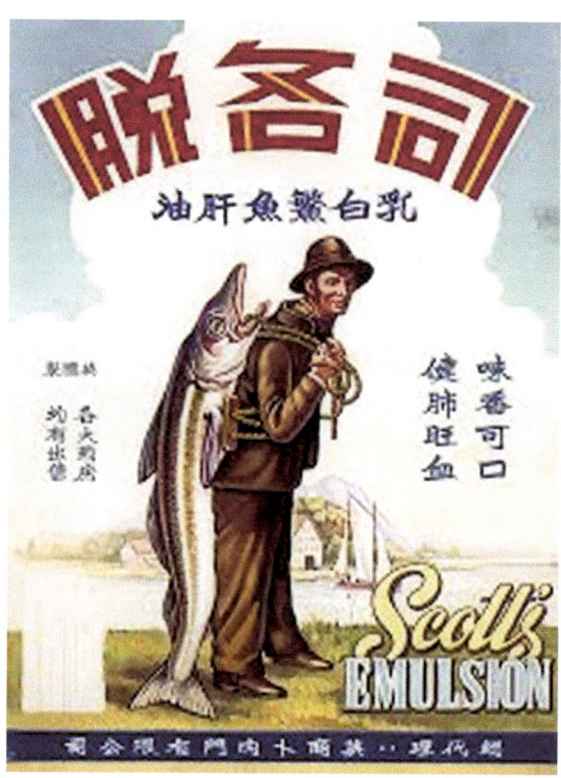

by menial labourers in the busy streets drew the pedestrians' attention in Central and Wanchai districts in the 1870s. Watson's Soda Water became the talk of the town as soon as it was marketed. As a result, the colony's hotels and restaurants soon stocked up icy cold orange or lime-flavoured bubbling drinks as novel drinks, much to the liking of their patrons. Wealthy Chinese merchants served Watson's icy-cold Holland Water in the hot and humid summer months instead of the popular Oolong Tea. Local retail and manufacturing chemists such as Dakin Dispensary, Koeffer Dispensary and others soon followed suit. In the following decade, A. S. Watson extended its Holland Water manufacturing capability to Manila in 1884 and Shanghai in 1886. A. S. Watson was also the first to market alcoholic and beverage drinks in ceramic jars, serving corporate and private banquets and parties from Shanghai to Singapore from the mid-1880s.

In 1892, Caldbeck, MacGregor & Co., a leading British wine, spirit and beverage importer in Shanghai, set up a Holland Water plant in Tilan Bridge (Tilanqiao), Hongkou. With its extensive retail, hotel and restaurant network throughout China, Calbeck MacGregor's Aquarius brand of Holland Water became another instant hit. This time, the Codd-neck bottle design and the manual labourer—drawn carts peddling up and down the Bund, the Shanghai International Settlements, and the French Concession drew crowds everywhere.[33] Consumers in Shanghai were once again fascinated by the design and the "mobile advertisements" of Acquaris Holland Water. Given the nature of Holland Water, cleansing, packaging, recycling, and transportation of the filled and empty glass bottles were daily supply chain challenges. As a result, regional soda water brands appeared in the market gradually in the first half of the twentieth century (Table 5.2).

In 1902, British merchant Balin Baldhan formed the Universal Mineral Water Company in the British Concession in Tianjin. Crystal Ltd. was founded as a separate company to manage the Crystal brand of Holland Water by Universal, which was produced in the Shanhaiguan area of Hebei province, the following year. Within the city of Tianjin, Crystal Holland Water was transported on bicycle carts and along the railway line across Northern China. Twenty years later, the Crystal brand of Holland Water gained nationwide coverage when it was served as a national beverage at the wedding banquet of Aisin-Gioro Puyi (溥仪, 1906–1967), the last emperor of the Manchu Qing dynasty, in the Forbidden City, Beijing. Baiwangmiao Aerated Water, Beer and Soya Sauce Ltd. was founded in Mukden, Northeastern China in 1922. Its Baiwangmaio brand became the regional brand soon after its launch. Shanghai was reckoned as the most creative city in China in the 1920s.

Soon after WWI ended, when the sugar supply became steady again, A. S. Watson launched the Chocolate Soda flavour Holland Water in Shanghai (Fig. 5.16). The new Holland Water aroused discussion among the young and trendy who became loyal consumers of Watson's brand of soft drinks. In 1927, China's Holland Water market

Table 5.2 Leading brands of locally produced soda water, 1876–1927

Leading brands of soda water manufacturers in the late nineteenth and early twentieth centuries in China

Year of production	Location	Brand	Company
1876	Hong Kong	Watson's	A. S. Watson & Co. Ltd
1886	Shanghai		
1892		Acquaris	Calbeck, MacGregor & Co. Ltd
1902	Shanhaiguan (Near Tianjin)	Crystal	Universal aertaed water, beer
1921	Mukden (Shenyang)	Baiwangmiao	Baiwangmiao Aerated Water, Beer and Soya Sauce Ltd
1927	Hong Kong, Shanghai	*Coca Cola*	Licensed by A. S. Watson & Co Ltd

Credit Transformation from Colonial Chemist to Global Health and Beauty Retailer: A. S. Watson, [Shanghai's Modern Pharmaceutical Industry] etc.

reached a new height. Coca-Cola appointed local bottlers to market its brand of Cola Holland Water in the three major regional markets of Northern, Eastern and Southern China, in Hong Kong and Shanghai by A. S. Watson, and the Capital and Tianjin region by Crystal Ltd. After a false start with a problematic local brand name, Coca-Cola changed its marketing tactic with the Chinese name Kekou Kele (可口可乐,'*Pleasing to the Mouth, Pleasing to the Heart*'). The brand colour was another bonus, with a red background in white characters representing festivities and happiness in traditional Chinese culture. Shanghai's top actress, Ruan Lingyu (阮玲玉) was the poster star (Fig. 5.17).[34]

Fig. 5.16 A. S. Watson's brand of *Chocolate Soda,* Shanghai @ 1926. *Credit* Hong Kong Society for the History of Pharmacy

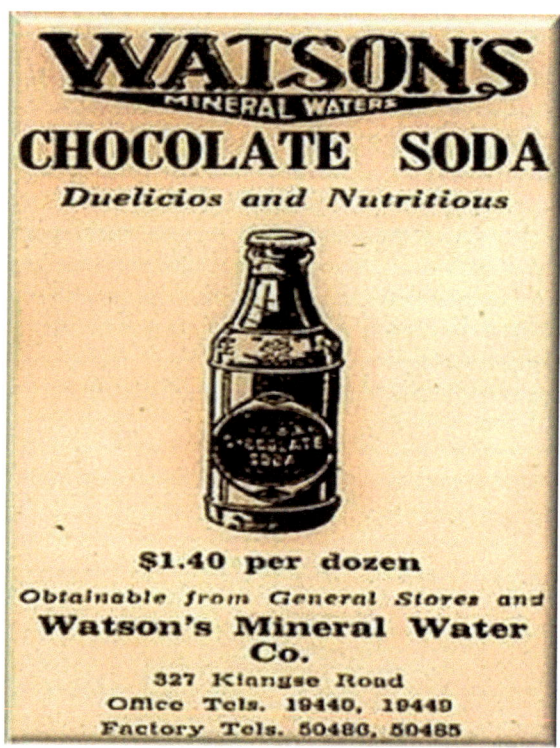

Fig. 5.17 Coca Cola
advertisement with
Shanghaiese actress Yuan
Lingyu as brand influencer.
Credit Hong Kong Society
for the History of Pharmacy

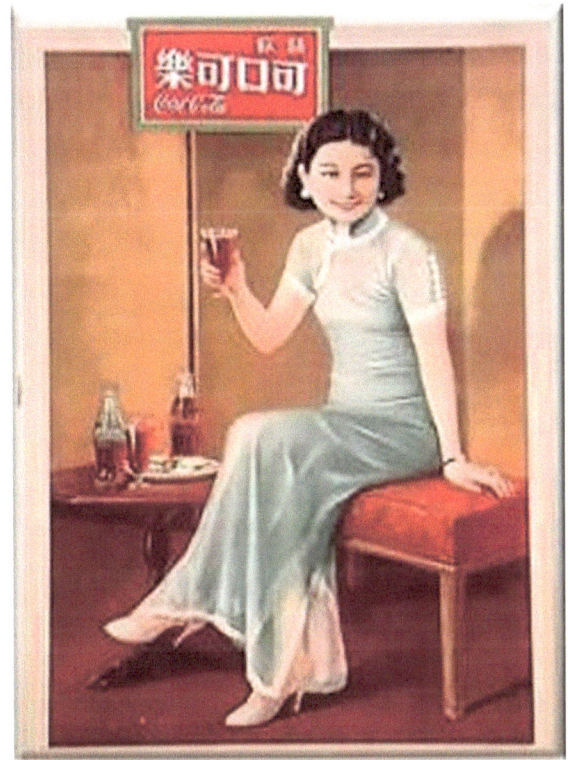

Notes and References

1. The proceeds of these narcotic drugs undoubtedly financed the scientific development of the
    modern pharmaceutical industry, as in the case of E. Merck and Bayer of Germany.
2. Many youths of Ningbo, a treaty port in the Zhejiang province, left their hometown to work
    as apprentices of western chemists in Shanghai. They learnt the dispensing skills at these
    western chemists and began to compete directly with their former employers by rolling the
    same "opium cures" in the early 1890s. Typical examples included Gu Songquan of Shanghai
    Dispensary who was the dispensing assistant of the British Dispensary owned by Mactavish
    and Lehmann, and Zhuang Lingchen of Laou Teh Kee owned by J. Llewellyn who opened the
    Great China Dispensary in the late 1880s.
3. Chiu, *Transformation from Colonial Chemist,* 12.
4. Krishnamrti, C., and Rao, C., "The Isolation of Morphine by Serturner", *Indian Journal
    Anaesthesia* 60, no. 11 (2016): 861–862. Accessed 29 September 2023.
5. E. Merck's branch in the US became independent from its German parent during WWI and
    it was later renamed as Merck Sharpe Dohme when the company merged with Sharpe and
    Dohme in 1953.
6. Castelow, Ellen, 'Opium in Victorian Britain", *Historic UK*. January 26, 2015. https://www.
    historic-uk.com/HistoryUK/HistoryofBritain/Opium-in-Victorian-Britain/.
7. International opium commission, report of the international opium commission, Vol. I,
    minutes of the proceeding, Shanghai, China, February 1 to February 26, 1909: 68.

Accessed 29 September 2023. https://www.unodc.org/documents/data-and-analysis/Studies/100_Years_of_Drug_Control.pdf.

8. "Opium cures", Classified advertisement by Laou Tek Kee, Shun Pao, 12 March 1874: 7. Accessed 29 September 2023. https://archive.org/details/shenbao-1874.03.12/page/n2/mode/1up?view=theater

9. Chiu, *Transformation from colonial chemist*, 11.

10. "A Century of International Drug Control", (Vienna: United Nations on Drugs and Crimes, *2008*), 7–25, esp.: 23–25. Accessed 29 September 2023. https://www.unodc.org/documents/data-and-analysis/Studies/100_Years_of_Drug_Control.

11. Chiu, *Transformation from Colonial Chemist*, 9–11.

12. Reins, T., "Reform, nationalism and internationalism: the opium suppression movement in China and the Anglo-American Influence, 1900–1908", *Modern Asian Studies* 25, no. 1 (1991), 101–142.

13. Zhou Yongming, *Anti-drug Crusades in Twentieth Century China: Nationalism, History and State Building*, (New York, Rowan & Littlefield 1999), 30.

14. Chiu, Patrick, Henry Humphreys (1867–1943): a visionary in retail pharmacy in colonial Hong Kong, *Pharmaceutical Historian, London,* Volume 48/3, 2018:77–78.

15. Opium dross is the opium residue collected from the used opium smoking pipes which contains 30–50% of the contents of opium due to incomplete combustion of prepared opium.

16. "Letter of opium farmers to colonial treasurer, 24 May,1893", *The Hong Kong Government Gazette*, 16 September 1893: 970–971. Accessed 29 September 2023. https://sunzi.lib.hku.hk/hkgro/.

17. Chiu, *Transformation from Colonia Chemist*, 13.

18. Reiss, Suzanne, *We Sell Drugs, The Alchemy of US Empire*, (Berkeley and Los Angeles: University of California Press, 2014), 16–53, esp. 24.

19. Jepson, Michael, from secret remedies to prescription medicines: a brief history of medicine quality, Stuart Anderson (Ed.), *Making medicines: a brief history of pharmacy and pharmaceuticals*, (London: Pharmaceutical Press, 2005), 231–232.

20. Advertisement, "Purify the Blood", *The North China Herald, Saturday*, 21 June 1851: 1. https://archive.org/details/north-china-herald-1851.06.21/mode/2up.

21. *Secret Remedies: What They Cost and What They Contain, Based on Analysis Made for the British Medical Association*, (London: British Medical Association, 1909): 170–185, esp.175, 180. https://wellcomecollection.org/works/y8hzb7a3/items?canvas=183.

22. Santonin, an active roundworm purgative derived from the plant *Artemesia cina,* was cultivated in Central Asia. It was a popular anthelmintic used in the nineteenth century and the first half of the twentieth century in Europe and North America, until it was replaced by piperazine in the 1950s.

23. "Santonium" *(Santonin)*, British Pharmacopoeia, (London, General Council and Registration of the United Kingdom, 1864), 127–128, 321–323.

24. Star Talbot was among the few Eurasians such as Sir Robert Hotung (1862–1956) who had the language skills and bicultural background to crisscross the Chinese and Western business worlds in the late nineteenth and early twentieth centuries.

25. [Shanghai's Modern Pharmaceutical Industry], 233.

26. Ningbo was one of the five treaty ports listed in the Treaty of Nanking in 1842. Located 220 km (140 mi) south of Shanghai, Ningbo's export industry dates back to the seventh century. Since the mid-1850s, waves of Ningboese youths migrated to Shanghai and settled there and overseas. The Ningboese diaspora included the late Chiang Kai-shek, a former leader/president of the Republic of China (1928–1975), Tung Chi-Hwa, and Carrie Lam, the first (1997–2005) and 4th (2017–2022) chief executives of the Hong Kong SAR, Morris Chang, the founder and former chairman (1987–2018) of Taiwan Semiconductor Corporation, Yoyo Ma, world renowned cellist, and many others.

27. Chang Ning 张宁, "Nao wei yisheng zizhu—Cong ai luo bu noozhi kan jindai zhongguo shnnti guan de bianhua" 脑为一身之主: 从「艾罗补脑汁」看近代中国身体观的变化, [From Heart to Brain: Ailuo Brain Tonic and the new Concept of the Body in Late Qing China],

[Bulletin of Institute of Modern History, Academia Sinica] 70, no.1 (2011), 1–40. Accessed 29 September 2023. https://www.mh.sinica.edu.tw/FileUpload/80/2011_張寧_腦為一身之主.pdf.

28. Dr Liang Peiji (梁培基, 1875–1947), a native of Canton, was a medical doctor who graduated from the Canton Hospital in 1897. In the late nineteenth century, malaria was an epidemic in that miners and outdoor workers became infected during the humid summer months. The loss of productivity and delay in shipment of minerals and construction projects led to a tremendous demand for anti-malarial drugs. Liang set up the Liang Peiji Pharmaceutical Factory in 1902 and produced a quinine and liquorice pill "Liang Peiji Fever Pills" (*Liang Peiji Falang Yao*) for miners and outdoor workers. Liang's antimalaria remedies were popular with tin miners and rubber plantation workers in Southeast Asia too. At the peak of its business in the 1910s, the Factory exported a million packs per annum of its antimalarial remedies to the Straits Settlements.

29. Farmer, Hugh, 'The Hongkong Ice Company Ltd, 1880–1919', The Industrial History of Hong Kong Group, July 25, 2016. Accessed May 5, 2023. https://industrialhistoryhk.org/hongkong-ice-company-1880-1919/.

30. Chiu, *Transformation from Colonial Chemist,* 13–14.

31. Ge Yuanxu, (葛元煦, *Huyouzaiji,* 沪游杂记), [Shanghai Travel Notes],Shanghai Guji Chubanshe, 上海古籍出版社, [Shanghai Classics Publishing House] 1940, 40; org.pub. 1876.

32. Torpedo-shaped bottles, also known as Hamilton bottles, were used for soda water from the 1840s onwards. These were oval-shaped, sealed with a piece of cork and held by a metal wire like the champagne bottle. The bottle was designed to lie flat so that the cork was kept wet during transportation and storage. The cork would not dry out and crack.

33. The Codd-neck bottle was designed and patented by Hiram Codd in 1872. The bottle neck had a piece of marble ball and a rubber gasket to seal it by the pressure of the carbon dioxide gas released from the carbonated water when placed upside down. The bottles were used until the 1930s when eventually replaced by a single—use metallic cap, crimped over the mouth of the bottle over a thin cork pad. The latter formed a leak-proof seal and separetd the drink and the metal cap.

34. Ruan Lingyu was the Coca Cola poster girl in 1927. She was in a relaxing posture in a modern Chinese evening dinner dress (旗袍, *qipao*), with her right hand holding the Coca-Cola drink in a glass and her left hand resting on the couch.

Chapter 6
Pharmaceutical Education and Manpower Development

This chapter examines the history of pharmaceutical education since the mid-eleventh century of Song dynasty. Modern pharmacy education began at the Beiyang Military Medical Academy in Tianjin in 1908. The positive impact of formal pharmacist training became evident during the Second Sino-Japanese War (1937–1949), particularly in terms of the supply of army pharmacists and the mass production of drugs and surgical supplies. By 1949, ~ 3000 pharmacists had been trained, with two thousand receiving their education from local universities and colleges, and four hundred trained in Japan's pharmacy vocational schools.[1]

In the ancient world, apprenticeship to become apothecaries was the main route until the mid-nineteen century when modern pharmacy schools sprang up in Europe, Japan, the UK, and the US. In 1076, the Imperial Pharmacy of the Song dynasty in China started state pharmaceutical education to train apothecaries and assistants to support the social medicine policy initiated by reformer Minister Wang Anshi. As a result, by 1151, seventy state retail pharmacy stores in the name of People's Pharmacy were set up by the Imperial Pharmacy Department to provide standardized herbal medicines at affordable prices to the public.[2] Unfortunately, the public health policy on subsidized herbal remedies fell into disarray towards the end of the reign of Emperor Wanli (万历 r. 1563-1620).

In the western world, the U.S. was one of the earliest countries to advance the pharmacy profession in the first quarter of the nineteenth century. In 1821, sixty-eight apothecaries gathered in Philadelphia, Penn. to voice their concerns that unethical traders supplying adulterated, inferior quality herbs controlled the wholesale drug market.[3] The consensus among the participants was to establish the Philadelphia College of Pharmacy the following year with a formal curriculum to train chemists to prepare, dispense and sell medicines. Twenty years later, in the UK, a group of chemists founded the PSGB in 1841. Their objective was to set the professional standards of the pharmacy profession and seek the legitimate right to dispense and sell medicines to the public. The Society then founded its School of Pharmacy the following year. The latter conducted examinations and began to keep an official

© The Author(s), under exclusive license to Springer Nature Singapore Pte Ltd. 2023
P. Chiu, *A History of Western Pharmacy in China*,
https://doi.org/10.1007/978-981-99-8635-4_6

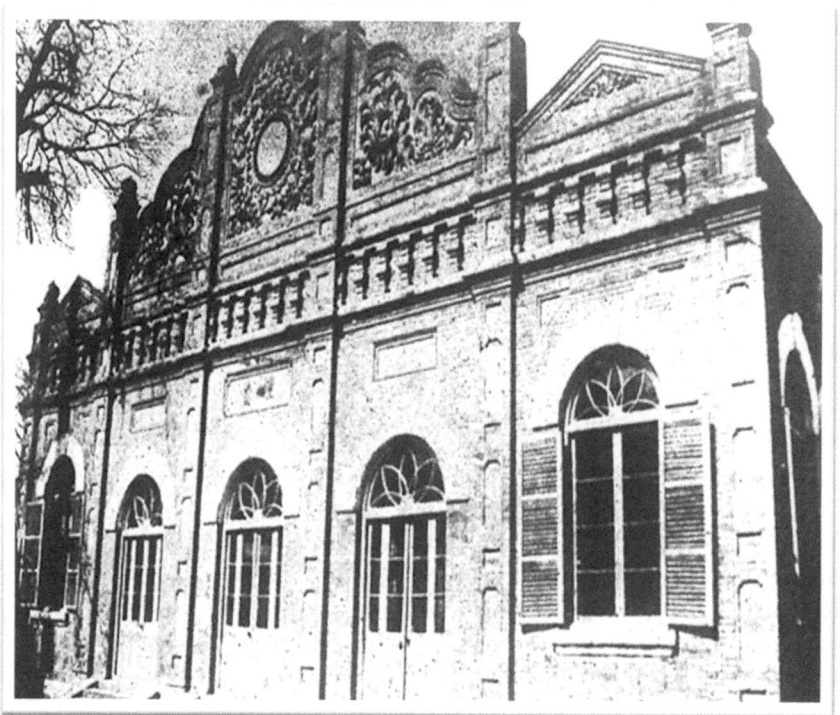

Fig. 6.1 Beiyang Military Medical School Assemby Hall, Tianjin, 1902. *Credit* Hong Society for the History of Pharmacy

register of pharmaceutical chemists in 1852.[4] The development of modern China's health system was gradual, with the informal training of local medical doctors by western medical missionaries in the last quarter of the nineteenth century. Official training of army medical and pharmaceutical personnel began in the first decade of the 1900s.

The loss of the First Sino-Japanese War and the signing of the 1895 Shimonoeki Agreement, which resulted in Taiwan's secession to Japan, served as a wake-up call to the officials and Confucian scholars of the Manchu Qing imperial court. They came to recognize that the Meiji Restoration in 1868 had transformed Japan from an ancient feudal society into a modern state on par with Western powers, offering a potential solution to China's long-standing challenges. Six years after the signing of the Agreement, Yuen Shikai, Governor of Chili and Beiyang Trade Minister, established the Beiyang Army Medical College in December 1902 (Fig. 6.1). However, it wasn't until 1907 that the School of Pharmacy, offering a formal 3-year pharmaceutical education following the curriculum of Japanese universities, came into existence.

Beginnings of Modern Pharmacy Education

Soon after the Convention of Peking was concluded between the Manchu Qing, Great Britain, France and the Russian Empire after the Second Opium War in 1860, active dissemination of western medicine and pharmacy practice commenced. Western missionaries began promoting Christianity, and enterprising chemists and traders marketed "opium cures" and proprietary medicines in the treaty ports.

Japan's Meiji Restoration was a 45-year journey from 1868 to 1912 during which the country launched its modernization and industrialization initiatives and adopted political, economic, scientific, and military models from western countries.[5] Three years after the First Sino-Japanese War in 1898, Zhang Zhidong (1837–1909), then Viceroy of Hunan, Hubei and Guangdong Provinces and a member of the Grand Council of the Manchu Qing court, advocated modernization of education in his publication of "Exhortation to Learning" (Quanxue Pian). The Boxers Movement (1900–1901), the most humiliating conflict with the Eight-Nation Alliance in the capital city of Beijing, was the final nail in the coffin of the Keju (imperial civil service examination system), whereby the old Confucian teachings were the only means of education and appointment of state officials. [6] The Manchu Qing imperial court organized the last Keju examination in 1904 in Kaifang, Henan province. After that, the Manchu Qing government stepped up its drive to send students to Japan and western countries to learn STEM subjects, Science, Technology, Engineering and Mathematics.

By 1906, 15,000 Chinese students had gone to Japan to attend higher learning institutions.[7] The provincial governments or wealthy families of the same clanship offered scholarships to students who passed the screening examinations and then went to university or vocational schools in Japan. A smaller number went to study in the US, and even fewer went to Europe and the UK. Therefore, the period from 1904 to 1914 was one that Japan had a lead in its medical and pharmaceutical influence on China's higher education. Japan was chosen as the country of learning and a model of industrial modernization by China's reformists because both countries shared the same Buddhist religion, Confucian culture and customary practice, and a similar written language. Moreover, the proximity of Japan was another consideration of parents who saw it as the priority instead of the modern states in Europe, the UK, and the US. Most importantly, Japan was far less costly and more accessible for the Manchu Qing officials to monitor the young minds.

From the 1880s to the end of WWII in 1945, the Meiji reformers and their subsequent followers in Japan emphasized the study of chemistry and immunology in its pharmaceutical education. This policy successfully produced chemicals, drugs, vaccines, and exports of narcotic drugs, including "opium cures" to Asian countries. The Imperial University of Tokyo, renamed the University of Tokyo after WWII, was the only university that offered a 4-year pharmaceutical manufacturing degree, established in 1877. All others pharmacy schools, including the privately funded Tokyo University of Pharmacy and Life Sciences, presented a 3-year pharmacy course. Both universities offered pharmacognosy as the core subject, whereas the former focused on research and chemical synthesis and the latter on compounding and mixing of prescription drugs.

Yuan Shi-kai (袁世凱, 1859–1916), Viceroy of Zhili and Minster of Beiyang, was authorized by Emperor Guangxu (光绪, r. 1875–1908) to build the Beiyang Military Medical School in Tianjin in 1902, which was renamed the Army Medical College (AMC) in 1906.[8] The appointment of Japanese academics as heads of the first two pharmacy schools helped chart China's initial academic development in pharmacy which was the German model of laboratory-based pharmacy education. The first intake of pharmacy students (P1) at the AMC began in 1908. It was initially a 3-year pharmacy course based on the Imperial University of Tokyo's pharmacy course curriculum with the core subjects of chemistry, pharmacognosy, formulation and manufacturing. The first batch of eighteen pharmacy students graduated in 1911,[9] and the Machu Qing military assigned AMC's pharmacy graduates to different units of the Army Medical Corps.

The Rockefeller Foundation sent a delegation to conduct a four-month survey and visited seventeen of China's medical institutions in 1914. The AMC was ranked the best among the five state medical institutions. In 1918, the AMC was relocated from Tianjin to Beijing and again in 1933 from Beijing to Nanjing. Dr. Heng J. Liu was also the de facto head of the AMC in 1934. Moody Meng, who became the head of the National Health Laboratories and the Central Hospital pharmacy department, assumed the official headship of the pharmacy department of the AMC in 1935. Meng introduced a year of on-the-job with rotational training for the fourth-year pharmacy students, involving two periods of six-months at the National Health Laboratories and the Central Hospital pharmacy department. Meng became the founding head and professor of the state-funded National College of Pharmacy (NCP) in Nanjing in 1936. The pharmacy diploma course was modelled after the School of Pharmacy of the University of London, where he graduated in 1924. The NCP was relocated to Chongqing in 1937 and he continued in his position until 1939.

With the outbreak of the Second Sino-Japanese War (1937–1949, "the War")[10] at the Marco Polo Bridge in Beijing on 7 July 1937, Chiang Kai-shek (蒋介石, Jiang Jieshi, 1887–1975) also assumed the headship of the AMC. The latter was relocated from Nanjing to Canton in September. Eight months later, the College moved again to Guilin, Guangxi and then to Anshun in Guizhou in 1939. While in Guiyang, the AMC's affiliated Pharmaceutical Manufacturing Institute (PMI), staffed by its academics and students, began producing sterile injectables, chemical weapons and consumables required for military and civilian uses until the end of the War. Dr Robert Lim (Lin Kesheng, Lim Kho-Seng, 1897–1969), another PUMC professor, became the Surgeon General of the Nationalist army and the first head of the National Defence Medical Centre (NDMC)—a merger of the College, Army Medical Reserve, and the Wartime Health Personnel Training Center in late 1946.[11] Lim's top priorities were to train more medical doctors and nurses to staff the urgently needed veteran hospitals to cope with acute illnesses and epidemics. His decision would result in nurses taking over dispensing in military and veteran hospitals instead of having a whole pharmacy department of the NDMC.

Pharmaceutical Missionaries and Pharmacy Colleges

Edwin Meuser (米玉士, 1880–1970) was born as a British subject in Elmwood, Ontario, and he graduated from the School of Pharmacy of the University of Toronto in 1904. Five years later, Meuser was sponsored as a pharmacist missionary by the Board of Mission of the Methodist Episcopal Church (MEM) of the US to work at the pharmacy department of the American Hospital in Chongqing in 1909. Meuser married Edna Speers (1883–1964), another Canadian Christian missionary, at the British Consulate in Chengdu in 1913 (Fig. 6.2).[12] Speers arrived in Zigong County, Sichuan, in 1908 and soon set up a boarding school there. She was a linguist and helped Meuser to translate the pharmacy lecture notes into Chinese during the class. The West China Union University (华西协和大学, WCUU) of Chengdu was founded in 1909 by the West China Educational Union (WCEU). The sole purpose of WCUU was to promote Christianity in West China which had a population of 100 million. The four founding partners were the American Baptist Foreign Mission Society, MEM, Friends of Foreign Mission Association, Great Britain and Ireland, and the General Board of Missions of the Methodist Church, Canada.

A medical college was opened by the WCUU in 1914 with Meuser as a pharmacy lecturer to medical students. Three-fourths of China's herbs were grown in Western China. Meuser was motivated to conduct research in crude drugs and start a pharmacy

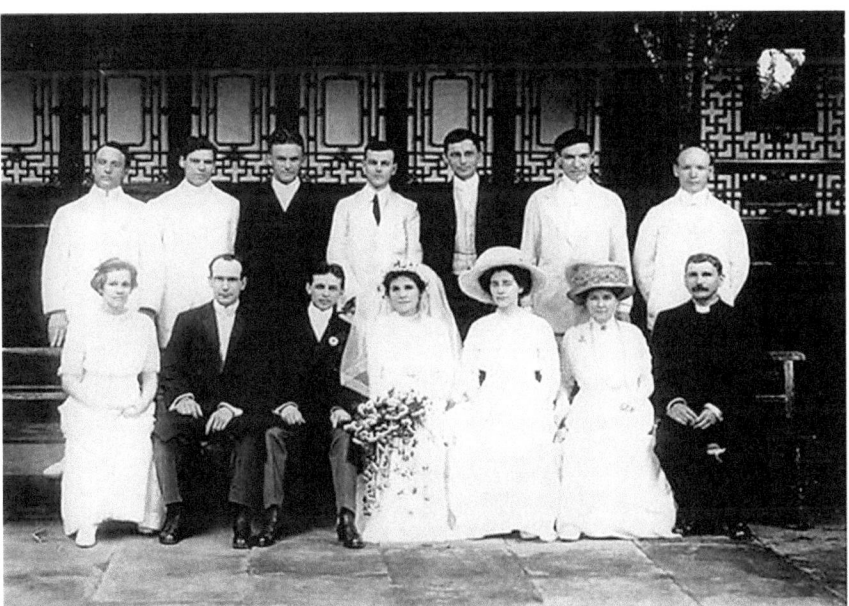

Fig. 6.2 Wedding photograph of Mr and Mrs Edwin Meuser and friends, British Consulate in Chengdu, 4 July 1913, Edna Speers (Mrs Meuser), centre, and Edwin Meuser 3rd left, 1st row. *Credit* Sichuan University West China School of Pharmacy

diploma course at the WCUU to train Chinese pharmacists in 1918 (Fig. 6.3). The anti-Christian movement of 1922–1927 united the Communist and the Nationalist Parties of China to reject the dominance of British and US Christian societies in providing education and medical service.[13] The "Recovery of Educational Rights" campaign reached a highpoint at the Seventh National Conference of the Students Union in June 1925. The student campaign was supported by both the communist and nationalist elements in the Nationalist government, in particular, the policy makers in the Ministry of Education (MoE) in Beiping and provincial bureaus of education. The consensus reached at the conference were:

> In the case of Fujian (Fukien province), this newly organized committee published a booklet and setup five objectives: (1) school administration and curricular should be entirely under the control of Chinese higher institutions; (2) there should be no religious education; (3) restoration of students' freedom, especially non-interference in their patriotic movements; (4) students participation in school administration; (5) the director of the school and the head of instructional departments should be Chinese.[14]

Pharmaceutical education at the WCUU was suspended from 1925 to 1931, and Meuser temporarily left Chengdu. It could have been a mixture of reasons that made Meuser feel unsafe to continue the pharmacy course, an increasingly anti-Christian movement and the intense fighting between the local warlords. Meuser returned to his wife's hometown in Saskatoon, Canada and took up the position as the acting head of the pharmacy department of the University of Saskatchewan. He undertook PhD studies in pharmacy at the University of Pennsylvania while concurrently serving as a professor at Saskatchewan. In-fighting between the warlords gradually improved after Generalissimo Chiang's success in the northern expedition. The Ministry of

Fig. 6.3 Edwin Meuser and students in dispensing class. c. 1920. *Credit* Sichuan University West China School of Pharmacy

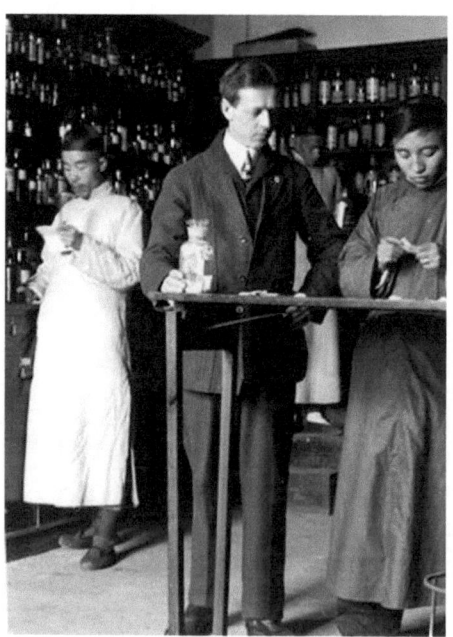

Education (the Ministry) promulgated the law on private schools on 29 August 1929 for nationwide execution. Only Chinese nationals could become members of board of governors, leadership of universities and normal universities (teacher training colleges), and faculty heads of academic colleges. It was what the Fujian provincial education commission had proposed a few years before, with minor changes.

Upon Meuser's return to Chengdu, he launched the BSc pharmacy degree course under the College of Science in the newly expanded WCUU in September 1932. It became a private university in 1933. A year later, the New York State University senate approved WCUU's pharmacy course as its external degree (Fig. 6.4). During the Second Sino-Japanese War (1937–1945), many WCUU pharmacy graduates join the Army Medical Corps. and a few pursued further studies in Canada and the US. In the academic year commencing October 1947, WCUU had 186 pharmacy students or 10% of its 1723 students. Of these, 104 were male and 84 were female students. Its alumni included key figures Zhu Yanru, Paul I. Sun, Chen Lanying, and Liu Shuchang in academia, hospital and retail pharmacy in China and aboard.[15,16,17,18] After forty years of living and working in Chengdu and Sichuan province, the Meusers returned to Willowdale, ONT., Canada, for retirement after the change of government in China in 1950. The School of Pharmacy of WCUU and its successor, Sichuan University were and have remained among the best run pharmacy schools in China since 1918.

Another Christian university in China that offered a pharmacy diploma course in 1920 was the Shandong (Shantung) Christian University (SCU), renamed in 1909. When founded in 1902, it was named Shandong Protestant University by consolidating the Shangdong Union Medical College and two other arts, science, and theology colleges in 1903 and 1904, respectively. In addition, a school of medicine was founded in 1911. In 1915, SCU adopted the Chinese name Cheeloo (齐鲁, *Qilu*)

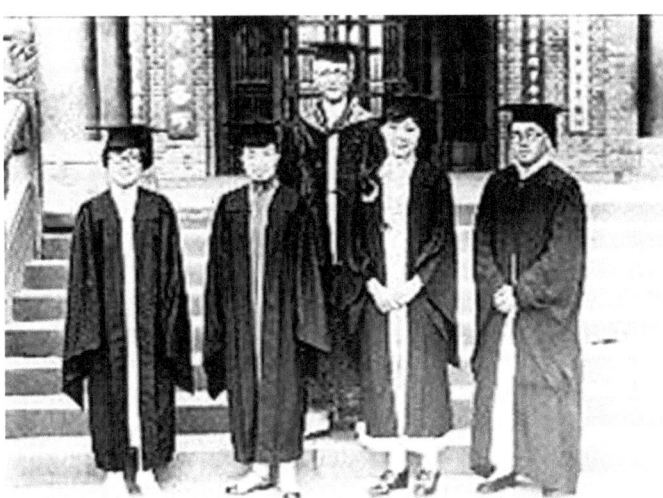

Fig. 6.4 Edwin Meuser and pharmacy graduates of WCUU and New York State University in 1934. *Credit* Sichuan University West China School of Pharmacy

University as the word "*Qilu*" is a synonym of Shandong. In 1919, SCU became a full-fledged university offering arts, science, medicine, and theology programmes. Reverend William Perry Pailing (帕林), a native of Birmingham, qualified as a pharmacist in the UK in 1909.[19] He subsequently completed his studies in theology at the University of London and became a pharmaceutical missionary with the Baptist Missionary Society.

Pailing joined the SCU's medical school as a pharmacist at the newly established hospital in Chinan (Jinan) and served as a part-time lecturer in the medical school and a hospital chaplain in 1915. Under the College of Medicine, the School of Pharmacy received its first in-take of a 2-year diploma course in pharmacy in 1920. He assumed the position of the founding head of pharmacy. Pailing, along with Dr Bernard Read and John Cameron, all British qualified pharmacists, were three of the four external advisors to the first edition of the Chinese Pharmacopoeia in 1930.[20] Like the other Christian universities, SCU became privatized in 1930 when the Ministry implemented the national law on "Regulations Governing Private Schools" in the previous year.

State Investments in Capacity Building

Moody Meng, the chief pharmacist at the National Health Administration (卫生署, NHA) and the official head of the pharmacy department at the AMC, founded the National College of Pharmacy (国立药学专科学校) (Guoli Yaoxue Zhuanke xuexiao, NCP) in Nanjing in July 1936. The opening ceremony was held on 17 September 1936 (Fig. 6.5).

His original intention was to establish a university college to offer a degree level of pharmacy studies with research and development capabilities. However, the policy of the MoE of the Nationalist government would only approve a vocational school to offer a diploma level of pharmacy studies. Meng's dream was gradually realized fifty years later with the several mergers of the NCP and smaller schools eventually resulted in the Chinese Pharmaceutical University in 1986. NCP's motto was "精业济群, Jingye Jiqun" (serving the masses through professionalism), and the badge contains the pharmacy symbols of a pestle and mortar and knowledge of a book (Figs. 6.6 and 6.7).

Although NCP could only offer a diploma course, Meng and his faculty decided to follow his alma mater's 3-year pharmacy degree course curriculum—the School of Pharmacy of the University of London. Meng introduced a 1-year pre-registration training in a hospital pharmacy and a pharmaceutical factory. A year later, the 2nd Sino-Japanese War erupted with the Japanese Imperial Army instigating a shooting incident at the Marco Polo bridge on the outskirt of Beijing on 7 July 1937. NCP promptly relocated from Nanjing first to Hankou, a district of Wuhan, and then eventually to Chongqing, the war-time capital, in the spring of 1938.

In the same year, Meng lost the support of his mentor and supervisor, Dr. Heng J. Liu, who was demoted to the Head of Health Services in June 1937. This was reportedly due to Chiang Kai-shek's disappointment in Dr. Heng J. Liu's failure to

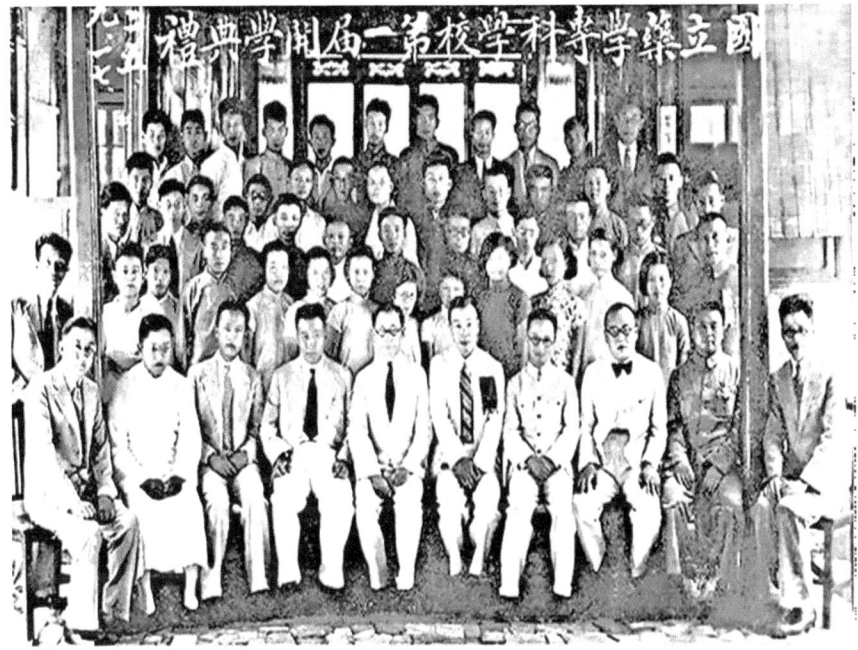

Fig. 6.5 Opening ceremony of National College of Pharmacy, Nanjing, 17 September 1936 Moody Meng, no-glasses, strike-tie, 5th on the right, front row. *Credit* Meng Zhaoyi and Meng Xianwei

Fig. 6.6 College Emblem. National college of Pharmacy in the upper row and pestle and mortar in the centre circle. *Credit* Meng Zhaoyi and Meng Xianwei

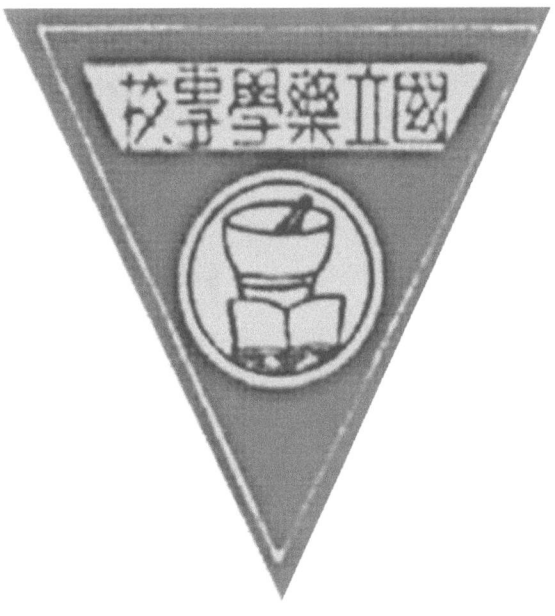

Fig. 6.7 College Badge.
National College of
Pharmacy in the outer ring
and pestle and mortar and
book in the inner circle.
Credit Meng Zhaoyi and
Meng Xianwei

restructure the AMC when he doubled up as the head in April 1935.[21] As a result,
Dr. Heng J. Liu resigned as the Head of Health Services six months later, in January
1938. Chen Lifu, the then Minister of Education who was a vocal opponent of
Dr. Heng J. Liu's policy to abolish Chinese medicine in 1929, immediately sacked
Meng and appointed Chen Siyi (陈思义), the academic head of NCP, as Meng's
successor from August 1938 until June 1945.[22,23] While in Hong Kong to operate
the Union Pharmaceutical Factory (协和制药公司, UPF) from mid-1938 to 1941,
Meng became acquainted with Arthur Bentley, a British pharmacist who was the
lecturer of the pharmacy course conducted at the University of Hong Kong.[24]

Prior to the Japanese occupation of Hong Kong on 25 December 1941, Meng
promptly shipped out and returned the production lines and inventory of drug stocks
and surgical materials to Chongqing. Meng continued to manage the pharmaceutical
plant and taught as a faculty member at the NCP. A month and a half after the
Japanese occupation of Hong Kong in late December 1941, Bentley fled Hong Kong
in and arrived in Chongqing a couple of months later. With Meng's introduction,
Bentley joined the NCP as a lecturer in the new academic year in August 1942.
As the degree course of NCP was similar to the British curriculum, Bentley had
a seamless transition there. A rotating chair occurred at NCP with Xue Yu (薛愚)
as the head for a year and for the other, Wu Rongxi (吴荣熙), who resigned from
the NDMC and joined the NCP in July 1947 until the end of October 1948. Guan
Guangdi (管光地,1904–1952) succeeded Wu in March 1949 until he died in June
1950.

Since NCP's inception in 1936, two hundred and eighty students graduated, with
the last batch in May 1949 before transitioning from the Nationalist to the Communist
government. Most NCP graduates stayed behind in China, with a few departing for

Hong Kong and some to Taiwan after Mao Zedong's Communist Party succeeded the Nationalist Party (aka *Kuomintang*) in October 1949. The NCP alumni of the Nationalist era also included Shen Jiachang (1921–2015), Peng Sixun (1919–2018), and Yuan Chengye (1924–2018), who all became pillars in the academic and industry sectors in Taiwan (Figs. 6.8, 6.9, 6.10 and 6.11).[25,26,27]

The late Madam Gu Jiheng (顾继衡, 1922–2022), a 1946 graduate of the NCP, was born in Taihu, Jiangsu province. Her family fled to Chongqing when the Japanese ransacked the Nationalist capital in the brutal six-week Nanjing Massacre from December 1937 to February 1938. After graduation from the NCP, Gu worked as a pharmacist at the Central Bank Dispensary in Nanjing. Towards the end of the civil war of 1946–1949, Gu relocated with the Nationalist Government to Taipei in May 1949 and worked with the Taiwan Central Bank Dispensary for twenty-seven years until her retirement in 1976. Gu then changed her career track and became an entrepreneur starting a successful health supplement import business in 1976 until 2022. She recalled her days at the NCP on the mainland in an interview:

> Moody Meng, the head of the National College of Pharmacy, was a fascinating teacher with a sense of humour, and students liked to attend his classes. A British lecturer, Arthur Bentley, arrived from Hong Kong in 1942. The campus of NCP was situated at the top of Gele Mountain in a tranquil environment in Chongqing. A former head and a professor of pharmaceutical chemistry of NCP, Wu Rongxi, also came to Taiwan and taught at the NDMC and National Taiwan University. He was also an entrepreneur and acted as the Taiwan distributor for Upjohn Pharmaceuticals. My school friend, Zhang Zhongliang (Cheung Chung Leung), went to Hong Kong soon after graduation in October 1946, and the Colonial British authorities recognized the NCP's qualifications.[28,29]

The Nationalist Government established Sun Yet-San No. 4 University (SYS4U) in Nanking in June 1927. It was a merger of several universities and colleges in the Jiangsu province, including the Jiangsu Medical University. The latter was renamed from the Jiangsu Medical College in Shanghai, founded in 1915, in 1925.[30] Three years later, SYS4U changed its name to the National Central University (国立中央大学). Its medical faculty, based and independently operated in Shanghai, became the Shanghai Medical College (上海医学院) in 1932. The first head of SMC, Dr. Fu Ching Yen (颜福庆, Yan Fuqing, 1882–1970), had graduated as a medical doctor at the St. John's University Medical School in Shanghai. He was subsequently awarded an MD degree at Yale University in 1909 and a post-graduate diploma at the Liverpool School of Tropical Medicine in 1910. Yen was the founder and director of the SMC from 1927 until 1940 and the founder of Sun Yat-sen (Zhong Shan) Hospital in Shanghai in 1937 Fig. 6.10.

Dr. Chu Heng-Pi (朱恒璧, Zhu Hengbi, 1890–1987) was the deputy head of SMC, who also doubled up as the head of its new faculty of pharmacy when founded in December 1936. Dr. Zhang Changshao (张昌绍, C.S. Jang, 1912–1967), a distinguished medical graduate in 1934, was appointed by Zhu initially as the lecturer in pharmacology for medical and pharmacy undergraduates. Zhang received a scholarship funded by the British Boxers Indemnity Fund and pursued a PhD at the University of London from 1937 to 1940. After a brief post-doctoral training in experimental pharmacology at the Harvard Medical School in Boston, Mass., Dr. Zhang returned to SMC in Chongqing as a professor in 1941.

SMC's affiliated teaching hospital, Sun Yat-sen Hospital, was opened on 1 April 1937. The 2nd Sino-Japanese War broke out three months later, on 7 July 1937, and the Japanese Imperial Army occupied Shanghai on 26 November 1937. SMC had two campuses. Shanghai was under the Japanese puppet government, the "Reorganized National Government of the Republic of China, 南京国国民政府", headed by Wang Ching-wai (汪精卫, Wang Jingwai, 1883–1944). Many of the SMC teaching faculty moved to Kunming, Yunnan, then to Gele Mountain in Chongqing in 1940 and continued as the original SMC under the jurisdiction of the Nationalist Government in Chongqing. From 1936, SMC's pharmacy department had a 4-year curriculum; the first three years were theoretical courses, and the fourth year was the pre-registration year. Annually, 10-15 students graduated who were assigned by the government to work in public hospital pharmacy departments. WWII ended in August 1945; the original SMC returned to Shanghai to resume classes in September 1946. In Shanghai, the fourth-year pharmacy students spent half a year in the pharmacy department of Zhongshan Hospital and half a year in a Shanghai pharmaceutical factory. In 1950, the Department of Pharmacy of l'Université Franco-Chinoise was absorbed into the SMC and, in 2000, it became the School of Pharmacy of Fudan University.

AMC's pharmacy course closely resembled the Imperial University of Tokyo emphasising research and development and industrial pharmacy. For the first 2 years, students attended classes in pharmaceutical chemistry, pharmaceutics, pharmacognosy, microbiology, and formulation. Third year students attended classes in one of the four subjects; pharmacognosy, forensics, pharmaceutical chemistry, and industrial pharmacy in greater depth and with hands-on experience. Final and fourth year students would undergo 1-year pre-registration training at an army hospital or at the AMC's in-house research laboratory.

In the late nineteenth and early twentieth centuries, the hospital pharmacy supervisor or the chemist shop owner would conduct training in dispensing for their assistants. Bernard Read soon initiated pharmacy assistant training, based on the two-tier British qualifications of the chemist and druggist, and pharmaceutical chemist minor and major examination model when he joined the UMC in 1909.[31,32] The same applied to the Civil Hospital in Hong Kong and the retail chemist shops of the British Dispensary and Lao Teh Kee in Shanghai.

The first vocational training school for hospital pharmacy dispensers, Beijing Vocational Pharmacy School (BVPS), was approved by the Beijing Health Bureau (BHB) in early 1929. The North China Pharmaceutical Association (NCPA), in conjunction with the individual pharmacy staff of the PUMC Hospital, including Moody Meng, Tu Wang-ting and others, opened its first class in April 1929. Meng in the 1910s and Tu in the 1920s were trained in-house as pharmacy technicians by the Hospital pharmacists, respectively. They were also the founding members, among others, of the NCPA. Meng advanced his pharmacy studies in the UK in the early 1920s and qualified as a pharmaceutical chemist in 1924. He rejoined the PUMC Hospital as the assistant pharmacist to John Cameron, who supported the BVPS and allowed three of his senior pharmacy staff to become part-time lecturers of the BVPS.

The BHB provided a room as the premises in Qianliang Hutung, a 40 minute walk from the PUMC Hospital site, for running the vocational course in 1929. However, with the success of the evening class, the BHB allocated a closer location and larger premises within a 15-min walking distance from the PUMC Hospital 3 years later. The duration of the BVPS course was extended to 2 years in 1933. NCPA's pharmacy dispenser course, which provided lectures from 2 to 3 h on weekday evenings, was aimed at those assistants who had completed their 5 years of high school and were working in the hospital or retail pharmacy sector. In 1933, Tu was appointed as the volunteer head of the BVPS by the mayor of Beijing. Tu continued his work as a senior pharmacy technician at the PUMC Hospital until 1942 when the hospital was closed down during WWII. Three voluntary lecturers who were the senior pharmacy technicians of the PUMC Hospital taught four of the five subjects in the evening class. John Cameron, the pharmacy supervisor of the PUMC Hospital, provided some of the teaching material and these included the Qualitative Chemical Analysis Tables, 1929; Posological and Percentage Tables, 1929; Special Short Course in Practical Pharmacy, 1930; and Elementary Quantitative Analysis for Pharmaceutical Students, 1930.

Inspired by the BVPS, other provincial vocational pharmacy schools opened in Nanjing in 1931, and Shanghai in 1936. For example, the Shanghai Vocational Pharmacy School opened simultaneously with the Shanghai Medical College Department of Pharmacy in 1937.

Since the foundation of the Republic of China in 1912, the Ministry's policy-makers, unfortunately, had left out the education and training of Chinese medicine pharmacists and technicians altogether. The National Institute of Chinese Medicine (中央国医馆, Zhongyang Guoyi Guan was founded in 1930 with the support of Chen Guofu and Lifu brothers and began to set Chinese medicine academic standards, unified disease terminology, compilation and review of the Compendium of Materia Medica, and textbooks. Many Chinese medicine schools opened for formal training soon afterwards. However, the first Chinese Medicine Vocational pharmacy school opened in Beijing to train dispensers of Chinese medicine pharmacy on the eve of the change to the Communist government in September 1949. Formal training of Chinese medicine pharmacists began in 1956 when Chinese medicine universities and colleges started to enroll students en masse.

Reversing the Gear in Pharmaceutical Education

With remarkable wartime achievements as the Director of the Chinese Red Cross Medical Relief Commission from 1937 to 1943 and Deputy Surgeon General of the Nationalist army from 1944 to 1945, Robert Lim was promoted to Lieutenant General in the Nationalist army and Surgeon General of the Republic of China. In late 1946, General Chen Cheng, the Chief of Staff of the Armed Forces, appointed Lim National Defense Medical Center (国防医学院, NDMC) President. After the opening of the new premises of the NDMC in the Jiangwan district of Shanghai in June 1947, Lim immediately reviewed the future of military education and the permanent location of the NDMC. With General Cheng Chen's support, Lim reached a consensus with the Ministry of Defence. His preliminary decision was to terminate the four-year pharmacy curriculum in the next academic year of 1947/1948. Instead, they aimed to cease the PMI operations and train more pharmacy technicians instead of pharmacists by organizing a 5-year diploma course for grade nine junior high school graduates. In addition, Lim argued that the NMDC would need the support of the US in rebuilding China after the War and could use the resources to train more nurses to perform multiple functions, including dispensing. The late King Ming-lu (金明儒, Jin Mingru, 1926–2021), a P34 (1948) class student who became the head of the Department of Pharmacy at the NDMC in Taiwan from 1974–1980, told what he knew of the historical development in "reversing the gear of pharmaceutical education":

> The reorganization of the NDMC in April 1947 hurt the pharmacy department. The original faculty of pharmacy became a unit of the newly formed Department of Medical Technology. Li Chenghu became the Chief of the Pharmacy Unit in June. Soon after the reorganisation announcement in April 1947, General Chen Cheng, Chief of Staff of the Armed Forces, held a town hall meeting with the academic staff and students and articulated his change decision. Even though his military career was at high risk and was highly likely to be court-marshalled, Professor Wu Rongxi, the original Head of the Pharmacy Department, petitioned General Chen to reconsider his decision and not to downsize the Pharmacy Faculty. Chen was furious about Wu's disobedience and reportedly said, "We initiate revolutions and not as the target for revolutionary change."

> The NDMC's pharmacy students immediately went to the capital Nanjing and teamed up with the students of the NCP to form the "National Pharmaceutical Students Association" (NPSA). They jointly held demonstrations at the Ministry of Education (MoE) in May. MoE officials asked the students to proceed to the Ministry of Defence (MoD) to lodge their complaints as they initiated the change. The NDMC officials further dropped hints to the students that it would be unwise to challenge the decision of the MoD as a military institution, and it would also be a rash decision to protest there. The students were so scared that they disbanded halfway to the MoD. Seventy years from then, the decision to reverse the progress in pharmaceutical education remained a mystery to me![33]

It was perhaps due to the intensive media reporting of the demonstrations and petitions by the NPSA that they drew strong support from academics and pharmaceutical experts, and the public's sympathy. It was also critical when the ruling Nationalist government escalated the civil war with the Communist's Red Army. General Chen promptly reversed the unpopular decision, which was rare in the Nationalist army because discipline was the cardinal law in military education. The newly appointed Head of the Pharmacy Department, Wu Rongxi, and several lecturers immediately resigned from their faculty positions. This incident was most embarrassing to the Nationalist army as a challenge to an issued order was subject to a court marshall. (See separate section) The Department of Pharmacy was reinstated in the next academic year of 1947/1948. By early 1949, the Nationalist army was fighting a rapidly losing civil war with the Red Army of the Chinese Communist Party (CCP). Accordingly, three batches of the academic staff and second-year students of the thirty-fourth pharmacy class (P34) of the NDMC retreated with the Nationalist government from

Shanghai to Taipei on 16 February, 16 March, and 4 May 1949. Classes were held off-site in Taipei before the new premises of the NDMC were ready in September 1951.

After a two-week Shanghai campaign launched by the Red Army on 12 May, the city fell into the hands of the Communists on 27 May 1949. The campus of the NDMC located in Jiangwan (Kiang Wan), on the outskirts of Shanghai, was taken over by the new Communist government. However, the majority or 475 of the faculty members and students of the NDMC, stayed behind, and it was merged with the East China Medical College as the Second Military Medical University (SMMU) in 1951.

Some former heads, teaching staff and graduates of the Department of Pharmacy of the NDMC during the Nationalist era had remarkable careers. They contributed to developing the mainland's and Taiwan's academic, hospital and industrial pharmacy sectors. They included Zheng Shou (1896–1982), Major General Zhang Pengchong (1882–1968), Li Weizhang (1910–1998), Lou Zichen (1920–1995), Xi Nianzhu (1927–), and King Minglu (1926–2021) (Figs. 6.8, 6.9, 6.10 and 6.11).[34,35,36,37,38,39]

Fig. 6.8 Major General Zhang Pengchong, P15 1910–1988), director of pharmacy, Nationalist Army, Republic of China. 1949. *Credit* Alumni Association of NDMC

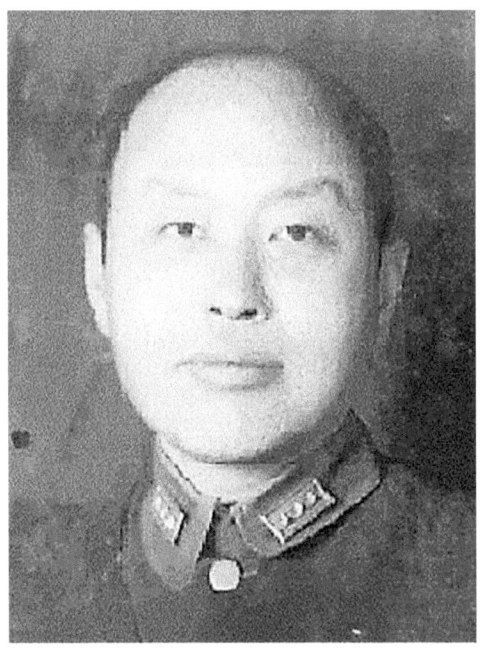

Fig. 6.9 Commader Li
Weizhang, P15 (1910–1968),
Director of pharmacy,
People's Liberation Army,
1949. *Credit* Alumni
Association of NDMC

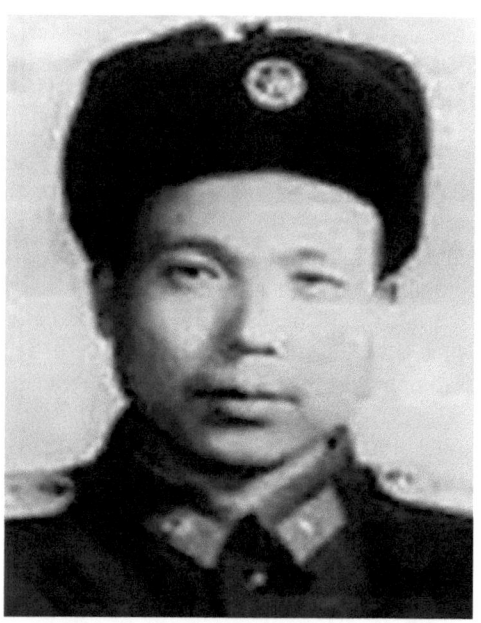

Fig. 6.10 Dr Lou Zhichen,
P24 (1920–1995) professor
of pharmacognosy, 1980s.
Beijing Medical College.
Credit Alumni Association
of NDMC

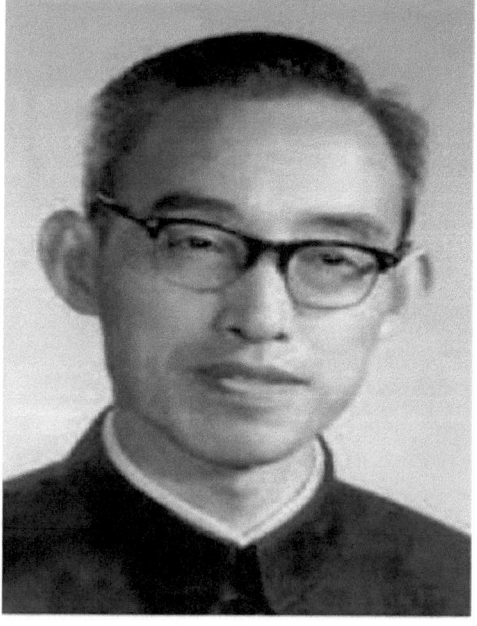

Fig. 6.11 Xi Nianzhu, P33 director of pharmacy @ 1980s Shanghai Medical College. *Credit* Alumni Association of NDMC

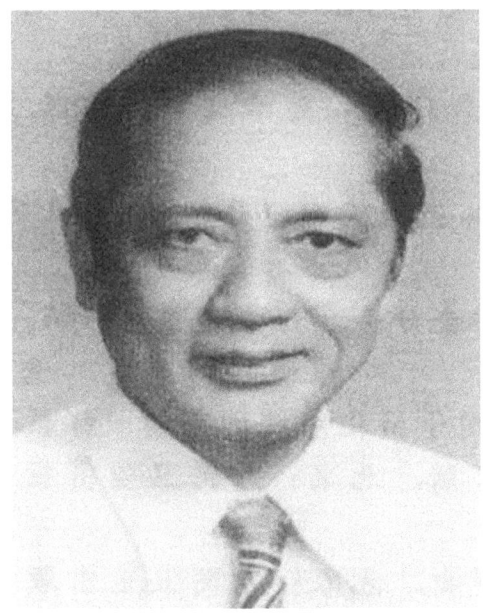

Although the Japanese pharmacy educators had a head start in 1907 at the AMC, the British and Canadian pharmaceutical missionaries established university pharmacy schools in Chengdu in 1919 and Jinan in 1920. Since then, in China there has been an ongoing shift in medical and pharmaceutical education and practice from Germany and Japan to Britain and North America.

From 1904 to 1949, about 2000 pharmacy students attended diploma courses at the 11 universities and colleges of pharmacy in China with 484 registered with the Nationalist government as qualified pharmacists These young pharmacists together with about 1000 pharmacy technicians trained at various vocational schools were serving in the academic, hospital, industrial, research, and retail pharmacy sectors in 1949 (Table 6.1). Almost all these pharmaceutical talents served in the young Communist state when founded on 1 October 1949. After a century of civil unrest, plagues, wars and revolutions, and domination by the Great Powers, China began a new chapter. These budding talents who graduated in the late Manchu Qing and early Nationalist era on the mainland became the backbone of modern China's medical and health system. They continued in leading the transformation of China's pharmacy system to meet the demands of its rapidly growing population (See the section on *Education Reform and Bench Strength of Local Talents* in Chap. 9)

Table 6.1 China's universities/colleges offering western pharmacy diploma/degree in 1949

Universities and colleges offering pharmacy course 1908–1949

#	Year	Original	1949	Now	Type	Head
1	1908	Beiyang Army College	National Defense Medical Centre	National Army Medical University	Public	Miyagawa Utsuo
2	1913	Zheiiang Medical College	Zhejiang Provincial Medical College	Zhejiang University	Public	Li Shenqi
3	1918	West China Pharmacy School	West China Union University	Sichuan University	Christian	Edwin Muser
4	1920	Shandong Christian University	Cheeloo University	Shandong University	Christian	W.P. Pailing
5	1929	l'Université Franco-Chinoise		Fudan University	Private	Song Wusheng
6	1936	National College of Pharmacy		China PharmaceuticalUniversity	Public	Moody Meng
7	1937	South Manchuria Medical College	National Shenyang Medical College	Shenyang Pharmaceutical University	Public	Yuan Shufan
8	1936	National Central University	National Shanghai Medical College	Fudan University	Public	Dr. Zhang Changshao
9	1943			Peking University Medical College was formed in 1938 with the pharmacy course launched in 1943. It became independent as Peking Medical College in 1952, and as a medical university in 1985. It then rejoined Peking University as a faculty in 2000	Public	Xue Yu
10	1944	National Zhejiang University		Zhejiang University	Public	Sun Zhongpeng
11	1949	Soochow University		Suzhou University	Private	Unknown

Credit The Prospect and Review of Pharmaceutical Education in China by Na Qi, Taipei Medical and Pharmaceutical Press, Taipei, 1969 (Chinese)

Notes and References

1. Naqi 那琦, *Zhongguo yaoxue jiaoyu zhi huígu yu qianzhan* 中國藥學教育之回顧與前瞻 [Review and Prospect of Chinese Pharmaceutical Education] (Taipei: Taipei Medical University, 1969): 196–216, esp. 203–204. Accessed 29 September 2023. http://libir.tmu.edu.tw/bit stream/987654321/26309/1.

2. Goldschmidt, A, *The Evolution of Chinese Medicine: Song Dynasty, 960–1200,* (London and New York, Routledge, 2009): 130–131.

3. In the early 19th century, Philadelphia, Penn. was the leading higher education centre in the U.S.

4. In 1988, the late Queen Elizabeth II granted the title "Royal" to the Pharmaceutical Society of Great Britain since its formation in 1841. The Royal Pharmaceutical Society of Great Britain (RPhC) accomplished its mission as a regulatory body for pharmacists in the UK when The General *Pharmaceutical Council* became the independent regulator for pharmacists, pharmacy technicians and pharmacy premises in *Great Britain in 2010.* The RPhC retains its role as the body representing the pharmacy profession in the UK.

5. From the mid-nineteenth century to the end of WWII in 1945, Germany was chosen as Japan's scientific and industrial development model, including medicine and pharmacy.

6. *Keju* is a system of choosing imperial court officials by merit rather than by birth in written examinations. It commenced in 605 CE during the Sui dynasty and underwent substantial changes with a formal, three-tier (prefecture, province and national) examination in the Song dynasty with the few successful candidates being awarded official positions. It was abolished in the final years of the Qing dynasty (1644–1911) in 1905. *Keju* was much criticized as a system to retain Confucian loyalty without challenging the status quo and stifling innovation.

7. Yamakawa, K., "Historical Sketch of Modern Pharmaceutical Science and Technology (Part 3)", *Pharmacist Jourrnal* (Japanese), 30. no. 1 (1995): 1–10.

8. The word *Beiyang* means Beijing and the coastal provinces and municipalities of Liaoning, Jinin, Shandong, and Tianjin. The dropping of the *Beiyang* name in 1904 upgraded the College from a regional one to a national medical institution.

9. The Army Medical College's pharmacy department had very high standards, and its core competencies were in pharmaceutical manufacturing and research and development. The first batch of 18 pharmacy graduates in 1911 was an exception as only a handful graduated at the AMC in subsequent years.

10. When Japan declared war on the US by attacking Pearl Harbour on 7 December 1941, the SJW became part of the Pacific Theatre of WWII.

11. Dr. Robert Lim was born in Singapore of Chinese descent. He graduated in medicine at the University of Edinburgh in 1919, taking a PhD in 1920 and a DSc in 1923. He was a Rockefeller Fellow at the University of Chicago in 1923–1924 and joined as the professor in physiology at the Peking Union Medical College from 1924–1937. During the Second Sino-Japanese War (1937–1945), he joined the Emergency Medical Service Training Centre and trained 13,000 paramedics. Lim became the Surgeon General in 1945 and the Director of National Medical Defense Centre in 1947. In 1949, Lim left China and assumed a full-time position as the Senior Research Fellow of the Medical Sciences Research Laboratory of Miles Laboratories (now Bayer) in 1951 until retirement.

12. The Canadian Federal Parliament passed the Canadian Citizenship Act in 1946, which officially granted fully independent Canadian citizenship to those born or naturalized in Canada. Prior to that, those born in Canada were British subjects under British rule.

13. The cause of the anti-Christian movement could have been a combination of the "New Culture" ideas on science and democracy, nationalism and communism. The Nationalist government eventually executed a policy of privatization of Christian universities in the late 1920s.

14. Yamamoto, Tatsuro and Sumiko, "The anti-Christian movement in China, 1922–1927", *The Far Eastern Quarterly* 12, no. 2 (1953): 133–147.

15. Zhu Yanru 朱廷儒 (1912–1998), graduated in 1937 and received a MS degree in pharmacy at Columbia University in 1951. After working as a pharmaceutical chemist in the US for four years, Zhu returned to China in 1955 and was appointed as a professor in pharmaceutical chemistry.

16. Paul I. Sun 孙博义 (1920–2020), graduated in 1942, and was a professor at the School of Pharmacy, University of Toronto.

17. Chen Lanying 陈兰英 (1921–2016), graduated in 1945 and was appointed as the chief pharmacist of the Peking Union Medical College Hospital in 1948. She was the pioneer in the formulation of total parenteral nutrition and initiated clinical pharmacy studies in China in the 1980s.

18. Liu Shuchang 刘素嫦 graduated in 1946, a co-founder of the West China Union University Hong Kong Alumni Association, and a fomer president of the Hong Kong Practicing Pharmacists Association.

19. William Pailing, passed his major examination, qualified and registered as a pharmaceutical chemist and a member of the Pharmaceutical of Great Britain in January 1909.

20. Bernard Read and John Cameron were pharmacists who worked for the PUMC and PUMCH in Beijing, and they served as the external advisors in the compilation of China's first national pharmacopoeia in 1930.

21. Yang Shanyao, 楊善堯 "Jiang zhongzheng yu kangzhan qianhou de junyi zhidu" 蔣中正与抗战前后的军医制度 [Chiang Kai-shek and Military Medical System in the Pre-and Post-2nd Sino Japanese War Period], Guoshiguan guankan, 国史馆馆刊 [*Journal of the National History Museum*] no. 12 (2015): 173–180.

22. Moody Meng was a protégé of Dr. Heng J. Liu and Meng's position as the head of NSP was terminated when he declined to join as a member of the Nationalist Party, which was a pre-requisite for university and college principals. Another theory was that Meng was a sympathizer of the Chinese Communist Party and was not keen to pledge loyalty to the ruling Nationalist Party.

23. Moody Meng continued his position as the chief pharmacist at the NHA and followed Dr. Heng J. Liu to set-up the Union Pharmaceutical Factory in Hong Kong in August 1939. Meng's registration as a pharmacist in Hong Kong was a simply a procedural one as he was a pharmaceutical chemist registered with the Pharmaceutical Society of Great Britain in 1924.

24. With funding by Song Ziwen 宋子文 (TV Soong), chairman of the Bank of China, who was the brother of Madam Chiang Kai-shek (蒋介石夫人宋美士玲, Mei-lin Soong), Dr. Heng J. Liu invited Meng to set-up the Union Pharmaceutical Factory 协和制药厂 (UPF) in Hong Kong in August 1939. UPS was to become a major producer of generic drugs and surgical supplies other than the PMI of AMC in the Second Sino-Japanese War of 1937–1945.

25. Shen Jiachang 沈家祥 (1921–2015), a graduate of 1942, completed his PhD degree in pharmaceutical chemistry at the University of London in 1949 and became a research scientist at the Northeast Pharmaceutical Works and a professor of the Shenyang Pharmaceutical College. The latter was upgraded to become Shenyang Pharmaceutical University in 1994.

26. Peng Sixun 彭司勋 (1919–2018), a graduate of 1942, completed his master's degree in pharmaceutical sciences at Columbia University in 1950. He became professor at the Nanjing School of Pharmacy and a member of the editorial board of the Chinese Pharmacopoeia.

27. Yuan Chengye 袁承业 (1924–2018), a graduate of 1948, completed his Associate PhD degree at the Soviet Pharmaceutical Institute in 1955 and was assigned to work at the Shanghai Institute of Inorganic Chemistry of the Chinese Academic of Sciences.

28. The late Cheung Chung Leung 张仲良, entered into the Register of Pharmacists entitled to practice pharmacy in Hong Kong in December 1946. *The Hong Kong Government Gazette,* February 22, 1957: 305.

29. Personal interview of Gu Jiheng 顾吉衡 with Patrick Chiu, at the Chinese Pharmaceutical Foundation, Taipei, 20 March 2018.

30. Shanghai was part of the Jiangsu (Kiangsu) province in the Manchu Qing dynasty until it became a centrally administered municipality governed from the Beiyang government of the Nationalist era in Beijing (Peking) and split from the Kiangsu province in July 1927.

After the successful Northern Expedition (1926–1928) led by Generalissimo Chiang Kai-shek, Shanghai was governed by the new Nationalist government which capital was relocated from Beijing (Peking) to Nanjing (Nanking). After the foundation of the People's Republic of China in October 1949, Shanghai has since been administered from the once again relocated capital in Beijing.

31. Kurzer, F., "George S V Wills and the Westminster College of Chemistry and Pharmacy: a chapter in pharmaceutical education in Great Britain" in *Medical History* 51, no. 4 (2007): 477–506. Accessed 29 September 2023. https://www.ncbi.nlm.nih.gov/pmc/articles/PMC200 2594/.

32. Zhu Zhu et al. 朱珠等 *Shìjì xiehe bainian yao shì: Běijīng xiehe yiyuan yaojì ke fazhan shì*, 世纪协和 百年 药事: 北京协和医院药剂科发展史 [A Century of Pharmaceutical Affairs of Peking Union Medical College Hospital: Historical Development of the Pharmacy Department] (Beijing: Peking Union Medical College Press, 2021): 136.

33. Zheng Shou 郑寿 (1896–1982), P3, a 1915 graduate, head (1929, 1933–1936), Chief Engineer of Southwest Pharmaceutical Factory in Chongqing (wartime capital of the Nationalist government).

34. Major General Zhang Pengchong 张郑翀 (1982–1968), P4, 1916 graduate, head (1937–1943), head of pharmaceutical chemistry, Shanghai Medical College.

35. Li Weizhang 李维祯 (1910–1998), P15, a 1933 graduate, chief pharmacist, MoH, People's Republic of China in 1949.

36. Lou Zichen 楼之岑 (1920–1995), P27, a 1946 graduate, received a scholarship from the British Boxers Indemnity Fund and a PhD from the University of London in 1950. Lou returned to Beijing and joined the as a pharmacy professor with the Beijing Medical College. Under his supervision, Tu Youyou later led the discovery of artemisinin (*Qinghaosu*) in the mid-1970s.

37. Xi Nianzhu 奚念朱 (1927–), P33, a 1949 graduate, head of pharmacy department, Shanghai Medical University (now Fudan University).

38. Jing Mingru (金明儒, King Minglu, 1926–2021), P34, a 1951 graduate, second head (1974–1981), Taiwan NDMC.

39. Naqi, [Review and Prospect], 196–216, esp. 200–201.

Chapter 7
Ethical Pharmaceuticals and Home-Grown Research and Development

This chapter traces the development of modern China's pharmaceutical industry in the very city of Shanghai. A notable contribution came from scholars who received Boxers Indemnity scholarships (庚子赔款留学奖学金) or state funding to pursue graduate studies in chemical technology and pharmaceutical sciences across Europe, Japan, the UK, and the US during the 1910s to 1940s (See the section on *Modernization with "New Cutlture" and "New Movement"* in Chap. 8). These individuals played a crucial role in the start-up as well as the large-scale production of novel chemical drugs such as neo-arsphenamine, porcine insulin, and sulphur drugs.

In the U.K. or the U.S., proprietary medicines containing one or more ingredients for treating minor illnesses such as chronic bronchitis, dermatitis, headache, indigestion, and other ailments, began flourishing in the 1850s. With the wide opening of the treaty ports, China's modern pharmaceutical industry started to grow in the late nineteenth and early twentieth centuries. In the early 1890s, entrepreneurial Chinese medicine dispensaries began to market imported "opium cures" and subsequently produced proprietary medicines including "opium cures" for their patrons. At the same time, dispensary technicians trained by western chemists in the International Settlement and the French Concession dispensaries or missionary hospitals in Shanghai and nearby cities sought investors to finance their dispensaries. These pioneers in modern drugs immediately rolled out the much sought after "opium cures" and created a vast network of retail drug stores competing with the Chinese medicine dispensaries. They gave birth to modern China's pharmaceutical "cottage" industry in the next six decades, from 1890 to 1949.

After the Boxers Movement, young students who had received the Boxers Indemnity Scholarships from the British, French, Japanese and U.S. governments studied chemical technology, mining, industrial engineering, medicine, pharmacy, pharmacology, and other scientific disciplines in their host countries. Some pursued advanced studies or undertook research work in the western pharmaceutical industry before returning to China in the 1920s and 1930s. These returnee chemical engineers and pharmaceutical scientists started producing high value, off-patented raw materials of neo-arsphenamine and sulphonamide drugs from scratch to treat sexually transmitted diseases and life-threatening infections in the mid-1930s.

Academic, and research institutions of medicine and pharmacy, and science and technology were relocated from the key cities of Beijing, Nanjing, and Shanghai during the War to the safe areas of Chengdu, Chongqing and Kunming in Southwest China, It is, however, public knowledge that local pharmaceutical manufacturers continued to operate in the early years between 1937 and 1941 in Shanghai., which was under occupation by the Japanese Imperial Army. Despite the lack of fermentation equipment, high-grade enzymes and standardized chemical raw materials of active substances, Shanghainese chemical engineers and pharmaceutical scientists were innovative enough to produce low-potency insulin and penicillin during the last years of WWII in 1944 and 1945 in the absence of imported ethical drugs. One significant achievement observed during the eight years of the War was the maintenance of a sound higher education system when the national universities were relocated to Chongqing and continued to operate unabated (See One Country, Two Pharmacy Systems in Chap. 9). As a result, some bright minds of the last batch of industrial engineers, medical doctors, pharmacists, research scientists etc. who graduated in the War years received their post-graduate training in the West from 1946 to 1949. The majority of them returned to China in 1950 to build a modern state.

Research of Ethical Pharmaceuticals

In the third quarter of the nineteenth century, retail chemists produced batch sizes of mixtures and creams and ointments in dozens in bottles and pots under their brand labels for sale to their patrons. They progressed initially as makers of "opium cures" and then continued with proprietary medicines. By the mid-1930s, some manufacturing chemists branched out into the ethical pharmaceutical market by targeting physicians who were prescribers or dispensing doctors in a hospital or clinic setting. Ethical pharmaceuticals are medicines of biological, chemical, or herbal origins prescribed by physicians under prescriptions in dosage forms such as capsules, tablets, powders and injections. National pharmacopoeia specifies the requirements of essential drugs commonly used in the country in drug monographs to ensure pharmaceutical manufacturers conform to such standards. Initially, few ethical drug manufacturers had in-house research departments in Shanghai, except for those entrepreneurial ones such as New Asia and Sine.

Yang's Chemotherapeutic Institute (Yang's) was a rare breed. It was primarily set up as a contracted research laboratory, subsequently becoming a specialty ethical pharmaceutical manufacturer of chemical drugs and health supplements. Yang Shunxun (杨树勋, Peter Shih-Hsien Yang) founded his research laboratory in Shanghai on 15 August 1937.[1] Yang, a southern Chinese Christian, was born in Teochew (Chaozhou), Prefecture of Canton (Guangdong Province), in 1899. The University of Chicago awarded him a PhD in chemistry in 1931. Yang continued his post-doctoral research in the chemical synthesis of anti-infectives in the US.

He married Zhang Juzhen (Jang Chu-chen), a Shanghai native, who graduated as a medical doctor from the University in 1933.

The Yangs returned to China in the same year. Yang worked as a professor and researcher, and his wife, Zhang, worked as a clinic physician at the PUMC in Beijing in 1933 until the couple decided to join Jang's family in Shanghai in 1935.[2] Yang was working initially as the Section Head of the Biochemical Laboratory, Institute of Chemistry of Academia Sinica (the IOC) and his wife, Zhang, as a physician at the Hongren Hospital. With the advance of the Japanese Imperial Army, the IOC relocated to Kunming, southwest China, far from the battleground, in April 1938. However, the Yangs stayed behind in Shanghai and set up their research laboratory in the occupied territory. Yang's first commercially researched drug product was the off-patent generic neo-arsphenamine, Neo-Sypharsan, a chemically synthesized second-generation arsenic compound for treating syphilis (Fig. 7.1).[3] Yang's partnered with Sine Laboratories & Co. Ltd. (Sine), originally a German founded pharmaceutical factory in Shanghai, to market the Neo-Sypharsan brand of generic neo-arsephenamine in China and Southeast Asian markets.

At the end of the Second Sino-Japanese War in 1945, US pharmaceutical companies exported their surplus pharmaceutical inventory to China, which nearly collapsed the fragile Chinese pharmaceutical industry. Yang's survived the influx of cheap drugs

Fig. 7.1 Neo-Sypharsan by Yang's for Syphilis. Marketed by *Sine Pharmaceutical, Shanghai. 1945. Credit* Hong Kong Society for the History of Pharmacy

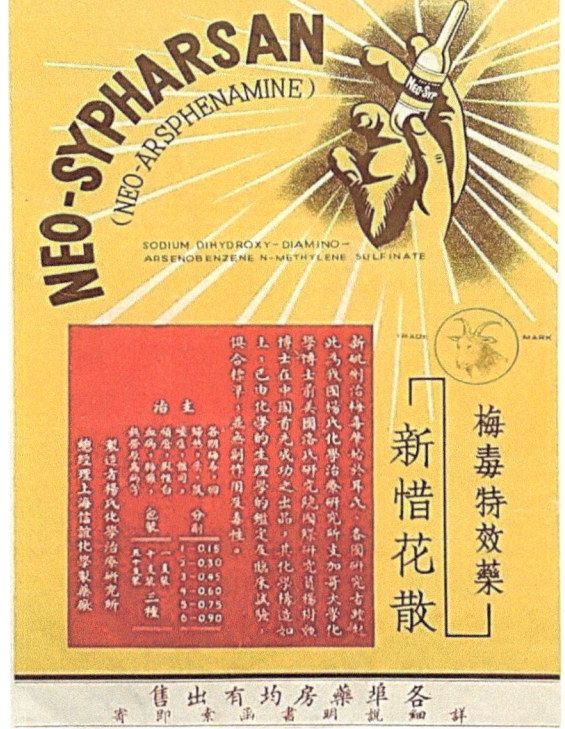

Fig. 7.2 *Pantramine*—An Essential Amino Acid Mixture by Yang's. @ 1948. *Credit* Hong Kong Society for the History of Pharmacy

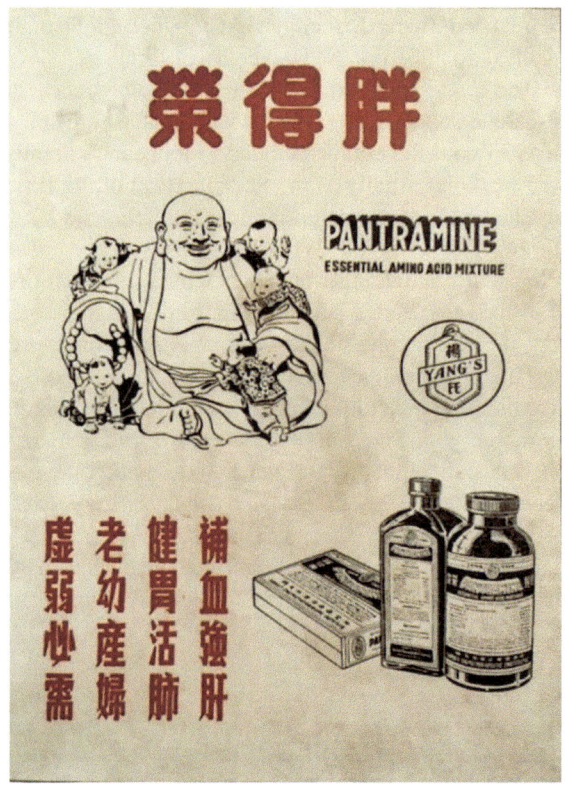

from the US. Yang minimized the adverse impact of dumping by US drug manufacturers by launching Pantramine (Fig. 7.2), a health supplement, instead of direct competition with established multinationals such as Eli Lilly, Pfizer, and Wyeth in 1948.

Koffer Dispensary (科发药房), among the western expatriate chemists operating in China from 1866 to 1949, was a fully integrated retail and manufacturing business based in Shanghai. Teophill Koffer, a Prussian chemist, opened Pharmacie de L'Union, a retail pharmacy in the French Concession in Shanghai, on 10 October 1866.[4] Five years later, Koffer departed for Hong Kong to succeed in his uncle's Medical Hall business in 1871. Another Prussian national, S Voelkel, acquired Pharmacie de L'Union from Koffer and retained the trade name of Koffer Dispensary. While in Hong Kong, Teophil Koffer who served as the chemist at the Medical Hall, otherwise known as the German Dispensary, located at 37 Queen's Road, Central (now Yu To Sang Building) acquired the business from his uncle on March 1, 1872. A.S. Schroder joined Koffer as a partner in Shanghai in 1905, and the corporate name changed to Voelkel & Schroeder Ltd. (V&K) with one million silver dollars as the registered capital. A customized package seal with a corporate name was used as the seal of dispensed medicine (Fig. 7.3). With the freshly acquired capital, V&K invested in industrial premises and modern production equipment to build an alcohol

Fig. 7.3 Voelkel and
Schroder package seal.
c.1910. *Credit* Hong Kong
Society for the History of
Pharmacy

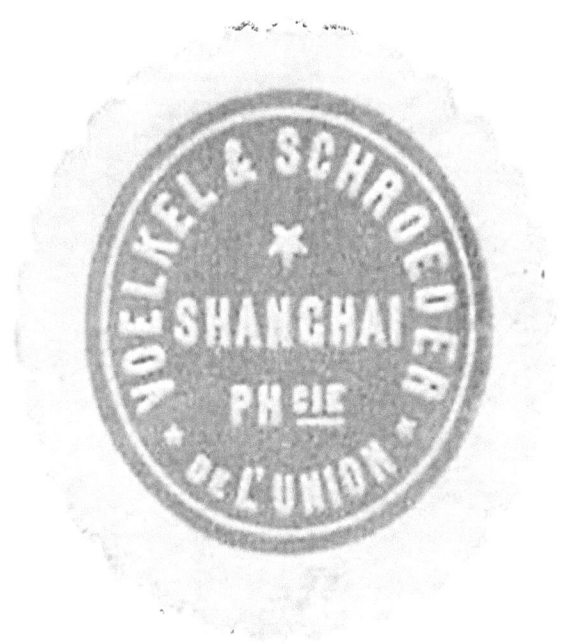

plant with two workshops. One workshop was for exclusively producing antiseptic and disinfectant solutions for hospitals and clinics. The other was to make elixir and tincture medicines for oral use.

V&K's pharmaceutical plant was in Changyang (Ward) Road in the Hongkou (Hongkew) District of Shanghai, in 1909. In the 1910s, Koffer and A.S. Watson's pharmaceutical plants, both installed with ultra-modern state-of-the-art distillation plants, were the most extensive western pharmaceutical manufacturing facilities in Shanghai and Hong Kong, respectively. Before they departed from Shanghai in 1914 to join the military in Germany. Messrs. Voelkel and Schroder transferred their Koeffer shareholdings to a fellow countryman, H Scholten. The latter was a man with a vision. He invited Chinese and US citizens to become shareholders of Koeffer to safeguard his interests before China joined the Allies in 1917. Scholten's move was to avoid the confiscation of Koeffer as enemy assets if Germany lost WWI.[5]

Business continued to thrive with new products launched in the 1920s and the Koeffer was incorporated with a paid-up capital of 579,600 Chinese Yuan in the US in 1928. By then, the German name of Koffer had been altered. The corporate name changed to Kofa American Drug Company, Federal Inc., U.S. Cornell Franklin, the senior partner of Franklin and Fleming Law Firm in Shanghai, owned 49.2% of Kofa & Co Ltd. and assumed the chairmanship of the board, The rest belonged to German and local shareholders, and the management held 2%. With injection of fresh capital, Kofa soon expanded into the production and export of Santal Anti-Gonorrheal Drug, and Absorbent Cotton (Figs. 7.4, 7.5 and 7.6). Soon after Japan declared war on the US on 7 December 1941, assets of Kofa, a US business entity, in Shanghai

Fig. 7.4 Santal Gonorrhoea Treatment Pills Flyer. c.1920. *Credit* Hong Kong Society for the History of Pharmacy.

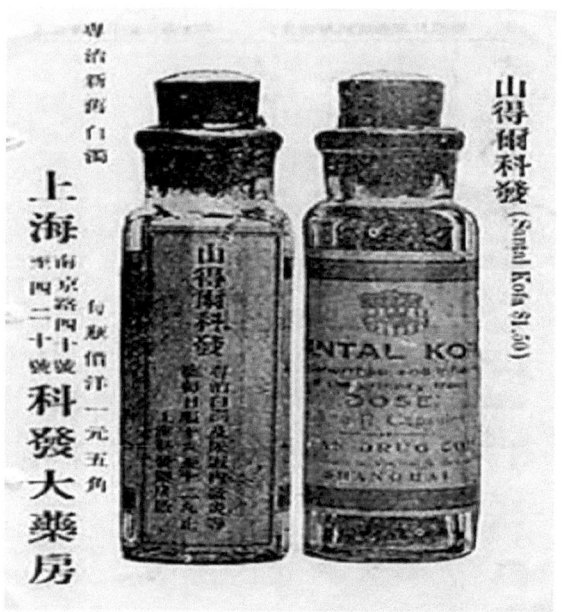

were confiscated and operated by Takeda, Japan's leading pharmaceutical company. At the end of WWII, the US Department of Justice confiscated the shareholding of Kofa's German equity holders and sold it to the Industrial Bank of China in 1946. The latter became the sole agent of Schering (now MSD) for the mainland market in 1947 until the Communist government nationalized Kofa in the early 1950s.[6]

Hypoule's (海普制药厂) humble beginnings could be traced back to Zhang Yuzhou's (張禹洲, YC Chang, 1903–1972) decade long work experience at Koffer Dispensary in the early 1920s in Shanghai. After graduating from high school in Shanghai, Zhang's first job was a student dispenser at the Paulun Hospital (宝隆医院) (renamed in 1910 in memory of the founder) in 1921 for a year. He then joined Scholten's Koffer Dispensary with rotations in counter sales and dispensing in its retail chemist shop and ampoule making and warehousing in its manufacturing plant from 1922 to 1929. While working at Koffer in Shanghai in 1925, Zhang received financial support from a physician friend to found Hypoule Chemical Works Ltd (now Haipu). Hypoule's mission was to become China's largest manufacturer of injection drugs.[7]

In 1929, Zhang resigned from Kofa, name changed from Koffer in the previous year, to become the full-time owner-manager of Hypoule. He soon set up a second company, Murray Drug Company, to import raw materials to produce generic medicines and medical supplies. In April 1936, Hypoule became a limited liability company and raised capital to expand its product portfolio and geographical coverage. When Shanghai fell under the Japanese Imperial Army on 12 November 1937, Hypoule halted its sterile injectable production and shipped out its inventory to Hankow (汉口, Hankou), a district of Wuhan, in Central China and

Fig. 7.5 Adsorbent cotton @ Late1930s. *Credit* Hong Kong Society for the History of Pharmacy

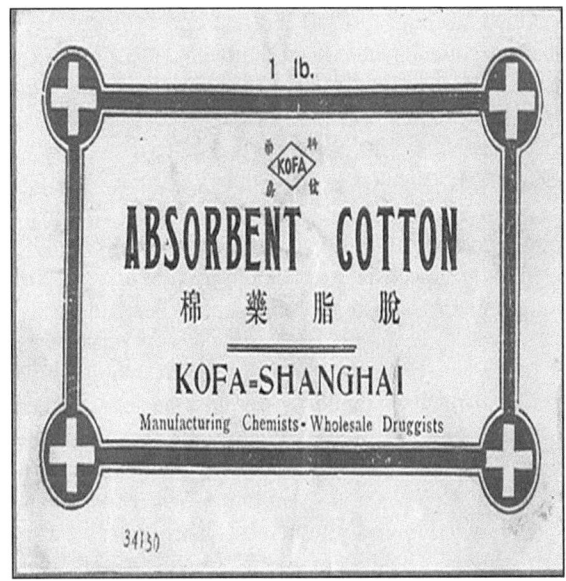

Fig. 7.6 Kofa corporate envelope, 1930s. *Credit* Hong Kong Society for the History of Pharmacy

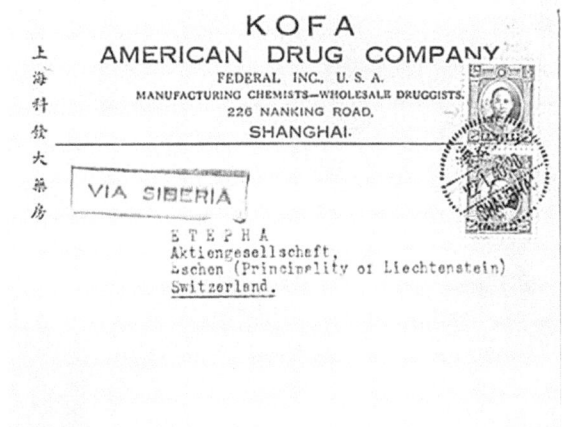

Chongqing in Southwest China. When on 20 March 1940, Wang Jinwei formed the 'Reorganized Government of the Republic of China', the puppet state governing the Japanese-occupied territories of China, established itself in Nanjing, whereas Chiang Kai-shek's Nationalist government relocated to Chongqing until the end of the War.

With a large customer base of physicians and hospitals in Shanghai and the eastern provinces of Jiangsu (江苏, Kiangsu) and Zhejiang (浙江, Chekiang) running out of injectable medicines during the Japanese occupation, Zhang felt that Hypoule, as the major ampoule medicine supplier, was obliged to serve patients on humanitarian grounds. Hypoule immediately formed a partnership with a glass factory in Shanghai and Zhang and his core team of managers returned to Shanghai with production resumed in August 1940. By the end of 1949, Hypoule was one of the leading pharmaceutical factories in China, with a portfolio of 159 products with a wide range of dosage forms, including tablets, tinctures, and syrups.

New Asiatic Chemical Works (新亚化学制药厂, Xinya Huaxue Zhiyaochang) was founded by the three partners; Xu Guanqun (许冠群, Kuan-Chun Hsu), an accountant, Zhao Rudiao (赵汝调, Yu-Tiao Chao), a pharmacist, and Tu Huansheng. Tu (屠焕生, Zhao Rudiao's brother-in-law), also an accountant, in May 1926.[8] They jointly invested 1000 silver dollars as start-up capital. A corporate logo was designed to position New Asiatic as a Star of Asia (Fig. 7.7). Xu and Tu were friends since their youth. Zhao spoke the same dialect of Wuchin (Wujin) county in Kiangsu province where the three came from. Zhao was a pharmacy graduate of Chiba University of Japan who possessed pharmaceutical manufacturing knowledge missing in Xu's venture. Together, the three started a business. Like other manufacturing chemists of the time, New Asiatic's first proprietary medicine, a short-lived "opium cures" pill, was produced in a store room in the neighbourhood of the French Concession in Shanghai. New Asiatic's Ten Drops Water for heat stroke became a "Star" product in the hot and humid summer. Its Distilled Water also became an all-season product for Shanghai's health conscious, growing middle class families.

In the early twentieth century, many pharmaceutical manufacturers produced their brands of toiletries. New Asiatic launched its personal care Peacock brand of tooth powder, toothpaste, and eau de toilette (toilet water) soon after Chiang Kai-shek kick-started the New Life Movement (新生活运动, "Xin Shenghuo Yundong") in Nanchang in 1934. New Asiatic rode along the hygiene and cleanliness slogans of the New Life Movement, a national neo-Confucius campaign to reenergize the lost

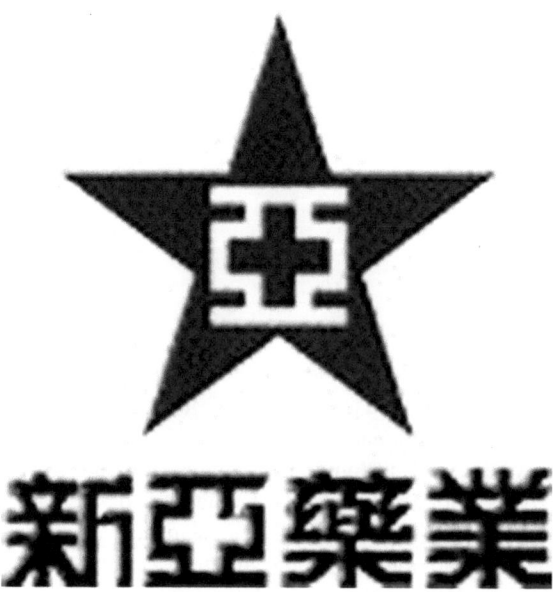

Fig. 7.7 New Asiatic Chemical Works corporate brand. C. 1920s. *Credit* Hong Kong Society for the History of Pharmacy

revolutionary spirit of the young Republic. (See the section on *Modernisation with "New Culture", and "New Life" Movements* in Chap. 8). The company successfully raised 5000 silver dollars and moved the factory to 24 Fengyang (Burkill) Road) in the second quarter of 1927.[9] In October of the same year, New Asiatic conducted a new round of fundraising of 5000 silver dollars and incorporated as a limited liability company, New Asiatic Chemical Works Ltd. (Xinya Huaxue Zhiyao Youxian Gongsi), with a cumulative registered capital of 10,000 silver dollars. With positive cash flow, New Asiatic purchased their first set of sterile distilled water equipment from Japan and leased additional premises for an ampoule filling station at Lane 586 (Sanfengli) of Chengdu North Road to mass produce ampoule injectables.

By now, Hypoule and New Asiatic were the only two sterile pharmaceutical manufacturers in China which had gained significant market share from the more expensive imported European and US brands. The Great Depression caused by the stock market crash in New York suddenly struck in October 1929, leading to cash flow issues as banks tightened business credits in Shanghai. New Asiatic was no exception. New Asiatic's increasing toiletries sales to the retail drug stores and neighbourhood sales counter came with mounting credits extended to the wholesalers. New Asiatic faced the problem of lacking further financial resources to extend credit to the medical clinic physicians for its sterile ampoule injections. New Asiatic promptly completed its third financing round with 50,000 silver dollars as registered capital in 1930. In August, New Asiatic leased the premises of 714 Huaian (Markham) Road to open a packaging glass factory for medicines, ampoules, and other glass instruments with a fully integrated pharmacaeutical and medical device plant in Shanghai.

The new plant's first product was a nutritional supplement, Precious Youth (宝青春), for beauty-conscious female consumers, launched in 1932. Other health supplements rolled out in subsequent years included Livemin, Placemon, and Hormspermin. Over-the-counter drugs had Panadin, Magsolin, Follimon, Tancnol and Sinasbin (painkiller for headaches and toothaches). Following the path of western pharmaceutical companies Bayer, Hoechst and others, New Asiatic was an early pharmaceutical company to promote its products by publishing the *"Journal of New Medicine"* (新医学杂志) for medical professionals in 1932 and *"Healthy Home"* (健康之家) magazine for the rapidly growing middle-class consumers in Shanghai in 1936. The 18 September Incident of 1931 in Shenyang (奉天, Mukden), northeast China, was regarded by many as the prelude to the second Japanese invasion of China in July 1937.[10] As a result, anti-Japanese sentiments were raised nationwide in the following years and boycotts of imported Japanese products boosted New Asiatic's brand of toiletries sales for female consumers in Shanghai and the rest of China. With increasing imports of Hoechst (now Sanofi)'s Neo-Salvarsan in the 1920s, the only clinically effective drug for syphilis available, Xu actively expanded the company's production and set up a printing plant and a carton factory for the eventual roll-out of the generic version of neo-arsphenamine.

The latter was a second-generation and improved version of arsphenamine (606 as commonly known by the medical profession), an arsenic drug discovered by Paul Ehrlich to treat syphilis in 1912, and with a wider safety margin Then, as an entrepreneur, Xu invited Zeng Guangfang (曾光方, K.K. Tseng), a pharmaceutical research scientist who graduated from the Imperial University of Tokyo, to start the New Asiatic Research Institute in 1935. A year later, Zeng launched the first product of the Institute; an intravenously administered neo-arsphenamine. New Asiatic's neo-arsphenamine injection quickly replaced the higher priced Neo-Salvarsan marketed by Hoechst.

Within ten years, New Asiatic grew from three employees in a store room with a capital of 1000 yuan to become the first large-scale pharmaceutical factory in Shanghai and China. New Asiatic's registered capital also increased to 500,000 yuan, with over 400 employees and an annual revenue of 1 million in 1936. In the same year, New Asiatic invited distinguished medical doctors, including Dr. Fu-Ching Yen (颜福庆, Yan Fuqing, 1882–1970) and Wu Lien Teh (伍连德,Wu Liande, 1879–1960), to become investors and members of the supervisory board. Other renowned scientists who worked for New Asiatic included Qian Siliang (钱思亮, Chien Shih-liang, 1908–1983), later President of the Academia Sinica (中央研究院) in Taiwan and National Taiwan University (台湾大学), who worked for New Asiatic's Shanghai Plant in the 1930s.[11] In 1937, New Asiatic issued another round of shares to finance a second chemical plant in Beijing. Zhao Juhuang (趙橘黃, Jue-Huang Chao, 1833–1960), elder brother of Zhao Rudiao, relocated to Beijing as the resident director of New Asistic's new plant there. He developed the lime method in Shanghai when working with the Academica Sinica's Institute of Chemistry and mass-produced ephedrine with simple equipment for domestic and export markets in 1938. New Asiatic successfully raised $500,000 in Hong Kong in November 1941, only six weeks before the Japanese occupation of the Colony on Christmas Day 1941 (Fig. 7.8). The New Asiatic Board of Directors then postponed its local operations until after WWII. In February 1945, New Asiatic launched the Sino-Penicillin Injection brand with advertisements in local newspapers, including Shun Pao and its 25 June 1945 edition (Fig. 7.9). It was, however, the first pencillin made locally by a privately owned pharmaceutical company in China.

After the War ended in August 1945, Hsu travelled to Hong Kong in December with his brother Henry Kuan-ying Hsu (许冠英, Xu Guanying) to escape charges of wartime collaboration with the Wang Jingwai puppet government. They also revitalized their business there which stopped during the Japanese occupation of Hong Kong. They set up New Asiatic's regional office in Hong Kong, serving the Southeast Asia market and diversified their investment into the banking and property development sectors there. Hsu's younger sister, Hua, graduated from the Sino-French University in Shanghai with a degree in pharmacy. Her brother-in-law Zhao Chixiong (赵墀熊, 1914–1999) graduated from the Imperial University of Riku with a master's degree in pharmacy. Both helped Hsu's business in Hong Kong and later in Taiwan. Like many pharmaceutical companies, New Asiatic also faced bankruptcy and underwent financial restructuring when surplus drug inventory from the US flooded the China market at a fraction of the cost of local drugs in 1946. As a result, New Asiatic laid off two-thirds or 700 of its 1000 employees in 1947.[12] At the invitation of the People's Republic of China's government, Xu returned to Shanghai to resume his position as the Chairman of the New Asiatic Board of Directors in September 1950.

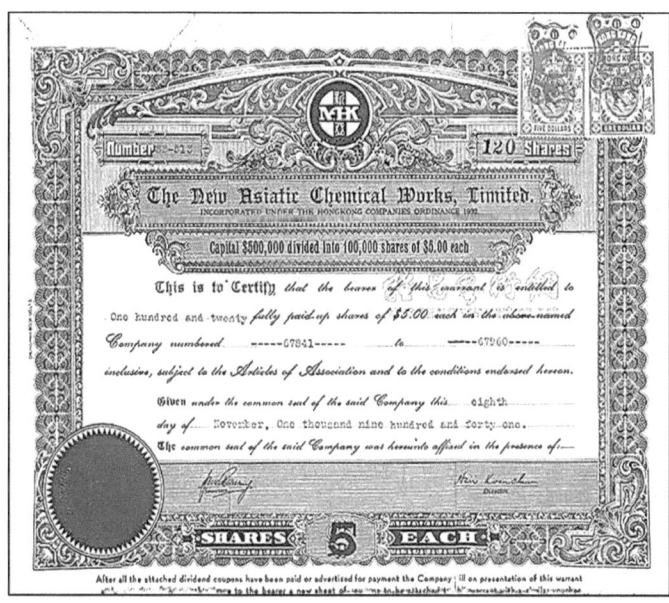

Fig. 7.8 Share certificate of the New Asiatic Chemical Works Limited issued on 8th November 1941. *Credit* Hong Kong Society for the History of Pharmacy

Fig. 7.9 Announcement of launch of Sino-Penicillin by the New Asiatic Institute for Biological Research in 1945. Advertising pitch: the world's ideal antibiotic: Sino-Penicillin. Shen Pao, Shanghai, June 25, 1945. *Credit* Hong Kong Society for the History of Pharmacy

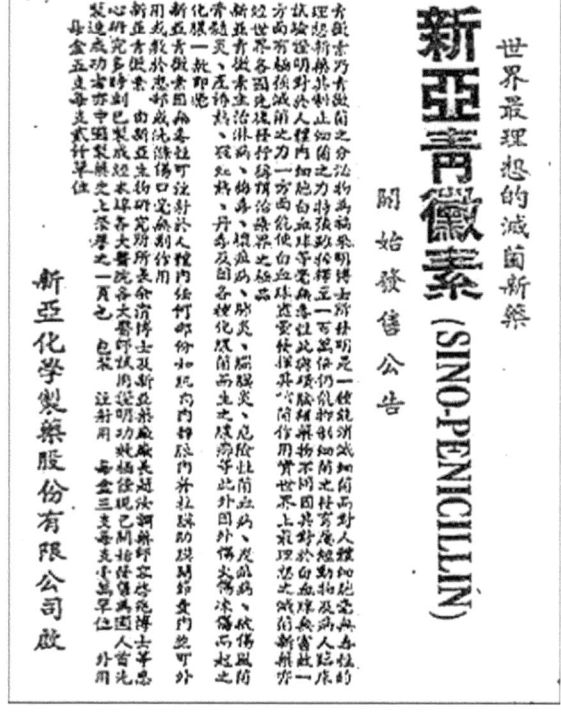

Another German pharmaceutical company that changed ownership in the 1930s was Sine Pharmacy—Deutsch Apotek GmbH (信谊药房, Xinyi). Max Joffee (霞飞), a German national of Russian descent, founded Sine at 746 Avenue Joffre (Huaihai Road) in the French Concession of Shanghai in 1916. Sine successfully launched Vita-Spermin, an oral and injectable vitamin, in 1918. Vita-Spermin alone contributed 50% of Sine's revenue in the next several decades (Fig. 7.10). In 1924, Joffee founded Sine Laboratories & Co. Ltd. with help from He Jikang (何子康, Ho Chi-kang), a pharmacist who had worked at the *Xiangya* (Hunan-Yale) Hospital in Changsha and the Voelkel & Schroder in Shanghai. In 1930, the Bao Guochang (包國昌, K.C. Bao) and Bao Guoliang (包國亮, K.L. Pao) brothers held the majority ownership, while Joffee held a minority shareholding. The Bao brothers increased their investments and expanded Sine's production capacity to serve domestic and overseas markets. As a result, many new products launched in and after 1932 included Aciflavin to treat sore throat, Glucocal health supplement, Thiazon anti-inflammatory ointment, and Zymasun digestive enzyme. The most significant product launched was Neo-Sypharsan in partnership with Yang's in 1937.

Joffee exited the business at the beginning of the War in 1937, and Sine became a Shanghaiese-owned pharmaceutical company. The Haolisheng (好力生) brand of Flounder Fish Oil Vitamin A and D Supplement, and Thiazon (Sulfathiazole) Tablet and Liquid for infections were instant hits when launched in 1938 (Fig. 7.11). In 1939, Sine established a local branch in Singapore to promote Vita-spermin and Zymasun for the Southeast Asia markets (Fig. 7.12). By 1940, Sine had over 300 employees working in its four factories manufacturing drugs, glass, adhesive medical plaster and vaccines in Shanghai. Its profits soared from $82,900 in 1938 to $576,578 in 1940.

Fig. 7.10 Sine Laboratory trade mark, c. 1930s. (Shade background with White Characters of Sine). *Credit* Hong Kong Society for the History of Pharmacy

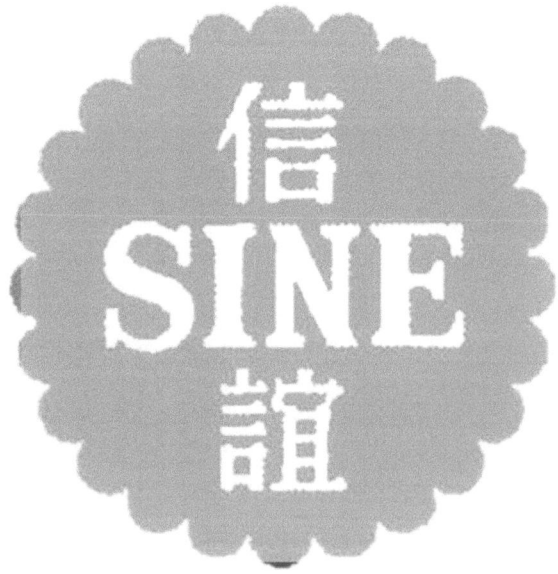

Fig. 7.11 Vita-Spermin supplement by Sine Laboratory, Shanghai. c. 1930. *Credit* Hong Kong Society for the History of Pharmacy

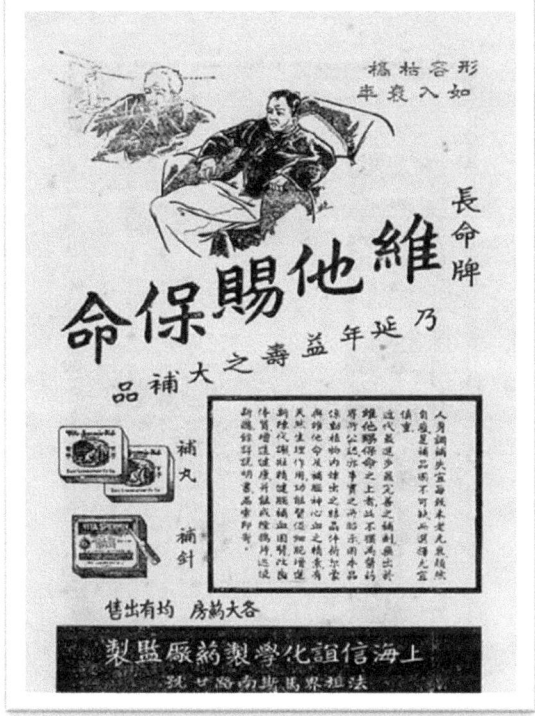

Under the Bao brothers' leadership, Sine became modern China's leading chemical and pharmaceutical company. During the period from 1924 to 1942, Shanghai became the incubation centre for ethical pharmaceutical manufacture in modern China (Table 7.1).

War-Time Pharmaceutical Production and Changshan

From 1937 to 1942, western medicines manufactured in the United Kingdom and the United States were transshipped through Hong Kong to Vietnam and detoured to Myanmar for onward delivery to the inland provinces of China. After that, air shipments were made to Yunnan and transferred for further deliveries to Chongqing, the wartime capital, and nearby regions. The birth of China's state-own pharmaceutical industry can be traced back to the Second Sino-Japanese War (1937–1945). The Nationalist government then stepped-up production during the War (Table 7.2). It is worth mentioning that Chinese medicine practitioners in Nanjing formed the Chinese Medicine Ambulatory Hospital (中医救护医院, "CMAH") to care for the wounded soldiers soon after the 7 July 1937 Marco Polo Bridge Incident in Beijing

Fig. 7.12 Flounder Fish Oil (Vit-A and D). Supplement by Sine Laboratory, c. 1938. *Credit* Hong Kong Society for the History of Pharmacy

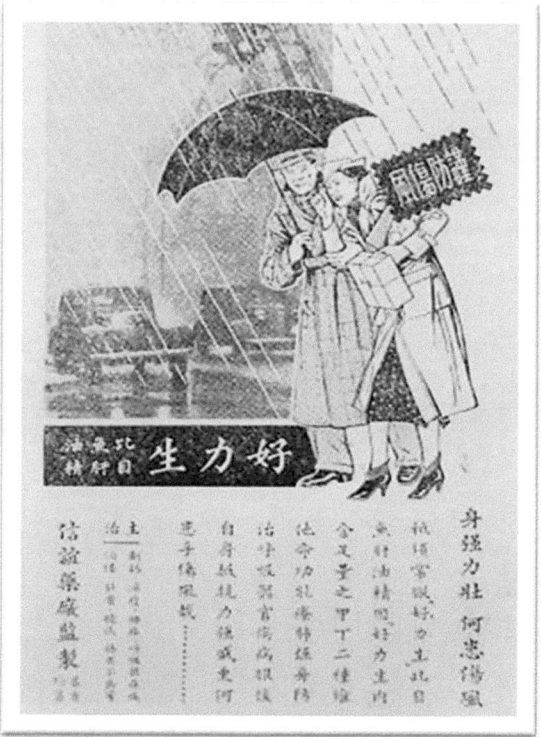

when Japan launched its second war of attack on China. In addition, the CMAH founded the Chinese Medicines Workshop (中华制药厂, CMW) to produce packaged herbal medicines for the Nationalist army once it moved to Chongqing in 1938. The CMW became the first state-funded China Pharmaceutical Factory (中国制药厂, CPF), supported by the Chen Guofu (陈果夫) and Lifu (立夫) brothers, both senior members of the Nationalist government, in 1943. It produced modern dosage forms of herbal remedies of tablets, injections, and wound dressings.[13]

Importing pharmaceutical raw materials to China was cut off soon after Japan occupied Canton on 21 October 1938. Nevertheless, Hong Kong played a critical role as an entrepot before the surrender of the British military to the Japanese imperial army on 25 December 1941. Song Ziwen (宋子文, Tse-ven (TV) Soong), the chairman of the Bank of China, the de facto central bank, raised a million dollars in US currency to purchase the production equipment and the UDCL premises near the former Kai Tak Airport in Kowloon in 1939. Dr. Heng J. Liu, the former head, and Moody Meng, the retired chief pharmacist of the NHA, were appointed as the CEO, and production director of The Union Drug Company Ltd. (协和制药有限公司, UDC, Xiehe Zhiyao Gongsi). With his British qualification as pharmaceutical chemist, Meng registered as a pharmacist with the UPC in Hong Kong in 1940 (Fig. 7.13). The UC produced a range of pharmaceutical preparations, sera,

Table 7.1 Key Ethical Pharmaceutical Manufacturers in Shanghai, 1923–1949

#	Year	Pharma enterprise	Owners	Location	Remarks
1	1924	Sine Laboratory	Dr Max Joffe and He Zhikang (Ho Chi-kang)	746 Avenue Joffre (Huihai Road)	Sine Pharmacy—Deutsch Apotek GmbH was founded by Dr Max Joffee at 746 Huaihai Road (Avenue Joffre) and was launched in 1916 Since 1930, the Bao brothers have led the company and become the leading pharmaceutical company in China
2	1925	Hypoule (Haipu)	Zhang Yuzhou	Avenue Road (Beijing West Road)	The first injectable drug manufacturer in China
3	1926	New Asiatic Pharma- cetical	Xu Guan Qun	Rue des Lieutenant Petiot (Chengdu South Road)	The second injectable drug manufacturer in China and the first glass syringe manufacturer A research institute was established in 1935 and the most significant pharma factory until 1946
4	1931	Jiufu Pharmaceutical Ltd	Wong Chu-Chiu	710 Avenue Edward VII (Yanan East Road)	Jiufu Pharmaceutical Ltd. first product was *Bailingji* (百龄机) launched in 1931. The best product—Lekofu Milk Extract, was a top selling nutritional supplement for 50 years
5	1942	Taishan Chemical and harmaceutical	Huang Daren	359 Connaught Road (Kangding Road)	Production of antibacterial lipoamides and saccharin

Source Author's Compilation

Table 7.2 Key state-owned pharmaceutical enterprises, 1935–1938

Year	Location	Ministry/ institution	Administration/ bureau	Unit name	Scope and range of products
1935	Nanjing	Interior	NHA	Narcotics Management Office	Relocation of narcotics production and supply base from Nanjing to Chongqing in 1937 Expansion to serve the frontier in 1943
1938	Chongqing	Interior	National Institute of Chinese Medicine	Chinese Medicine Factory	Research, development, and production of *Changshan*, a Chinese Medicine malarial drug
1939	Anshun, Guizhou	Military Commission	Army Medical Corps	PMRI	Sterile injectables and infusion solutions, chemical weapons and military and civilian pharmaceutical supplies
1940–1949	Hong Kong	Bank of China	China Assets Ltd	UDCL	Liquid and solid dosage forms including glass ampoules
1944–1949	Chongqing	Interior	National Health Administration	No. 1 Pharma Factory	100 employees, 40 + products, located back to Nanjing in 1946

(continued)

Table 7.2 (continued)

Year	Location	Ministry/ institution	Administration/ bureau	Unit name	Scope and range of products
				Central pharma factory	Produce anaesthetic ether, calcium gluconate injection, and diagnostic reagents Relocated to Shanghai in 1946
1945–1947	Shanghai	Executive Yuan	Post-war assets custody commission		Take-over of Japanese pharma enterprise; Fu Shou Pharma Factory in Shanghai and NE region. Chinese government after the War

Source Author's Compilation

glass ampoules and sterile drugs for the military and civilian markets. Zhang Maolin (张茂林, Chang Mao-lin), former quality laboratory director of UDC recalled:

> In this unfortunate encounter, it was lucky that Dr. Heng J. Liu had the opportunity to transport a large stock of medicines produced in Hong Kong to China in time. Therefore, during the last few years of the War, the supply of drugs was excellent! Dr. Heng J. Liu was far-sighted in anticipating the Japanese move to Hing Kong.[14]

Meanwhile, the National Army Medical College (NAMC) relocated to Guiyang, an inland city of Guizhou province far from the Japanese Imperial Army. NAMC consisted of three departments, namely the Pharmaceutical Manufacturing Institute (药品制造研究所, PMI), the Sera and Vaccines Manufacturing Institute (血清疫苗制造研究所, SVI) and the Army Nutrition Institute (陆军营养研究所, ANI). The PMI was responsible for producing alcohol using locally sourced maize and sweet potato by fermentation and distillation methodologies with a 24-h, 7-day, all-year-round roster. Daily production of 95% purity alcohol was about 50 gallons for use as automobile fuel and as antiseptics by military hospitals, clinics and retail pharmacies.[15] From 1940 to 1945, the battlefield hospitals received a steady supply of included sterile infusion solutions of 500 ml Normal Saline, Dextrose Solutions, and 20 ml Dextrose 50% Injection. Small-volume injectables, including procaine, emetine, atropine, quinine, strychnine, calcium chloride, and calcium gluconate injections were produced.

In addition, over 50 non-sterile liquids and solid dosage forms were made, including camphor tincture, iodine tincture, Brown mixture, liquorice tablets for common illnesses, and medical dressing and plasters for wound care. The PMI also produced glassware for medicinal and laboratory uses, including flasks, containers,

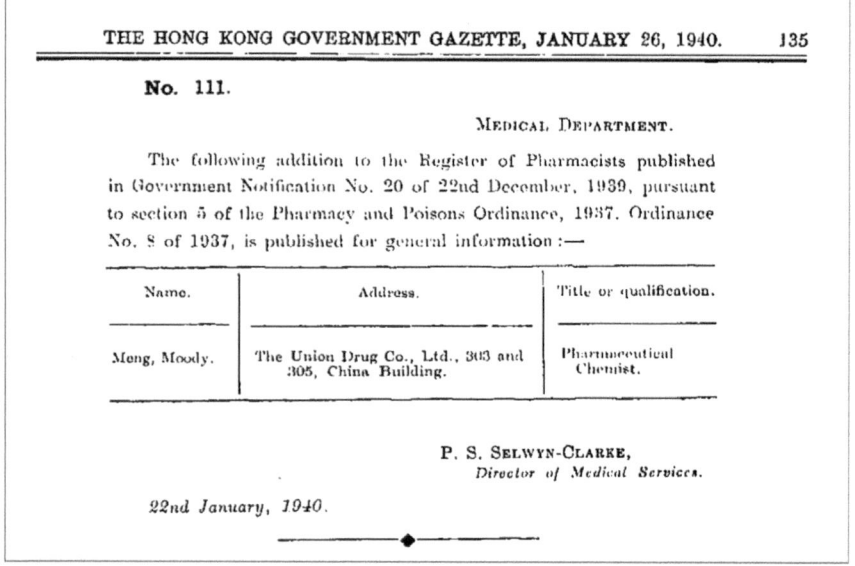

THE HONG KONG GOVERNMENT GAZETTE, JANUARY 26, 1940.   135

No. 111.

MEDICAL DEPARTMENT.

The following addition to the Register of Pharmacists published in Government Notification No. 20 of 22nd December, 1939, pursuant to section 5 of the Pharmacy and Poisons Ordinance, 1937. Ordinance No. 8 of 1937, is published for general information :—

Name.	Address.	Title or qualification.
Meng, Moody.	The Union Drug Co., Ltd., 303 and 305, China Building.	Pharmaceutical Chemist.

P. S. SELWYN-CLARKE,
Director of Medical Services.

22nd January, 1940.

Fig. 7.13 Pharmacist registration record of Moody Meng of The Union Drug Co. Ltd. in Hong Kong. *Credit* Hong Kong Government Gazette

measuring cups, test tubes, balances and scales, filtration funnels, bottles, ampoules and pharmaceutical pipettes. Under the SVI, the NAMC's pharmacy faculty and student volunteers developed and mass produced many high quality vaccines for preventing and treating typhoid, cholera, and smallpox. Malnutrition and vitamin deficiency frequently occurred in the army units during the War.[16] The ANI undertook research and recommended the processing methods of coarse noodles and rice to optimize its nutritional value and prevent vitamin deficiency diseases such as night blindness and beriberi. The ANI also held nutrition classes and recommended protein-rich soya food products to the army catering units.[17]

In 1943, the NHA publicized the "Provisional Standards Chart of Wartime Medical and Pharmaceutical Products" (战时医药和药品临时标准表), which listed 114 essential drugs, of which ten were not cultivated or produced in China, and another ten were Chinese materia medica freely available. Among the Chinese materia medica, commonly used raw materials such as orange peel, camphor, pepper, berberine, gall, gentian, liquorice, polygala, rhubarb, talc, and ginger were included in the wartime formulary. By then, over 50 domestic pharmaceutical manufacturers in the southwest and western regions supported by the central and provincial governments and the NAMC could produce some or all these products.[18] During the War, the Nationalist army fighting the Japanese Imperial Army in the inland provinces was severely short of one critical drug—quinine. As a result, malaria caused more deaths of soldiers than combat in the hot and humid months in the southern provinces of China. In addition, millions of refugees fled from the central regions to the southwestern areas of Szechuan and Yunnan faced similar health hazards. At the same time, the Japanese military successfully halted the export of quinine from Java when they occupied the Dutch East Indies (modern-day Indonesia) from March 1942 to September 1945. Sakata Takashi explained the supply situation of quinine during WWII in Asia:

> In 1940, more than 90% of the world's production of quinine, the single most important anti-malaria drug, was manufactured from cinchona bark produced in the Dutch East Indies, mainly Java. Accordingly, the Japanese occupation of the Dutch East Indies in March 1942 more or less brought the entire supply of quinine under the control of Japan.[19]

Finding a local solution to prevent and treat malaria in southwestern China for civilians and the Nationalist army became an urgent issue. China started cultivating cinchona trees in Yunnan province in the early 1930s with only one-third of the average annual 100-tonne volume to meet its demand during peace time. Hence, the search for an alternative supply of indigenous bencao effective against malaria began well before the War. Chen Guofu, Head of Nationalist Central Party School, was sourcing herbal remedies used by the natives of Yunnan province to treat cadets infected with malaria. Changshan (常山), genus *Dichroa febrifuga,* came to his attention by word-of-mouth of Chinese medicine practitioners in the Southwestern Region (Fig. 7.14). In view of the intensifying War and the severe shortage of quinine, soon after Dr. Zhang Changshao return to China in 1942, he was invited by Chen Guofu, who organized a Changshan clinical trial team, to join as the clinical investigator. Zhang was a young clinician and pharmacologist who graduated with a PhD from the University of London in 1941. He then received further training in clinical pharmacology at the Harvard Medical School in the US. It was the most important project under the Scientific Research on Nationally Produced Drugs Programme (国产药物科学研究计划) during the War years.

Zhao Chenggu, the pharmaceutical scientist of the changshan project team, promptly isolated the active compound, dirchrone, from changshan, which was effective against the malarial parasite. Dr. Zhang Changshao completed his changshan clinical trial on the Central Party School's clinic with thirteen malarial patients in Chongqing in late 1942. The clinical study was based on the "Reversed Order Programme" (反向顺序计划) instead of the established 4-phase protocol. Despite changshan's high potency in its anti-malarial activity over quinine, its highly toxic side effects quickly halted the continuing research and development of changshan. While the Changshan clinical study did not come to fruition, however, more Chinese clinicians and scientists have gained solid experience in the identification, isolation, and purification of the active ingredients in Chinese materia medica like what K.K. Chen did in 1925 at the PUMC. In addition, they have also mastered the clinical trial exercise for future drug development.

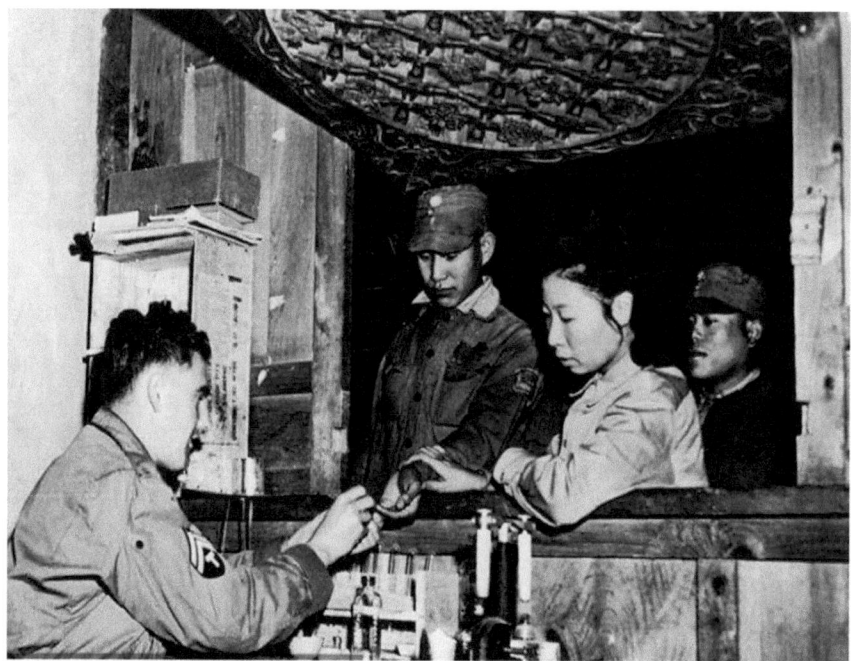

Fig. 7.14 Collection of blood specimens for diagnosis of malaria infection of Nationalist Solider in Chongqing, by US Navy Medical Corp. Technician. C. 1944. *Credit* Hong Kong Society for the History of Pharmacy

State and Private Research Institutes

After the foundation of the Republic of China on 1 January 1912, the priorities of the newly established NHA under the Ministry of the Interior in Beijing were for the development of qualified human resources, including registration of medical practitioners, pharmacists, and nurses; the regulatory control of narcotic drugs and pharmaceutical manufacturers; and the quarantine controls to prevent epidemics and vaccine production.

Soon after the successful Northern Expedition in Nanjing in 1928, the Nationalist government initiated long overdue institutional reforms by forming the Ministry of Health (MoH). Chiang Kai-shek, head of the Nationalist government, upon advice from widow, Madam Soong Ching-ling (Song Qingling 1893–1981), appointed Dr. Heng J. Liu, former medical superintendent of the PUMC, as the Deputy Minister of Health in Nanjing in 1929 and then Minister in 1930 to oversee the development of a public health system with four administrative divisions covering medical administration, public health, epidemic prevention and general administration, and four functional institutions - the Central Epidemic Prevention Bureau, the Central Hospital, the Shanghai Port Quarantine Service and the Central Hygienic Laboratory (the Laboratory). The Bureau was the only original institution in place from 1919. It was an extension of the North Manchurian Plague Prevention Service founded by Dr. Wu Lien Teh in 1909. The Service continued to play a significant role in producing sera, vaccines, and calf lymph for supply to provincial health departments, and in anti-epidemic campaigns and sudden outbreaks of tuberculosis, as in the case of the flooded areas of the Yangtze River in 1931.

Dr. Heng J. Liu doubled up as the director of the Central Hospital when the latter was completed in the capital, Nanjing, in 1929. The Laboratory was a new division of the MoH established in Shanghai on 1 March 1929. Its functions were to conduct chemical and pharmaceutical analysis, bacteriological and pathological examinations, and laboratory-based research. The MoH reorganized as the National Health Administration in 1932. The Central Hospital became separately administered as the Central Health Facilities and Laboratories (the Laboratories) under the National Economic Commission. Dr. Heng J. Liu continued as the head of the NHA, and the Laboratories, which expanded, with eight departments and specialty laboratories.[20]

In 1941, the role of the Laboratories changed to that of the US model of the National Institutes of Health. The Pharmaceutical Chemistry Department (PCD) was reorganized into three laboratories in the same year, each responsible for nutrition, pharmacology, and pharmaceutical analysis. The latter would qualitatively analyze medicines purchased by the central government's Pharmaceutical Management Committee (PMC) for wartime supply and distribution of drugs. After WWII, the PCD was again restructured as the Food and Drug Administration (FDA) and officially opened in Shanghai in 1947. Ma Jiahua (馬基華, George Ma), the pharmacy director of the Central Hospital since 1936, doubled up as the first director of China's FDA director. Ma was a qualified pharmacist and received a PhD from Columbia University, New York. The interaction of the state and the private sectors in the young Republic in the 1920s and 1930s was not what we usually practice today, For instance, Dr. Heng J. Liu, head of the NHA was concurrently the director of the privately owned PUMC with the blessing of the Nationalist government. Frequent movements from one institution to the next or from the private to the public sector and vice versa were regular for other ministers.

Dr. Bernard Read, dubbed the "Father of Pharmacology" in modern China, was a British pharmaceutical missionary who joined the UMC as a lecturer in chemistry and pharmacy in 1909. After the Rockefeller Foundation's CMB acquired the UMC in 1915, Read's position became an associate professor in physiology at the newly renamed PUMC Read received a scholarship from the CMB to study biochemistry and pharmacology at Yale University in the United States in 1916, successfully obtaining an MS degree in 1918. He returned to the PUMC, continued his teaching position, and undertook pharmacological research on bencao. In 1922, Read received a second scholarship from the CMB and returned to Yale University to pursue his PhD research on the drug metabolism of chaulmoogra oil, the only herbal drug effective in treating leprosy. It was in both CMB and Read's interest to develop the Pharmacology Department to become a centre of excellence in the research of Chinese materia medica.

After Read received his PhD in 1924, he returned to the PUMC the following year and assumed the position of professor and chairman of the Department of Pharmacology in January 1925.[21] Five years later, Dr. Heng J. Liu, and Editor-in-Chief of the Chinese Pharmacopoeia Commission, invited Read as one of the four external advisors to the editorial board of the first edition of the Pharmacopoeia in 1930. (See the section on *The 1930 Chinese Pharmacopoeia* in Chap. 8). He was a founding member of the Chinese Physiology Association in 1926.

Read left the PUMC on 1 April 1932 when he felt that the Christian character was being lost in the programmes of the institution, as its affiliated PUMC Hospital became a private hospital with only a small sector serving the underprivileged.[22] He joined as head of the Division of Physiological Sciences, the newly founded Henry Lester Institute for Medical Research, Shanghai (上海雷氏德医学研究院, the Institute), a unit of the Lester Chinese Hospital (now Renji Hospital).[23] In conjunction with other Chinese collaborators, he translated volumes 12–50 of the Compendium of Materia Medica published by Li Shizhen in 1596 into English between 1931 and 1941. The Institute's activities in 1940 were reflected in an article published in the 4 October 1941 edition of the British Medical Journal:

> The annual report for 1940 of the Henry Lester Institute of Medical Research, Shanghai, describes continued widespread activities, despite restrictions imposed by the war. Fifty-eight original papers were published during the year under review. Many cases of nutritional deficiency were investigated, chiefly beriberi and pellagra. During the latter part of the year a study was made of more than a hundred cases of ariboflavinosis. Various types of eye lesions were found; also mouth lesions and seborrhoeic dermatitis. The eye lesions responded most rapidly to riboflavin treatment, signs and symptoms beginning to recede within 48 h.

> Experiments were carried out on some four hundred children in a refugee camp to test the efficacy of soya bean powder mixture. This substance contains soya bean powder, sugar, starch, sodium chloride, and calcium carbonate. After a period of four months, it was found that children fed on this mixture showed greater growth and suffered less sickness than control children fed on an ordinary diet.[24]

Read declined an opportunity to take up a teaching post in the US before the Japanese occupation of the International Settlements of Shanghai in December 1941. The Japanese later interned him at the Longhua (龙华, Lunghua) Internment Camp in Shanghai until the end of the War in August 1945. Read remained in Shanghai after the War and became the director of the Henry Lester Institute when the then director and his friend, Dr. Herbert Gastineau Earle, passed away in 1946. He translated and published a book entitled "Famine Food" (救荒本草) in 1946. This important work details edible plants' nutritional value during ancient China's famine. Read had been closely associated with the PUMC for 31 years, with 22 years in academia in Beijing. All along, Read retained a relationship with the PUMC as a member of its board of directors between 1936 and 1944. Read lived and worked in China for forty years and became an expert in bencao. He was actively involved in the research and teaching of experimental pharmacology. He died in Shanghai on 13th June 1949 after a long illness.

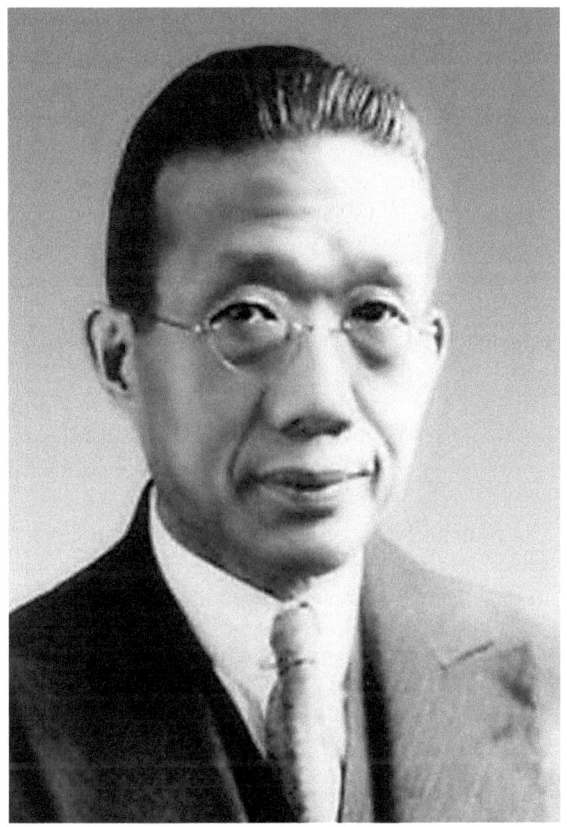

Fig. 7.15 Zhao Chenggu, founding director of National Institute of Materia Medica, @ 1925. *Credit* Peking Union Medical College Archive

Zhao Chenggu was another China's most prominent pharmaceutical scientist in the twentieth century (Fig. 7.15). He pioneered the research and development of modern drugs in China from the mid-1920s and was dubbed the "Father of Pharmaceutical Chemistry" in Modern China. Zhao received a scholarship from the Jiangsu provincial government at twenty-one to study in the U.K. in 1905. He first attended a matriculation course in science subjects, then graduated with a B.Sc. degree in chemistry from the University of Manchester in the U.K. in 1910. He then completed an M.Sc. degree at the Swiss Federal Institute of Technology in Zürich in 1911 and a Doctor of Science degree at the University of Geneva, Switzerland, in 1914. After working as a research scientist and lecturer at the University for another two years, Zhao joined Poulenc Frères as a researcher in France in 1916. He discovered a new process in the synthesis of procaine a couple of years later, and the company promoted him to a unit head of the research department until his return to China in 1922.

After a short stint as the chemical technology professor at the Nanjing Senior Teachers College and the chemistry professor at Southeast University from 1923 to 1924, Zhao joined the PUMC as an associate in the Department of Pharmacology, conducting pharmaceutical chemistry research in Chinese medicine, on 1 September 1925. His job was to follow up on the work in ephedrine after it was rediscovered by K.K. Chen in 1925. Zhao worked under Bernard Read, the Department head, to isolate active compounds such as ephedrine and pseudoephedrine. [25] His work on ephedrine contributed substantially to K.K. Chen's commercialization of ephedrine at Eli Lilly. Zhao became an authority in the chemical analysis, identification and synthesis of ephedrine and one of its salts, pseudoephedrine, has been used as a vasoconstrictor for cold remedies for a century.[26] He received the China Foundation Scientific Research Prize twice, in 1927 and 1930, for remarkable achievements in his studies and isolation of active principles from Chinese herbal remedies. PUMC promoted Zhao to assistant professor of pharmacology in 1930, and he continued his work there until 30 June 1932. Zhao left the PUMC six months after Read moved to Shanghai in April 1932. He then joined as the founding director of the newly established the National Institute of Materia Medica. The latter was one of seven institutes formed under the National Academy of Peiping (NAC) on 1 September 1932 (Chart 7.1).

In March 1933, the Japanese crossed the Great Wall in Beijing in a surprise attack.[27] Zhao promptly relocated the Institute to Shanghai, into the School of Pharmacy of the Sino-French University building, as most of China's ethical pharmaceutical houses were in Shanghai. In the spring of 1936, the Institute moved into a four-story building at 395 Route Wukang (Ferguson) Raod in the French Concession, sharing the building with the Institute of Radium. By then, Zhao had three assistants and three trainees, with each pair serving the medicinal chemistry, pharmacology, and pilot production sections. The latter produced batches of ephedrine, haemostatic agents, chaulmoogra oil and Vitamin B complex. While in Shanghai, Zhao consulted the Institute's panel of local and overseas advisors, including clinical and basic pharmacology researchers, namely K.K. Chen, the research director of Eli Lilly in the U.S., and Wang Jingxi, Chu Hengbie, and C.S. Jang. The latter had a joint Changshan project with Zhao during the War years in 1942.

Zhao published singly or jointly with Chinese and western collaborators over 40 original research papers in leading experimental research journals including *Nature*, *Scientists* in the 1930s and 1940s. Read wrote as a peer reviewer on Zhao's research activities in a 1938 edition of the Chinese Medical Journal:[28] By far the best chemical work is that published by Zhao. The more important work of Zhao has dealt with the isolation of the active principles detected in Chinese materia medica based on established pharmacognosy protocols (Table 7.3). He stayed behind in Shanghai during the War and had close academic friends from his earlier days when studying in Europe. By then, they had become officials in charge of public health and higher education in the puppet Wang Jinnwei regime. He did not yield to their persuasion or pressure to join the puppet government in Nanjing nor had any official position in Shanghai. Zhao was therefore not charged with war crimes when the Nationalist government returned to power in September 1945. Zhao continued his work in the newly founded People's Republic of China in 1949 until his retirement in the mid-1960s. He passed away in 1966 in Shanghai.

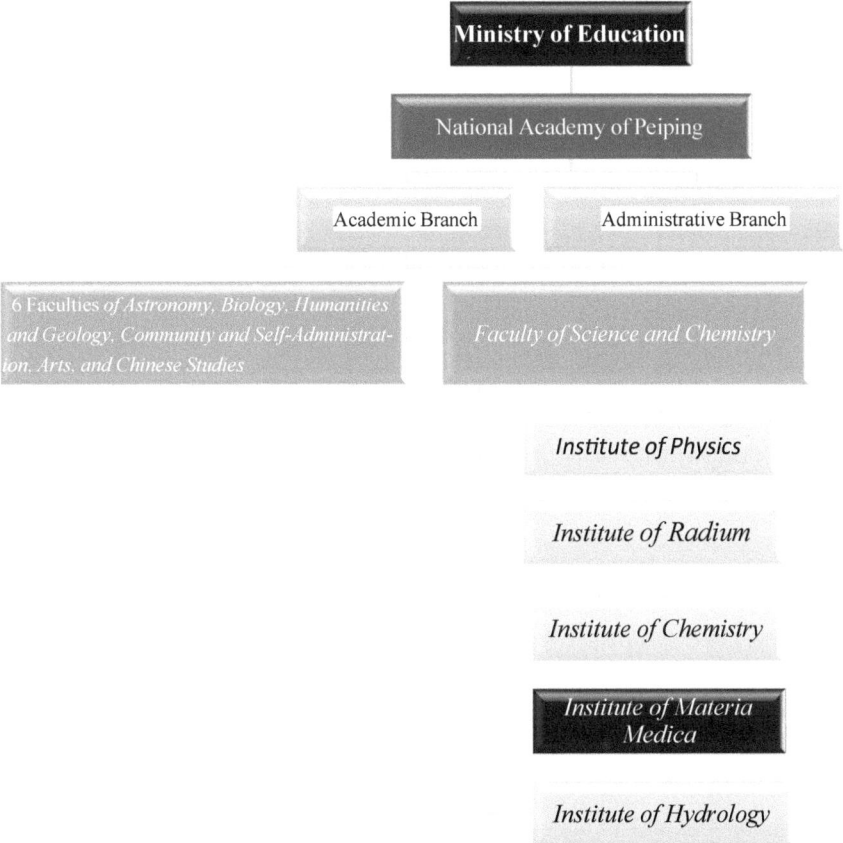

Chart 7.1 Organization structure of the National Academy of Peiping, 1936. *Credit* Shanghai Institute of Materia Medica, Chinese Academy of Sciences

Zhao Juhuang (赵橘黄, Chao Jue-huang, 1883–1960) was a distinguished pharmacognosist in modern China. He first graduated with a diploma from the Tokyo School of Pharmacy in 1907. He was a founding member and honorary secretary of the Chinese Pharmaceutical Association, formed by Chinese students studying pharmacy in Tokyo in the same year. Zhao then completed his studies and graduated with a higher diploma in Pharmaceutical Sciences from the Imperial University of Tokyo in 1909.[29] He joined the Tongmenghui (同盟会, Chinese United Alliance), a revolutionary organization led by Dr. Sun Yat-sen (孙逸仙又名孙逸仙, 1866–1925), to topple the Manchu Qing dynasty in 1910. After Dr. Sun Yat-sen declared the foundation of the Republic of China on 1 January 1912, Zhao joined the Department of Health of the Beiyang government from 1912 to 1918. Zhao then changed his career track and became a pharmacognosy professor and researcher at the Zhejiang College of Medicine and Pharmacy from 1919 to 1929. In the next 5 years, Zhao joined as a full-time researcher at the Institute of Chemistry of Academia Sinica in Nanjing

Table 7.3 Important Chinese Materia Medica Research Studies of Zhao Chenggu, 1927–1936

Year	Botanical name of Chinese materia medica	Active principles
1927	Illicium religiosum, Sieb	Sikimitoxin
	Rhodedenum	Two toxic principles
1928	Corydalis ambigua (1929, 1929, 1933, 1934),	13 Alkaolids,
1931	G.elegans	4 alkaloids, koumine, kouminicine, kuominine and, kouminidine
1932	Fritillaria roylei	Premine and peiminine
1933		Fritimine
1934	Ephedra sinica	Ephedrine and the volatile oil
	Chrysanthemum Erariacefolium	Chrysanthine and chrysanthene
1935	Datura stramonium	Neural principles
	Mu Fang Chi	Two alkaloids
1936	Triptergium wilfordis	Pigments and sugars

Credit 1938 Edition of Chinese Medical Journal

from 1930 to 1934. In 1935, Zhao moved back to Beijing and became a researcher at the Institute of Physiology of Academia Peiping until 1937.

When the Institute relocated to Kunming in 1938, Zhao decided to stay in Beijing and joined Asiatic Chemical Works as the director of their Beijing Workshop, responsible for producing ephedrine from 1940 to 1946. Zhao's research work in pharmacognosy gained recognition from his peers Dr. Bernard Read and Koichi Kimura, an expert in medicinal plants of Japan. After the War, Zhao resumed his teaching position as a professor in pharmacognosy at the Beijing Medical College from 1946 until 1960, when he passed away. Li Nan and Wan Fang summarized the rediscoveries of Chinese materia medica during the 1920s and 1930s:

> During the Republican era, western science and technology positively impacted the scientific research on Chinese medicine in China. Several sub-specialties of pharmacognosy, pharmacology, and pharmaceutical chemistry were gradually developed which were closely related to those scholars and pharmaceutical scientists who had returned from studying abroad. Zhao Juhuang (1883–1960), who studied in Japan, was a pioneer of Chinese pharmacognosy. In particular, he and Xu Bojun (Hsu Bo-jun), a professor of pharmacy at Zhejiang Medical College, compiled the "Modern Pharmacognosy, Volume One", which became the masterpiece in China's pharmacognosy studies.

> Some western trained academics and scientists pursued a "total westernization" approach in their research of Chinese materia medica. They categorized certain indigenous herbs of China under the taxonomy of similar botanical herbs ex China, leading to inaccurate conclusions and a negative impact on Chinese medicine.[30]

The War allowed the small pool of Chinese intellectuals, who had achieved recognition in their respective spheres in academia, industry, and research to optimize their outputs with limited resources and solidarity. Together, the research institutes they worked towards common objectives, as in the case of changshan (Table 7.4). They also jointly laid a foundation to shape China's modernization of its pharmaceutical industry. Other than the Nationalist army which had the PMI as its pharmaceutical production base, the Red Army's China Pharmaceutical Factory in Yanan also produced Morphine Hydrochloride Injection for pain relief of the Chinese Communist Party military forces in 1941. While the War was a tragic event, it nonetheless transformed the traditional Chinese pharmaceutical practice of compounding and mixing into modern pharmaceutical dosage forms by adopting modern pharmaceutical technologies and formulation techniques. The Chinese medicine dosage forms of *gao* (pastes), *dan* (pellets), *wan* (pills) and *san* (powders) became creams and ointments, granules, tablets and sterile injections within a few years by the establishment of the state-own CMF, PMI, and UPC in Chongqing.[31]

Table 7.4 State and private pharmaceutical research organizations, 1917–1938

Year	Ministry/ organization	Institute	Location	Scope and research direction
State-owned research institutes				
1929–1937	Education	Institute of Materia Medica, National Academy of Peiping (IMM)	Beijing	Research of active drugs of Chinese medicine Founded in Beijing in 1932, with Zhao Chenggu as the founding director and the IMM was relocated to Shanghai in 1933 1950, IMM changed its name to Shanghai Institute of Materia Medica and became part of the Chinese Academy of Sciences
1930	Industry	The Pharmaceutica Institute, (TPI) Central Industrial Laboratories	Shanghai	Research of pharmaceutical raw materials, improvement of production techniques, and isolation and identification of pharmaceutical substances Founded in Shanghai in 1930, and Dr Peter Yang was the founding director of the Biochemical laboratory of TPI in 1933 Relocated to Chongqing in 1937 and Yang stayed behind in Shanghai. (See below) 1957 was re-established as the Shanghai Institute of Pharmaceutical Industry

(continued)

Table 7.4 (continued)

Year	Ministry/ organization	Institute	Location	Scope and research direction
1932	National Economic Commission	Central Health Facilities and Laboratories	Nanjing	Founded in 1932 and was headed by Dr. Heng J. Liu In 1933, its name was changed to Central Health Laboratories and relocated to Chongqing in 1937 Returned back to the capital in Nanjing in 1945 and then to Beijing in 1950
Private foundations				
1917	China Medical Board (CMB), Rockefeller Foundation	Peking Union Medical College (PUMC)	Beijing	Founded as Union Medical College (UMC) with a seeding fund by Emperor Cici in 1904 and managed by the London Missionary Society until 1916 In 1917, the China Medical Board acquired the UMC and changed its name to PUMC with its new hospital wing completed in 1921 Active drug research of Chinese medicine conducted in 1924 with KK Chen rediscovered ephedrine with clinical efficacy in asthma from ephedra Zhao Chenggu became a faculty member of the Pharmacology Department and worked closely with the head and professor, Dr Bernard Read, in 1925

(continued)

Table 7.4 (continued)

Year	Ministry/ organization	Institute	Location	Scope and research direction
1932	Henry Lester Foundation	Henry Lester Institute of Medical Research	Shanghai	Founded in 1932 with Dr Bernard Read, previously head and professor of the PUMC, as the first director of its physiology department. The other two departments were pathology and clinical with the latter based in the Renji Hospita (previously called the Chinese Hospital), founded by Dr. William Lockhart of the London Missionary Hospital in 1844 Main functions were the study of Chinese medicine and also pharmacology
Commercial research laboratories				
1938	Peter Yang	Yang's Chemotherapeutic Institute (YCI)	Shanghai	Founded by Yang in 1938 when the TPI relocated to Chongqing, and he decided to stay in Shanghai and opened the YCI

Source Library of Institute of Modern History, Academia Sinica, Taipei

Notes and References

1. [Shanghai's Modern Pharmaceutical Industry], 1987, 177.
2. [Shanghai's Modern Pharmaceutical Industry], 1987, 233.
3. Neoarsenphamine is the generic name of Neo-Salvarsan, the "magic bullet" which was an improved version of Salvarsan or "606", discovered by Paul Ehrlich, the Nobel Laureate, in 1912. Hoechst of Germany (now Sanofi) marketed both Salvarsan and its successor, Neo-Salvarsan in the 1910s. Penicillin, the first broad spectrum semi-synthetic antibiotic with a wide safety margin, was launched in the last year of the WWII to save limb amputations and life-threatening infections for soldiers with gunshot wounds in Europe.
4. The German states were united by Prussia into the German Empire and its citizens have been called Germans since 1871.
5. During World War I (1914–1918), the Allies, formed an international military coalition of countries including France, the United Kingdom, Russia, the United States, Italy, and Japan, against the Central Powers consisting of Germany, Austria-Hungary, the Ottoman Empire, and Bulgaria.
6. [Shanghai's Modern Pharmaceutical Industry], 196–197.
7. [Shanghai's Modern Pharmaceutical Industry], 127.
8. [Shanghai's Modern Pharmaceutical Industry], 274–275.
9. Burkill Road (now Fengyang Road 凤阳路) in Shanghai was named after Albert Robson Burkill (1839–1913) who was the Chairman of the Shanghai Municipal Council in from 1897 to 1898.

10. The Japanese Imperial Army invaded Shenyang (Mukden), Northeast China on 18 September 1931 by claiming the Japanese controlled South Manchurian Railway 南满铁路 line was under attack by the Nationalist army. The incident is called the "18 September Incident 九一八事变 or Shenyang (Mukden) Incident".

11. Lo, York, *New Asiatic Chemical Works: Pharmaceutical Star*, The Industrial History of Hong Kong Group, 9 December 2019 (Traditional Chinese). Accessed 29 September 2023. https://industrialhistoryhk.org/new-asiatic-chemical-works.

12. [Shanghai's Modern Pharmaceutical Industry] 1987: 287–288.

13. Pi Kuoli, 皮国立, *Gailiang yu daiyong: Kangzhan shí zhongyao juese de zai sikao* 改良与代用: 抗战时中药角色的在思考 [Improvement and Substitution: Rethinking the Role of Chinese Medicine during the Anti-Japanese War." *Workshop on Mutual Learning between China and the West: The Introduction of Western Pharmacy and the Evolution of Chinese Pharmacy* Symposium, Department of History, Shanghai University, 11 February 2023.

14. Chang Maolin, 張茂林 Wang Hepeiyyao 王何佩瑶,"Xihe Zhiyaochang" 协和制药厂 [Union Drug Co. Ltd.], *Liuruìheng boshì yu zhongguo yiyao ji weisheng shìye* 刘瑞恒博士与中国医药及卫生事业 [*Heng J Liu and Medical and Health Development in China*], Liu Sijin 刘似锦 (Ed.), (Taipei:.The Commercial Press,1989), 72.

15. Cheung Lian 张丽安 *Zhang Jian yu junyixuexiao—Jianshu kangzang shiqi junyi jiaoyu* 张建军医学校—兼述抗战时期军医教育 [*Zhang Jian and the National Army Medical* College] (Hong Kong: Cosmos Books 2000), 231–295, esp. 231–251, 286–287.

16. Cheung, [*Zhang Jian*], 248.

17. Cheung, [*Zhang Jian*], 242.

18. Pi Kuoli, [Improvement and Substitution] 2023.

19. Sakata, Takashi, "Japanese Diplomatic Policy and Differences in the Handling of Quinine Supply by the Japanese Government during World War II", *Bulletin of Ishinomaki Senshu University,* no. 31 (2021):125–147. Accessed 29 September 2023. https://www.researchgate.net/publication/349915323_Japanese_Diplomatic_Policy_and_Differences_in_the_Handling_of_Quinine_Supply_by_the_Japanese_Government_during_World_War_II/link/6065357692851c91b194623f/download.

20. The eight departments and specialty laboratories of the Central Health Facilities and Laboratories were: Pharmaceutical Chemistry Department (PCD), with three specialty laboratories of Chemical, Pharmaceutical Research, and Pharmaceutical Manufacturing; Bacteriology; Parasitology; Sanitary Engineering (for Fresh Water Supply); Maternal and Infant Health; Health Education; Medical Social Service, and Health Statistics.

21. Shanghai was chosen as the location to set up the newly founded Food and Drug Administration in 1947 instead of the Nationalist capital Nanjing. This was primarily due to the close proximity to the large number of pharmaceutical factories located there.

22. Bowers, *Western Medicine,* 168.

23. Bowers, *Western Medicine,* 168.

24. *Henry Lester Institute Shanghai, British Medical Journal,* October 4, 1941:476. Accessed May 5, 2023. https://www.ncbi.nlm.nih.gov/pmc/articles/PMC2163011/.

25. Chou, T.Q., and B.E. Read." Isolation and Comparative Action of Ephedrine, and Pesudoephedrine from Ma Huang (Ephedra vulgaris, var. helvetica)". *Proceedings of the Society for Experimental Biology and Medicine,* Society for Experimental Biology and Medicine, New York, April 1926, V. 23:618–620.

26. Chou, T.Q. "Preparation and Properties of Ephedrine and Its Salts". *Journal of Biological Chemistry,* American Society for Biochemistry and Molecular Biology. September 1926, V70:109–113.

27. The military intrusion by the Japanese Imperial Army across the Great Wall in Beijing eventually led to the Japanese incited incident at the Maro Polo Bridge and the beginning of the Second Sino-Japanese War on 7 July 1937.

28. Read, Benard E.," Chinese: A Review of Some of the Work of the Last Decade", *Chinese Medical Journal* 53, No. 4 (1938): 353–362.

29. Biography of Zhao Yuhuang 赵黄, "Zhongguo yaoxue hui bainian shi 1907–2007", 中国药
学会百年史, 1907–2007 [Centenary History of Chinese Pharmaceutical Association, 1907–
2007] (Beijing: Chinese Population Publishing Company, 2008), 264.
30. Li Nan, 李楠, Wan Fang 万芳, "Jindai xifang kejì yinjin dui minguo shiqi zhongyao xueshu
zhi yingxiang". 近代西方科技引进对民国时期中药学术之影响 [The Influence of Modern
Western Science and Technology on the Academic Studies in the Nationalist Era of China],
Proceedings of the 18th Conference of National History of Pharmacy and, Professional
Committee of the History of Pharmacy, Chinese Pharmaceutical Association, Hefe, Anhui
Province, 13th–15th November 2015:239–240.
31. Pi Kuo-li 皮国立, "Guoyao huo 'doiyong xiyao? Zhan shí guochan yaowu de zhizao
yu yanjiu" 「国药」或「代用西药」?战时国产药物的制造与研究 ["Chinese Drugs" or
"Western Medicine Substitutes": Manufacture and Research of Domestically Manufactured
Drugs in Wartime], Journal of Chinese Medicine 30, no. 2 (2019): 27–47, esp. 32. Accessed
29 September 2023. http://ejournal.nricm.edu.tw/jcm/30/30-2-2.pdf.

Chapter 8
Modernity, Pharmacy Law, and The Chinese Pharmacopoeia

This chapter delves into the "Modernity Drive" championed by Dr. Sun Yat-sen and embraced by the educated elite, including academics and professionals with western education. The movement garnered significant support from university students, college students, and the burgeoning middle class. Systemic institutional reforms and the initiation of the "Abolish Chinese Medicine" campaign by young doctors trained in the West occurred concurrently in early 1929 which the MoH officials faced challenges from various stakeholders, including proponents of Chinese and western medicine, retailers and wholesalers of materia medica, and modern drug, and politicians from different ideological spectrums. The publication of the Chinese Pharmacopoeia in 1930 played a crucial role in consolidating the position of western medicine and pharmacy as a cornerstone of the modern healthcare system.

The seeds of modern medicine and pharmacy were sowed at the beginning of the nineteenth century when Dr. Pearson of the EIC began mass vaccination of smallpox to the residents of Canton and Macau in 1805. So, what made China suddenly realize the urgent need for industrialization and the adoption of new technologies and sciences in the 1920s? The defeat of the Manchu Qing empire in the Second Opium War (1856–1860) awakened the senior court officials, including senior officials Zeng Guofan (曾国藩, 1811–1872), Zuo Zongtang (左中堂, 1812–1885), Li Hongzhang (李鸿章, 1823–1901), Zhang Zidong (张之洞, 1837–1909) and others to consider the imminent change. With blessing from the "Old Buddha"—Empress Dowager Cixi who initially ruled jointly with Empress Cian (慈安太后) from 1861 to 1881 and then independently until she died in 1908, and Prince Yixin (奕钦亲王, 1833–1898), these senior court officials pursued the "Self-Strengthening Movement" strategy in 1861 as inspired by Wei Yuan (魏源, 1794–1857) a close counterpart of Lin Zexu (林则徐).[1] The objective was to upgrade its defense capability to be at par with the western imperial powers.

But unfortunately, the Movement was a total failure after a 35-year experiment as it only addressed the "hardware" issue and was short of a change of mindset. What Dr. Sun Yat-sen described in his "Three Principles of the People" (三民主义,

P. Chiu, *A History of Western Pharmacy in China*,
https://doi.org/10.1007/978-981-99-8635-4_8

San Min Zhu Yi) as the basics of nationalism (民族, *minzu*), rights of the people (民权, *minquan*), and people's livelihood (民生, *minsheng*) were totally lacking. The defeat of the Manchu Qing military in the First Sino-Japanese War of 1894–1895 was a shock. A neighbour in the East China Sea, who had adopted the Chinese language and cultural practices since the seventh century Tang dynasty, won the war against its former "cultural" master. A fresh debate on what Japan did right in its Meiji Restoration (明治维新, 1868–1889) resulted in a consensus that the complete overhaul of its political and educational systems had yielded remarkable results within two decades. Kang Youwei (康有为, 1858–1927), an imperial court official from Canton, was empowered by Emperor Guangxu to initiate the Reform Strategy (戊戌变法) in 1898. Kang recalled his first visit to Hong Kong in 1887:

> The magnificence of the mansions of the Westerners, the cleanliness of the streets, and the patrols by police officers, all within the laws and regulations promulgated to administer the city in an orderly and proper manner, were not the ancient barbarians we learnt from history.[2]

Still, once again, the Reform Movement (改革运动) lasted only 100 days. The turning point occurred when the Boxers Movement ended in disaster. However, they eventually introduced a mandatory education system in 1905, followed by the national census from 1908 to 1911. The Manchu Qing military commanders took the lead in opening the Beiyang Military Academy of Medicine in Tianjin in 1902. Thomas Cochrane of the UMC seized the opportunity to open a showcase western medical school and hospital in 1906 in Beijing. As a result, Bernard Read became the first full-time pharmacist and lecturer at the UMC Hospital in 1909. By now, Dr. Sun Yat-sen and his followers could no longer wait for a regime change. The Republican Revolution started a fresh chapter on 10 October 1911 in China's journey to modernity. Sun advocated his middle-of-the-road Three Principles of the People as the national strategy to unify the country.

Modernization with "New Culture" and "New Life" Movements

After years of debate on the Self-Strengthening Movement strategy, China's first attempt at modernization began in 1865 with the formation of the Jiangnan Machinery Bureau (江南机器制造总局, "JMB") to produce military ordnance, which soon branched into shipbuilding. Then, the China Merchants Corp. (招商局, "CMC"), the first shipping company, was incorporated in Shanghai in 1872. From 1872 to 1875, the Manchu Qing court sent four groups of 30 students per group, a total of 120 young and talented school children, most of them from Canton and Shanghai, to receive western education in the US. Six years after the last batch of young students went to the US, the original 15-year western education programme to train future engineers and scientists in the US was cut-short in 1871 as many young students opted for a liberal and democratic life. Some even gave up their Manchu hairstyle of shaved head and braid to short back and sides and their dress from long robes to a bowtie, shirt, and jacket. However, the change was too much for the Manchu Qing court officials to accept. In their eyes, the experimental western education programme was a total failure.

The loss of the First Sino-Japanese War in 1895 was a severe blow to the fragile Manchu Qing empire. It revealed the JMB and CMC's state sponsored projects were not cost-efficient as both corporations were managed like the civil service and were not result oriented. Moreover, the Manchu Qing court officials had still not realized the ancient feudal system with an elitist scholar official top-down approach was stifling innovation and productivity. In hindsight, the First War with Japan should never have begun with blind faith. One of the early symbolic changes to modernity driven by Dr. Sun Yat-sen after the Republican Revolution was to change Chinese men's appearance and attire. The newly founded Nationalist government promoted a new national identity by means of hair style and attire (See the section on *New Chinese Identity to Serve the Masses or a Privileged Few,* Chap. 9).

Despite the Old Buddha's decree in endorsing the termination of foot binding in February 1902, a cruel but widespread antiquated customary practice for girls from upper class families since the eleventh century, old habits die hard. Dr. Sun Yat-sen, the provisional president of the Republic, reaffirmed the abolishment of foot binding in March 1912 which eventually eradicate this millennial practice within a couple of decades through public education. In the mid-to-late nineteenth century, Europe, the UK and the US had begun secondary education for children to become responsible members of civil society. Moreover, public and private universities and colleges were founded to groom the next generation of civic leaders. Japan's visionary politicians adopted as early as 1872 and constitutional monarchy in 1885.[3] By 1900, Japan's literacy rate was only half of Britain's and the Netherlands' 95%, but it was two-and-a-half times higher than China's (Chart 8.1).

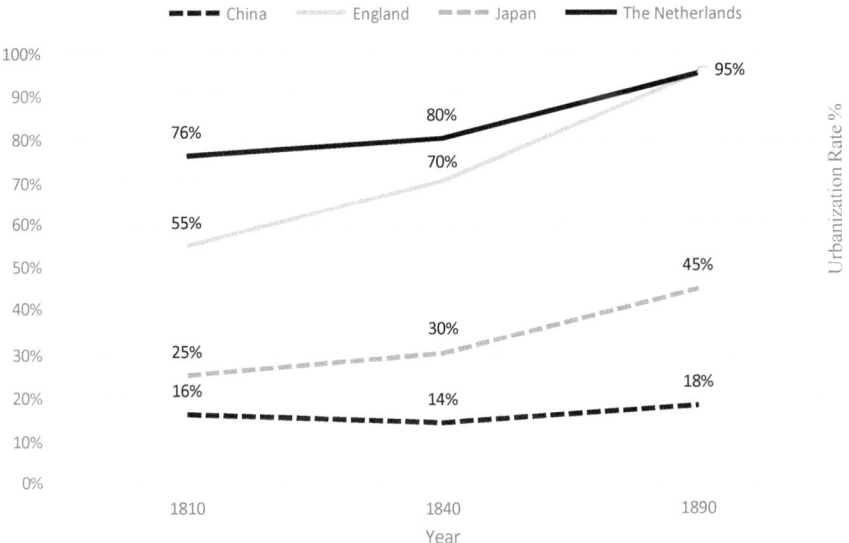

Chart 8.1 Literacy rates of China, England, Japan, and the Netherlands. *Credit* Robert Allen, "Progress and poverty in early modern Europe", *The Economic History Review*, LVI, 3 (2003)

In China, the transition from a feudal, agrarian society to a modern, industrialized state with the introduction of public education came in 1906, starting thirty-four years later than Japan. This was due to the Manchu Qing emperor and his Confucian court officials holding conservative views on the Keju which had sustained ancient China's senior civil service system for over a millennium. The Manchu Qing government's education of health professions, including pharmacists, industrial chemists and engineers, began in 1907, half a century later than the U.K. or the U.S. and a quarter of a century later than Japan. Systematic higher education started with local scholarships at the provincial level at the turn of the twentieth century (See the section on *Education Reform and Bench Strength of Local Talents* in Chap. 9).

The Boxers Indemnity scholarships awarded to Chinese youths to study aboard in France, Japan, the UK, and the US came later. These scholarships provided the talent for China's modernization when the students pursued graduate studies and postgraduate research programmes in medicine, pharmacy, science and engineering in leading European and US universities in the 1910s to 1940s. The late Manchu Qing dynasty and successive governments did commit investments to infrastructure and transportation networks, but with limited results. This was due to a weak treasury, frequently plagued by wars and revolutions, flooding, and epidemics, unable to finance China's sizeable geographical region and a population of thirty-five times that of Japan at the turn of the twentieth century.[4] Also, only 10% of China's 450 million people lived in urban areas in the first half of the twentieth century (Chart 8.2).[5] Five years after Dr. Sun Yat-sen declared the foundation of the Republic of China in 1912, animosity between the Northern and Southern leaders of the Republican Revolution intensified to an extent beyond reconciliation. In July 1917, two separate presidencies and military governments co-existed, one in Beijing and the other in Canton, with respective provincial governors loyal to each other's faction until Chiang Kai-shek's successful Northern Expedition in 1928. During this chaotic period, laws and regulations were separately promulgated by the two independent governments, each claiming their right to represent China.

The much-needed nationwide institutional reforms declared in the revolution in 1911 all evaporated. The modernity drive, also known as the New Culture Movement (新文化运动, *Xin Wenhua Yundong*, 1915–1923), was led by young intellectuals who had recently graduated in Japan and the US. Chen Duxiu(陈独秀), Hu Shi (胡适) and Lu Xun (鲁迅), the three founders and their followers of the New Culture Movement, embraced anarchism, liberalism, nationalism, and pragmatism. On the other hand, they abhorred traditional Confucian values and Buddhist and Daoist beliefs. Moreover, they attacked Chinese medicine as a pseudo-science. The New Culture Movement reached its climax on 4 May 1919 when students took to the streets with mass demonstrations to denounce traditional Confucian ideas and advocated western ideas, particularly science and democracy. After the 4 May demonstrations, Chen and Hu pursued a different route. Chen advocated communism and was one of the two founders of the Chinese Communist Party in 1921. Hu advocated liberalism and "Complete Westernization", yet he was an atheist and, at the same time, a staunch anti-communist. Chang Yu-fa, emeritus director of the Institute of Modern History

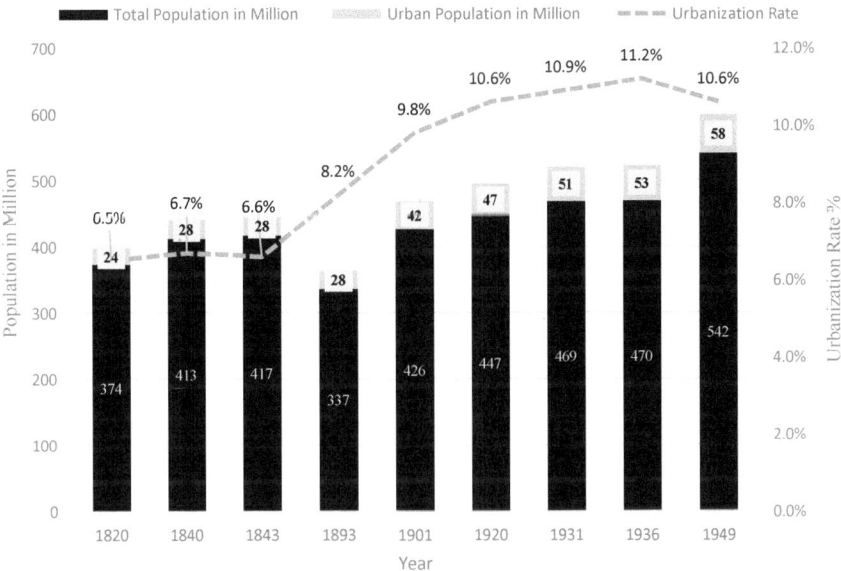

Chart 8.2 China's population, 1820–1949. *Credit* History of China's population, China Annual Report 1985

of Academic Sinica, articulated Dr. Sun Yat-sen's Three Principles of the People in addressing traditional values and western political thought:

> The trend of political thought in the 1920s was with that socialism on the left, liberalism on the right, and the Three Principles of the People were in between. The thought of the Three Principles of the People was created by Dr. Sun Yat-sen from the fusion of traditional Chinese (Confucian) thought and modern western thought.[6]

Chiang Kai-shek succeeded Dr. Sun Yat-sen when he passed away in 1925. Representing the Southern faction, he initiated the Northern Expedition (1926–1928) and successfully united with the dissenting warlord governors at the end of 1928. By then, the "Complete Westernization" camp within the Nationalist Party bureaucracy was gaining inroad in policy making. Public health, to transform the delivery of medicines to the masses, was a significant concern. The Song emperors were fully aware of what their subjects needed almost a millennium before. The main character in the speedy transformation of Chinese medicine was the Harvard educated Dr. Heng J. Liu, a graduate of medicine who became the medical superintendent of the PUMC Hospital at thirty-six in 1926.[7] Chiang Kai-shek appointed Dr. Heng J. Liu as the Vice Minister of the NHA in the government in the newly re-established capital of Nanjing in October 1928. Any policy change in public health would have a tremendous impact on all stakeholders down the supply chain. The stakeholders included patients as end users, Chinese medicine practitioners as prescribers or service providers, traditional pharmacists as drug storekeepers, wholesalers, and farmers of medicinal herbs. In short, this would be a "cultural revolution" without anyone being the winner if handled in a rushed and immature manner.

With blessing by Dr. Heng J. Liu, Dr. Yu Yan, a western medicine practitioner who graduated from Osaka Medical University of Japan in 1916, mooted the "Abolish Chinese Medicine" (废除中医) motion at the First Public Health Conference organized by the NHA in Shanghai from 23 to 26 February 1929. The participants were all western trained medical doctors who voted in support for the "Abolition Chinese Medicine" motion. But unfortunately, the NHA deliberately excluded Chinese medicine practitioners from participating at the Conference even though there were more of them than western medicine practitioners in the late 1920s.[8] The Chinese medicine practitioners soon organized a parade, supported by the public and politicians, three weeks later in Nanjing, on 17 March 1929. In response to the call of the people, the Chinese medicine practitioners, owners and employees of the Chinese medicine dispensaries, Chiang Kai-shek, the newly elected Chairman of the State Council vetoed the request by Dr. Heng J. Liu of the NHA to abolish Chinese medicine as a health discipline.[9] Another controversy in the modernization of pharmacological therapeutics—Chinese or western drugs—soon arose (see the section on *The 1930 Chinese Pharmacopoeia* in this Chapter).

Madam Angela Chen-Lin (陈林颖曾), the chairperson of Lifu Medical Research, Cultural, and Educational Foundation (the Foundation) recalled her discussion with the late Chen Lifu:

> While the intention to chart a course of modernization of China's public health system was long overdue, Dr. Heng J. Liu's "quick, sharp, shock" approach drew fire from the Chinese medicine practitioners, whose immediate reaction was to end the NHA's Conference motion. As a senior policy maker, Dr. Heng J. Liu also overlooked the fact that upgrade of a time-honoured Chinese medicine and materia medica practice could be complimentary in building a modern and sustainable health care system to serve both the urban and rural population of China.[10]

Chiang Kai-shek converted to Christianity on 23 October 1930, opening a new chapter of his life.[11] By 1934, Chiang felt the Nationalist party members was losing the spirit in implementing Dr. Sun Yat-sen's Three Principles of the People. Therefore, it was an opportune time to launch the Xin Shenghuo Yundong ("New Life Movement") to focus on Confucian values with healthy living in a "disciplined manner". Supported by his Christian wife, Madam Chiang Kai-shek (蒋宋美龄, Song Meiling), Chiang Kai-shek finally launched the New Life Movement in Nanchang, Jiangxi, on 19 February 1934.

Chen Lifu, who was in charge of the Nationalist Party's publicity machinery, issued the guidelines on Nationalist Party Members and New Life Movement (中国国民党党员与新生活运动, *Zhongguo Guomíndang Dangyuan Yu Xin Shenghuo Yundong*) in 1935. In his book, Chen articulated the transformation of the young Republic into a modern society by building a new identity with disciplines and yet retaining the good old virtues of Confucianism in the spirit of Sun's Three Principles of the People:

The foundation of the New Life Movement is "li" (礼, etiquette), "yi" (义, righteousness), "lian" (廉, integrity) and "chi" (耻, shame). As far as individuals are concerned, these virtues are the minimum conditions for a nation to be loyal to the country. For nation states, it is the strength of unity. So, it is said: "li, yi, lian, chi" as the four dimensions of the country; if the thinking is not open, the country will be destroyed. But, on the contrary, the country will be reborn when the four dimensions are fully explored.[12]

In support of Chiang Kai-shek's campaign to promote social good and well-being, Dr. Heng J. Liu of the NHA, published two books on *Xin Shenghuo Yundong Yu Gonggong Weisheng* (新生活运动与公共卫生, "New Life Movement and Public Hygiene"), and *Xin Shenghuo Yundong Yu Jiankang* (新生活运动与健康, "New Life Movement and Health") with the messages articulated to school children and workers. Posters published by the Political Education Department of the Military Commission of with Generalissimo Chiang Kai-shek's headshot displayed at the top left corner with clear messages of good hygiene and health habits were distributed to all channels of public institutions to reach the masses in 1935 (Figs. 8.1, 8.2, 8.3 and 8.4). Dr. Heng J. Liu eventually changed his mind and supported a resolution on "Equal Treatment for Chinese and Western Medicine" (中西医医师一视同仁) passed by the Nationalist Party Congress in 1935 and promulgated the law on "Chinese Medicine Ordinance" (中医条例) in 1936.[13] The long inactivity in making Chinese medicine a part of the public health system could be partly due to Dr. Heng J. Liu and his successors at the NHA, who were all western medical doctors and lacking the kind of sensitivities when dealing with Chinese medicine. They faced tremendous challenges in the promotion of biomedicine as a modern science in the prevention and treatment of diseases when Chinese medicine was viewed as part of cultural identity of the masses in China in the 1920–1930s.

On the pharmaceutical front, modernization of the formulation of Chinese materia medica was more of a direct result of the high profitability of "opium cures" which incentivized local entrepreneurs to imitate their former employers' success in the retail and manufacturing chemist sectors in the late 1880s. This happened in the absence of laws and regulations to protect intellectual property rights and standard-ization of drugs in the late nineteenth and early twentieth centuries until the Chaing Kai-shek's young Nationalist government was established in Nanjing in 1928 with a full agenda of institutional reform. (See the next section on *Pharmaceutical Legis-lation*). The timely supply of young returnee scientists after their overseas studies sustained the drive to push for new boundaries. Ephedrine and generic equivalents of neo-arsphenamine, insulin, and penicillin rolled out from the 1920s to 1940s, including the War period, provided an incubation period for the transition from a "cottage industry" to "modern pharmaceutical plants" producing modern drugs with pharmacopoeia standards.

Fig. 8.1 *Kitchen and toilet hygiene* poster. *Credit* Roy Delbyck

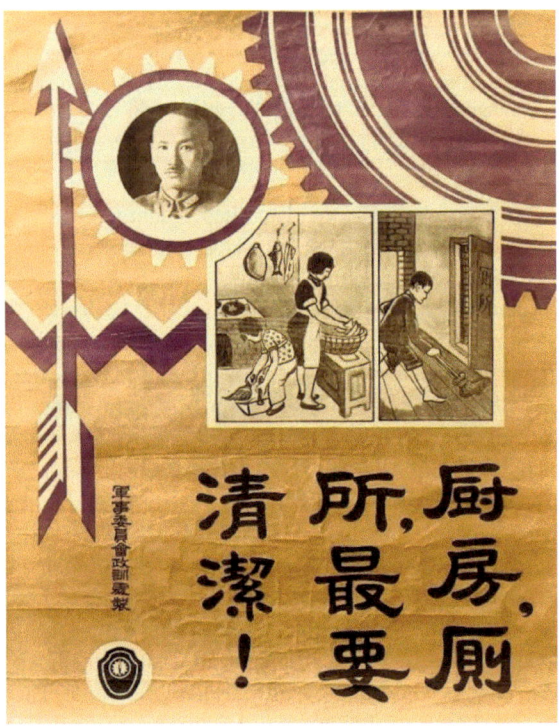

Pharmaceutical Legislation

The first piece of the national law governing the import of opium was a decree by Emperor Yongzheng (r. 1723–1755) in 1727. The import of medicinal opium was unrestricted upon payment of import duty. In contrast, import for the narcotic use of opium was punishable by exile to the borders of the Manchu Qing empire, i.e., the Tibetan or Xinjiang regions. In 1907, the Manchu Qing government took the adulteration of herbal medicine seriously and incorporated a criminal code in the new law which governs Chinese medicine apothecaries in the compounding and mixing of Chinese materia medica with substandard herbs. The National Health Administration (NHA) of the Ministry of Interior of the newly founded Nationalist government in 1912 had four departments with their expanded functions covering the sale, supply, and distribution of Chinese materia medica and western medicines, including review qualifications, registration, deregistration, monitoring and issuance of pharmacist licenses, supervision of pharmaceutical manufacturers, inspection and restriction of the sale and supply of poisons and dangerous drugs, and investigation of the drug formulary.

In the first eighteen years of the Nationalist era, politics between the regional warlord governments and the politicians who led the 1911 Republican Revolution

Fig. 8.2 *Do not spit* poster. *Credit* Roy Delbyck

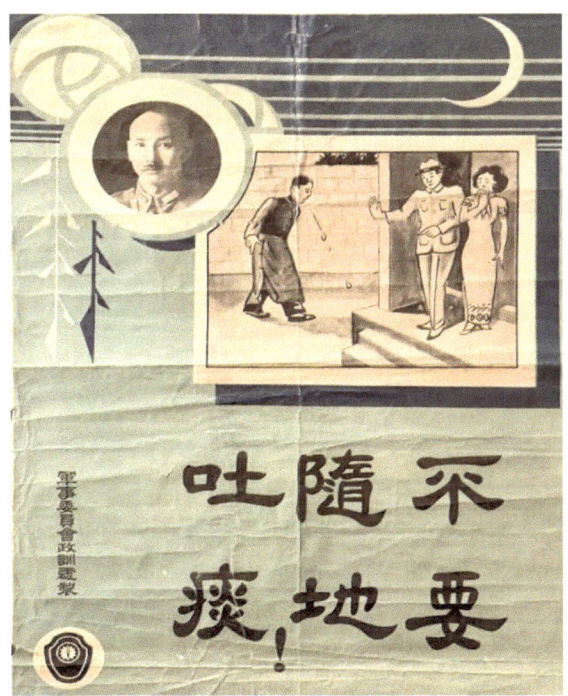

were often chaotic and in disharmony, affecting the introduction and implementation of pharmaceutical legislation across the country. Canton was the earliest and most successful municipal government to implement laws governing the registration of Chinese medicine dispensary practitioners, quality assurance of pharmaceutical products, and examining and testing of adulterated medicines. (Figs. 8.5 and 8.6).[14] Upon the unification of the warlords in October 1928, the Nationalist government in Nanjing promulgated a series of laws concerning the pharmaceutical industry and pharmacy practice to safeguard public health and promote fair trading from 1921 to 1944. These included the following laws and regulations (Table 8.1). In China's largest treaty port, the self-elected Shanghai Municipal Council opted for a *laissez-faire* approach with minimum laws and maximum freedom for traders operating in the International Settlements from 1863 to 1941. During these seventy-eight years, Shanghai became the centre of retail and wholesale chemists with duty-free import and distribution of "opium cures", branded proprietary and ethical pharmaceuticals. However, the single greatest challenge of the Nationalist government from 1928 to 1949 were the provincial governments' regional armed forces governed vast tracts of land, and they continued collecting tax revenues from the opium traders in the rural provinces although there was an official ban on opium cultivation and trading.

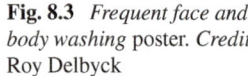

Fig. 8.3 *Frequent face and body washing* poster. *Credit* Roy Delbyck

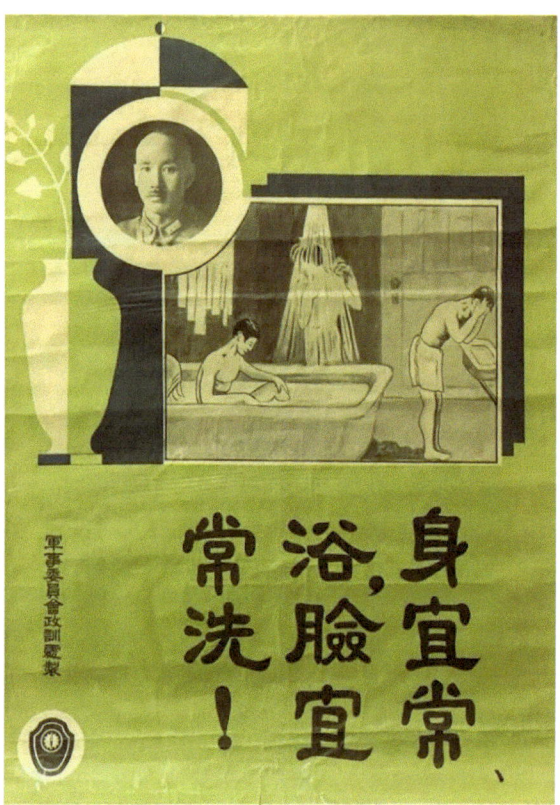

Intellectual Property Laws

Time-honoured brands, in particular herbal remedies dispensed or sold by reputable apothecaries for centuries in Beijing, Shanghai and across the country had been treated with the utmost respect by consumers despite the change of dynasties. These Chinese medicine apothecaries were well known for authenticity and quality in the selection and dispensing of each batch of their proprietary formulations. Tongrentang (同仁堂) was one of several Chinese medicine apothecaries that had a nationwide reputation. Founded in Beijing in 1669, it was regarded as the leading supplier of quality herbal remedies to the Qing imperial court. It became the appointed apothecary to Emperor Yongzhen in 1723. Only the high officials in the Qing imperial court, wealthy merchants, and the landowner class could afford Tongrentang and other branded medicines of reputable Chinese medicine apothecaries.[15] Tongrentang's motto, shown in its pair of large shop front wooden plaques, was "Despite the compounding and mixing of being complicated and time consuming, we dare not save on labour. Furthermore, although the taste (high quality) is expensive, we dare not substitute lesser-quality materials".

Fig. 8.4 *Free of vices* (prostitution, gambling, smoking and alcoholism) poster. *Credit* Roy Delbyck

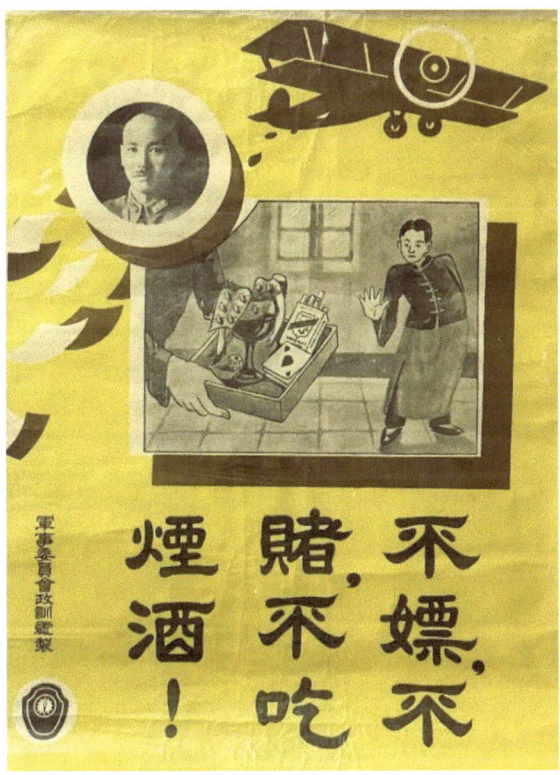

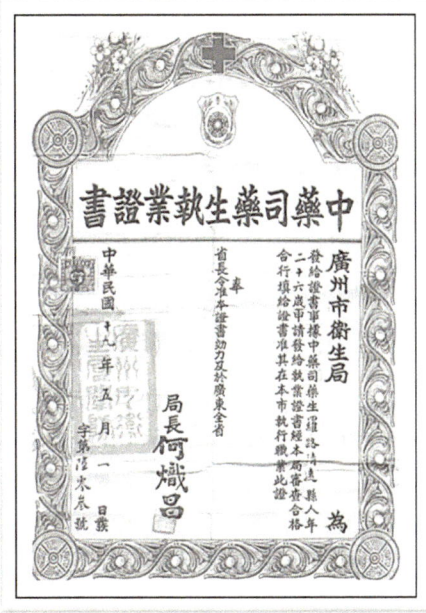

Fig. 8.5 Certificate of registration of Chinese medicine dispensary authorized practitioner by the Guangzhou health Bureau, 1930. *Credit* Hong Kong society for the history of pharmacy

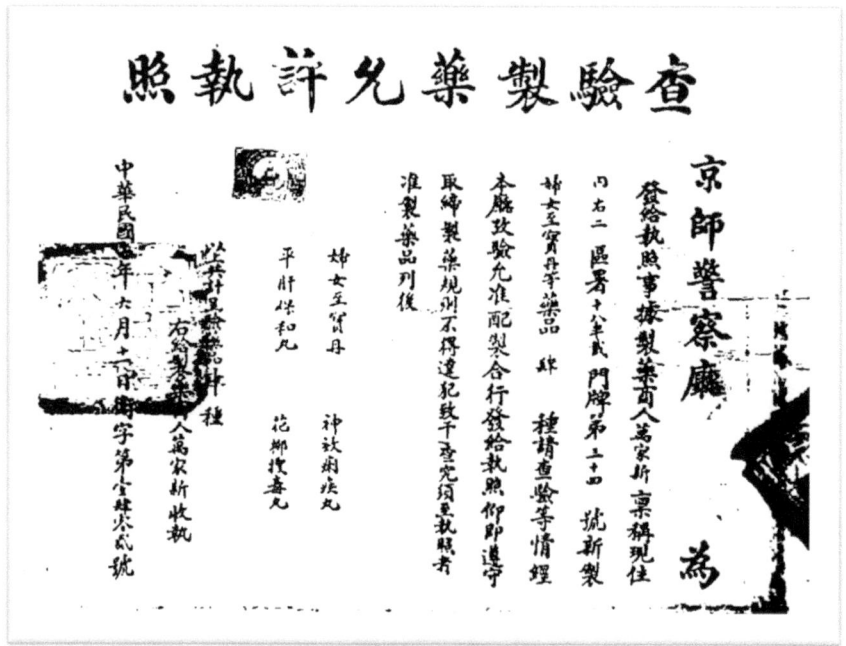

Fig. 8.6 Certificate of approval of pharmaceutical manufacturing by the capital police bureau, 1930. *Credit* Hong Kong Society for the History of Pharmacy

Table 8.1 Major laws concerning the pharmaceutical industry and pharmacy practice, 1928–1944

Year	Month	Laws	Mandatory implementation year
1929	January	Pharmacist registration regulations	1949
	April	Narcotics administration regulations (amendments)	1930
	August	Pharmaceutical manufacturers regulations	1930
1930	April	Proprietary medicines administration regulations (revised)	1930
1937	May	Bacteriological and immunological products administration regulations	1937

Credit Library of Institute of Modern History, Academia Sinica, Taipei

In China, intellectual property rights were a new concept in the nineteenth century. For example, in 1881, Zheng Guanying (郑观应), an entrepreneur owner of the Shanghai Machinery and Weaving Plant (上海机器布局), sought imperial approval for his proprietary weaving technology. As a result, Emperor Guangxu awarded the Plant a ten-year imperial patent right. With increasing imports of consumer goods including the proprietary medicines in the late nineteenth century, foreign powers were seeking protection of the trade marks of their exports to China. The Manchu Qing court officials responded by initiating intellectual property laws at the turn of the century. Sir Robert Hart of the China Maritime Customs (大清总税务司英籍赫德爵士) officially announced the draft of the first set of "Provisional Regulations on Trade Marks" (商标暂行条例) on behalf of the Manchu Qing government in August 1904.[16] However, the eight western powers, including Japan, could not agree on what sections favoured their respective countries, so the proposed law was shelved. As a compromise, a tentative arrangement was for the Shanghai and Tianjin Maritime Customs Administrations to accept the filing of notification of registration. Litigation on infringement of intellectual property rights soon arose in Shanghai as the market for branded proprietary medicines became red hot between local enterprises that were gaining market share from the original brands of imported drugs.

In 1913, the Ministry of Agriculture and Commerce (MoAC) of the newly established Nationalist government in Beijing established a trade mark registration preparatory office. However, Britain and Japan objected to China developing a new set of trade mark laws instead of the tentative arrangements. The archive materials of the Ministry of Foreign Affairs of the Nationalist government revealed that Japan and the UK were entangled in a trade dispute. During the "vacuum period", Japan exported many counterfeited British branded goods to China. It was a complicated diplomatic matter as Japanese companies had filed for notifications of trade mark registrations of those British brands not licensed by them with the Shanghai and Tianjin Maritime Customs Administrations. This Japanese trade practice seriously damaged British commercial interests and thus objected to the Chinese government promulgating a new trade mark law.[17] In the end, Japan backed down and agreed that "first-to-use" rather than "first-to-register" should be the principle for distinguishing genuine and counterfeit trade marks.

By early 1923, importers had filed over 1000 notifications and trade mark applications to the two Maritime Customs offices and the MoAC. They exerted mounting pressure on behalf of their overseas principals to protect their trade marks in China. As a result, the MoAC swiftly drafted the Trade Mark Law (商標法), passed by the Senate and the House of Representatives on 4 May 1923. The 1923 Trade Mark Law was the most comprehensive law containing forty-four articles and thirty-seven by-laws based on a first-to-use principle with a twenty-year validity period. These included the evaluation procedures, civil compensation for infringement and criminal penalties for counterfeiting trade marks. After the Northern Expedition in 1928, the unified Nationalist government established the National Registration Bureau the following year. It soon changed its name to the Trade Mark Office, which continued to use the Beiyang government's 1923 Trade Mark Law to process applications and resolved disputes. In 1929, the Trade Mark Office began reviewing and revising the 1923 Trade Mark Law, with the Legislative Yuan (立法院) passing the forty-article Trade Mark Law with forty implementation regulations. The law was enacted in 1930 with the same first-to-use principle and a 20-year validity.

The first court case involving a trade mark dispute between the two Chinese medicine herbal remedy brands of Jintan and Rendan proprietary Chinese medicine formulations arose soon after the establishment of the Beiyang government of the

Republic of China in 1912. Morishita Hiroshi & Co. (森下博, Morishita) of Japan developed the Jintan brand in 1905 as a red-colour pill. The word Jintan consists of two characters: "*jin*" (仁) for "benevolence" and "*tan*" (丹) for "pill". Morishita established an export department in 1907, with China as the primary overseas market. Three outlets of Morishita were set-up in the treaty ports of Shanghai, Tianjin and Hankou in the eastern, northern and southern regions in 1908, serving as sales channel of 4000 postal agencies in China in the following years. Morihita was responsible for business promotion in the provinces north of the Yangtze River, including Tianjin's treaty ports and Beijing's capital region. East Asia Company (東亞商社, EAC), Morishita's exclusive distributor, was responsible for provinces south of the Yangtze River, including the treaty ports of Shanghai and Hankou.

In 1908, Morishita and EAC filed for notification of the Jintan brand's trademark registration with the Tianjin Maritime Customs Administration (Fig. 8.7). The trade mark consisted of a man carrying a big moustache dressed in formal attire with an application number 10214 issued on 8 September 1908, and another one printed on cardboard with an application number 10909, also issued on 8 September 1908. In response to market needs, Huang Chujiu of the Great Eastern Dispensary soon developed his own Rendan brand through a separate company called Dragon and Tiger Company (龙虎公司, *Longfu Gongsi*) in July 1911 (Fig. 8.8).[18]

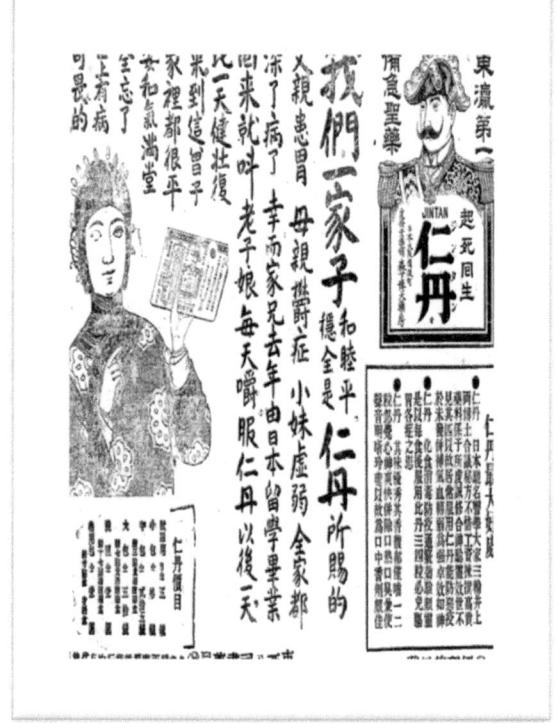

Fig. 8.7 Jintan (仁丹) newspaper advertisement showing its trade mark at the top right hand corner with a gentleman wearing a mustache, a hat and a formal attire. *Credit* Shun Pao, 18 July 1911, Page 7 of Second Edition

Fig. 8.8 Rendan (人丹)
flyer showing a "dragon" in
the top left hand corner and a
"tiger" in the bottom right
hand corner with the
characters of (人丹) in the
centre as its trade mark.
@1911. *Credit* Hong Kong
Society for the History of
Pharmacy

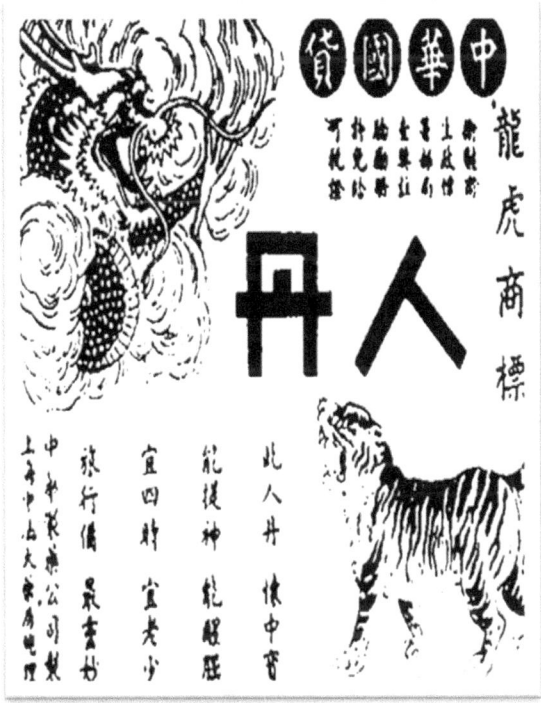

Morishita immediately registered its third trade mark containing the Chinese characters of China Jintan with an application number of 12,535 issued on September
6, 1911, two months after the official launch of Huang's Rendan in Shanghai. EAC,
acting on behalf of Morishita, lodged a litigation case against DTP's Rendan's
infringement of Jintan's trade mark rights in 1912. Rendan's Dragon and Tiger
design bore no resemblance to Jintan's formal attire design, although Morishita's
Jintan brand was the first to use the character "*jin*" (仁), which sounded phonetically
the same as "*ren*" (人) in Mandarin Chinese. However, it had a different meaning
than "*ren*" in writing. Both companies used the same character, "*tan*" and "*dan*" (丹),
written the same and with the same meaning, but it was a generic term of "pill" for
Chinese medicine in both China and Japan. The court case dragged on for a decade
until the Supreme Court in Beijing ruled Rendan was not infringing Morishita's
Jintan trade mark in 1927. Lee Puitak summarized his views:

> The main reason for the delay in the adjudication is not the case's complexity but that the
> United Kingdom and Japan have been opposing the trade mark law announced by China.
> The law violates the original trade agreements signed by China with the United Kingdom
> and Japan.[19]

In November 1935, the Nationalist government further updated the Trade Mark
Law; article one specified that the characters or words used in the trade mark should
include its phonetical translation. This change led to a flurry of litigation in the next

fifteen years by holders of foreign trade marks against owners of common pharmaceutical drug names used in the pharmaceutical market. Bayer's parent company, IG Faben, held effectively registered trade marks in both Chinese characters and English words of aspirin, Bayer Aspirin, and the blue-colour image of the aspirin tablet. Faben filed its trade mark registration with the Shanghai Maritime Customs Administration in 1922 and its successors in due course. In 1936, the National New Medicine Traders Association (全国新药业同业公会, NNMTA) and the Shanghai New Medicine Traders Association (上海市新药业同业公会, SNMTA) informed their retail chemist members not to stock up on Bayer Aspirin.[20] This was in response to Bayer's decision to distribute its pharmaceutical products, including Bayer Aspirin, directly to the provincial distributors instead of SNMTA's members.[21] NNMTA and SNMTA took IG Farben to court, and the litigation dragged on for a decade. Chang Ning (张宁) explained the decision of the Nationalist government:

> By 1930, the Chinese had built their pharmaceutical industry and formed a nationwide trade association. Intriguingly, the Chinese eventually won their case by persuading the Chinese government that aspirin had become a commonly used name for pain relief and thus lost the essential distinction of a trade mark. Though this seems to be a typical case of indigenous Chinese enterprise versus a multinational corporation, the events reveal the astonishing degree to which pharmaceutical companies, whether indigenous or international, rely on the state's power to protect their interests.[22]

From 1915 to 1949, the Republican government had promulagated a series of intellectual property laws and regulations which formed the basis for fair trade for all suppliers; local or foreign (Table 8.2).

The 1930 Chinese Pharmacopoeia

Since the first century CE, medicinal herbs that improve human well-being and treat illnesses have been recorded in *The Divine Farmer's Classic Materia Medica*. Ancient China's first official pharmacopoeia, Xinxiu Bencao ("新修本草"Tang Pharmacopoeia) was published in the early period of Tang dynasty in 659, and the last official pharmaceutical codex or formulary, Formulary of the Taiping People's Pharmacy (太平惠民和剂局方, *Taiping Huimin Heji Jufang*) was circulated in the late Song dynasty in 1208. In the next eight hundred years, attempts were made to compile national pharmacopeias by emperors of Mongolian Yuan, Ming, and Manchu Qing dynasties which unfortunately were either not released or distributed nationwide. Non-official dispensatories or formularies based on the previously published national pharmacopoeias and pharmaceutical codex were circulated by those Chinese medicine practitioners in the private sector. Some even gained royal accreditation but not as official pharmacopeias or formularies and a typical example is the *Bencao Ganmu* ("本草纲目", Compendium of Materia Medica) by Li Shizhen, which was published in 1596.[23] Li's Compendium became a recognized drug reference book for both domestic apothecaries and western natural scientists, including Charles Darwin (1809–1882) in the nineteenth century.

Table 8.2 Intellectual property laws, 1915–1949

Year	Key intellectual property laws and regulations	Implications
Copyright		
1915	Copyright Law promulgated by the Beiyang government	Protection of creative writing
1928	Exceptions including laws, court cases and rulings, public announcements. and speeches and those not of an academic nature were excluded	Academic freedom (use of materials for teaching, reference and footnotes with quotations of original sources allowed.)
	Submissions for copyrights would not be approved if in infringement of the Nationalist Party's ideology, and ruled as unsuitable by a court of law	Promotion of patriotic sentiments and the Three Principles of the People
	Lifetime protection for the copyright holder and 30 years thereafter for the successor of the deceased unless otherwise specified	Original translations had 20-year copyright but other translation versions not protected
	Fines of for different infringements ~ Unintentional infringement of copyrights, if found by a court of law	Unintentional infringement of copyrights, if found by a court of law
1944	Copyright Law Amendments	Further amendments in 1949
1949	Further amendments of Copyright Law	
Patent		
1912	Provisional regulations on incentivising artcrafts	Inventions or improvements of foods, beverages or drugs were covered except those which would lead to social unrests or have received prior approval
	Exclusive use for 5 years from date of approval	Short duration to allow growth of domestic industry
	Copycat or false claim of right of use will be subjected to criminal prosecution	Discourage abuse of law
1923	Provisional regulations on incentivising industrial products	
	"Exclusive right of sale" replaced "patent right"	
	Validity of 3, 5, and 15 years	Fair trade for all
1932	Patent law	
1939-1941	Patent law (amendment)	Extension of patent validity to 15 years
1944	Complete review of patent law	Foreigners or foreign companies were allowed to seek patent protection

(continued)

Table 8.2 (continued)

Year	Key intellectual property laws and regulations	Implications
Trade Mark		
1912	Provisional regulations	Trade Mark disputes arisen due to ambiguity of regulations
1923	Trademark law and regulations by the Beiyang (Peiyang) government	Each major country had own interests to protect and consensus not reached among Japan and Western powers Eight Nation Alliance
1930	Trademark Law	Promulgated on 6 May 1930 and became effective on 1 January 1931

Credit Library of Institute of Modern History, Academia Sinica, Taipei

Adulteration of imported and locally supplied chemical drugs by importers and wholesalers became a serious issue in the early twentieth century. Canton was the first municipality to regulate routine testing of Chinese materia medica and also registration of Chinese medicine dispensers in China in 1922, though with strong initial resistance from the druggists and herbal medicine traders. When the new Nationalist government was in place in Nanking in 1928 and the new laws and regulations including the 1930 "Narcotic Drugs Ordinance" were promulgated, a new momentum was gaining pace in the implementation of pharmacy laws and regulations.[24] With an increasing number of pharmacists and pharmacy technicians graduating annually from 1911 onwards, they initially relied on the Japanese Pharmacopoeia (JP) for quality standards of western drugs.

However, from 1916 onwards, more graduates attending pharmacy diploma courses returning from the US and later local university pharmacy graduates following a Canadian or UK curriculum, using the British Pharmacopoeia (BP) or the United States Pharmacopeia (USP) as reference guides, became more frequent. The BP, JP or the USP. are of great value in its drug monographs with detailed specifications on purity, identification, and testing methods.

The national pharmacopoeias aim to ensure that marketed drugs meet the national safety, efficacy and quality standards of respective countries. The same applies to pharmaceutical houses which mass-produce such formulations in tablet, and injectable forms. By the mid-1920s, the growing use of western drugs in the urban centres in China had led to challenges caused by unethical imports and trading of chemicals and raw materials for dispensing and production use of hospitals and generic drug houses. John Cameron, the pharmacy supervisor of PUMC Hospital, China's leading western teaching hospital at the time, faced the adulteration challenges and aired his views in the 1927 winter edition of the National Medical Journal:

> From our own experience, we have found that it is sometimes necessary to submit drugs to careful analysis before issuing them to the wards of our hospital or as prescriptions to our outpatient department. We have published elsewhere the results of our analysis, and these

prove that it is a mistake to accept chemical and drug stocks without verifying the contents of the bottles.[25]

A closer look at Cameron's earlier article on "Adulteration*s*", in which he reported that only one per cent of all the chemicals and drugs submitted to analysis showed any deficiency in purity when compared with the pharmacopeial monographs.[287] However, Cameron also wrote in a separate article on Morphine Hydrochloride BP which contained 15% phenacetin (an analgesic), and acid picric. The sample analysis contained about 90% potassium sulphate and 10% acid picric (Table 8.3).[26] The latter cases would give rise to a grave situation assuming all the smaller western clinical institutions and pharmacies numbering several hundred would receive adulterated or substandard drugs regularly. Most of them were ill-equipped with the necessary analytical equipment or reagents to test drug samples on a routine basis using the BP or USP as the reference standard. Cameron advocated in the professional journals that:

> What we want in China today is an official Chinese Pharmacopoeia which will contain a list of the chemicals and drugs used in medicine in this country with tests for their impurity, tests for their identity and characteristic descriptions of each added as a short monograph after the official name of the drug. Then it will be possible to publish an official Chinese Formulary which shall contain only items which are officially "Chinese Pharmacopoeia". And what is perhaps much more important in this country is that there will be an official standard of purity and strength established by law which prevents the sale of a chemical or drug below standard.[27]

The Nationalist government was firmly in place in Nanking, and the Ministry of Health was established in January 1928. Dr. Heng J. Liu, was appointed as the Vice Minister of NHA and later as Minister of Health. He also immediately acted as the Editor-in-Chief and appointed the editorial committee of the Chinese Pharmacopoeia (CP), composing 4 pharmacists of whom three were trained in Japan, one in the U.K. and one medical microbiologist trained in Japan, in January 1929 (Table 8.4). Dr. Heng J. Liu appointed Moody Meng, seconded from the PUMC Hospital to the Ministry as a reviewer and editor of the first CP on 1 January 1929. His tenure was initially for six months, which ended up being a 16-month assignment. The first edition of the CP was eventually published at the end of 1930 and released in 1931.

The difficulty in reaching consensus and compiling the Republic's first Pharmacopoeia was that western trained doctors and pharmacists were from all over the world and British, European, Japanese and US medical and pharmaceutical practitioners differed in their approaches to professional practice.[28] Hence, four external advisors of the Pharmacopoeia, including Bernard Read (British, PUMC), William Pailing (British, Shandong Christian University), John Cameron (British, PUMC Hospital) and Sasaki Motouji (佐木元治, Japanese, Head of Tokyo Health Laboratory) provided their invaluable inputs. The first edition of the Pharmacopoeia was based primarily on the 10th Revision of the 1926 United States Pharmacopoeia (USP X) with special reference to the latest editions of the British Pharmacopoeia and the Japanese Pharmacopoeia. Each Drug monograph provides the names in Chinese and Latin with descriptions, specifications, testing methods, reagents and

Table 8.3 Adulterated chemical drugs supplied by bona-fide chemical houses in the Europe or the US in 1926

Item	Drug	Content analyzed by PUMCH	USP drug monograph unless otherwise indicated
1	Opium	Only 5% morphine	9.5–10.5% when powdered opium dried at 60 °C
2	Cocaine Hydrochloride	Melting point of one sample was 8° above the maximum limit	182–186 °C
3	Iodoform B.P	4% sand found in sample	Labelled as Iodoform cryst. pursis B.P
4	Formaldehyde solution 40%	4% Solution of Formal-dehyde HCHO	Very weak smell on opening led to suspicion of aldulteration
5	Formuladehyde solution	Polymerized and only 30% strength only	Storage condition was critical as a 50% loss could occur if sotred in a courtyard in the cold winter months of December to February in North China
6	Acid: salicyl B.P	6% Sodium Salicyl as an impurity and the whole sample had a reddish tint	Colour should be white
7	Methly alcohol	14% actetone	Labelled as chemically pure
8	Sodium hydroxide	Contained 5% iron and was of a reddish colour, and shipped in a badly rusted 5 pound tin container	
9	Bleaching powder	60% available chlorine content	Desirability of assaying each batch for the preparations of Carrel Dakin solution
10		25% available chlorine content	
11	Saccharose (sucrose)	Contained some destrose but labelled as "extra pure"	Useless for the purpose for which it was acquired
12	Tragacanth Gum. owdered. B.P	Two samples were analyzed. One wa found to be about eight times stornger in suspending properties	Not able to account for this great difference in properties
13	Methylene blue tablets (sugar coated)	A sample was found to have burst the sugar coating	Stored in the pharmacy for 3 years
14	Quinine tablets	One batch was found to have a splinter of wood	The wood when examined microscopically was not cinchina bark

(continued)

Table 8.3 (continued)

Item	Drug	Content analyzed by PUMCH	USP drug monograph unless otherwise indicated
15	Green soap	One sample found to contain a small percentage of a highly smelling fish oil	
16	Lysol	One sample of this disinfectant was found not to be properly emulsified	It had to be heated before being used

Credit China Medical Journal, Issue 4, 1927: 345–347
Remarks A closer look at John Cameron's article on "Adulterations", he reported that only about one per cent of all the submitted chemicals and drugs showed any deficiency when referencing the pharmacopeial monographs

Table 8.4 Editorial board of the 1st edition of Chinese pharmacopoeia, 1930

#	Names	Profession	University	Country of graduation	Official position in the central/ municipal government
1	Heng J. Liu (1891–1961)	Surgeon	Harvard University	United States	Minister of health (1929–1930), Director general (1931–1936), National Health Administration
2	Yan Zhi Zhong (1889–1974)	Medical bacteriologist	Imperial University of Tokyo	Japan	Director, Medical Administration, MoH
3	Moody Meng (1897–1983)	Pharmacist	University of London	United Kingdom	Senior pharmaceutical specialist, MoH
4	Yu Dawang (1886–1956)	Pharmacist	Imperial University of Tokyo	Japan	Senior pharmaceutical specialist, MoH
5	Xue Yiqi (1884–?)	Pharmacist	Chiba Medical School	Japan	Secretary, MoH
6	Chen Pu (1897–1955)	Pharmacist	Imperial University of Tokyo	Japan	Head, health laboratory, Nanjing Municipality

Credit Hong Kong Society for the History of Pharmacy

standard solutions. The 1930 Chinese Pharmacopoeia contains 708 drug monographs, including 120 organic drugs, 197 inorganic drugs, 101 materia medica of which sixty belongs to Chinese materia medica, five biological products, and 285 pharmaceutical preparations.[29]

It was an open secret that the MoH eventually intended to eliminate Chinese medicine practice. The contents of the 1930 CP thus heavily skewed towards western medicines, which was an obvious move by the senior policymakers headed by Minister Liu. Only 60 or 8.5% of the Chinese materia medica out of the 708 drug monographs were included in the CP.[30] This was in stark contrast to the official policy of the Nationalist government of 1930 that both Chinese medicine and materia medica and western medicine and drugs would be treated in the same way. Every sector of the pharmacy profession, be it in retail, hospital, industrial or wholesale, saw the tremendous value of the Pharmacopoeia as it provided the official standard of drugs in the dispensing, import, sale, supply and distribution of medicines.

Some pharmaceutical manufacturers took advantage of referring their products meeting the standards and specifications of the Pharmacopoeia as an implication of the official endorsement by the Nationalist government. "Olinsol Disinfectant", presumably containing chloroxylenol, made by the International Dispensary (万国药房, *Wanguo Yaofang*) of Shanghai, advertised in the 7 July 1935 edition of Shun Pao (Fig. 8.9). "The Elephant Brand First Aid Epidemic Solution" advertisement, in the 15 August 1935 edition of Shun Pao by the Great Eastern Dispensary, also referred to the product with similar implications (Fig. 8.10). Inaccuracies in the 1930 CP were rectified soon after the War. Moody Meng was again responsible for updating the second edition, which was completed but not distributed by the Nationalist government before its exile to Taiwan in 1949. When Mao Zedong founded the People's Republic of China (PRC) on 1 October 1949, Moody Meng became the responsible official for compiling the first edition of the Pharmacopoeia of the PRC in 1953. The strategic shift in responsibility for providing medicine to the public from the medical missionaries to the state first arose when the Nationalist government established the MoH in 1928. Sean Lei articulated that the change resulted from the western trained practitioners being fascinated by the progressive health policies adopted by England and Russia after the First World War:

> To popularize scientific medicine in China, promoters had no choice but to rely on the state's political power. While the state appeared to emerge as the subject of medical history, the real actors in this history were mostly the Chinese practitioners of western medicine ......
> such as Dr. Wu Lien Teh, Dr. Heng J. Liu, Dr. Fu-ching Yen, and their western allies, John B. Grant, and the leading players at the Rockefeller Foundation.[31]

At the height of the Cold War in the 1950s, the Communist government actively pursued a self-reliance strategy with the adoption of Chinese materia medica as a complimentary health care system. While the first edition of the Pharmacopoeia of the People's Republic of China of 1953 retained western medicines as the basis of modern medicine, the second edition took a shift in 1965. (See the section of *One Country, Two Pharmacy Systems* in Chap. 9).

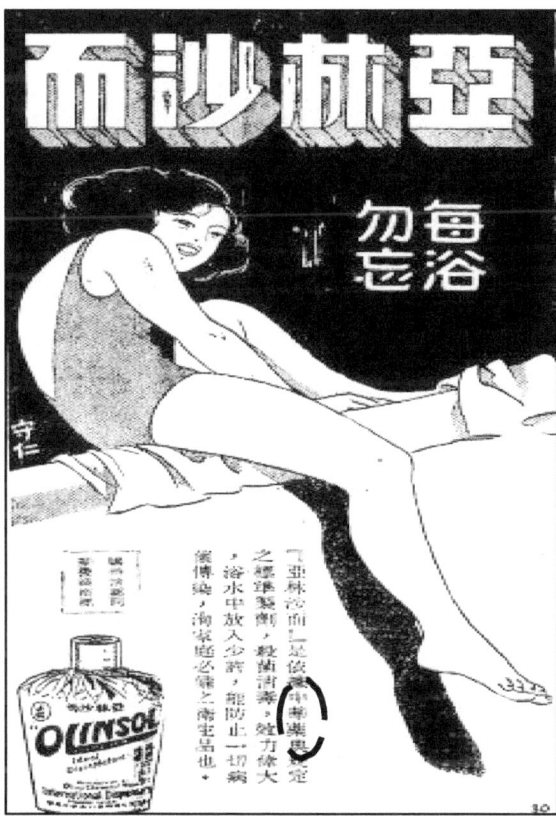

Fig. 8.9 Advertisement of the *Microscope brand Olinsol* Disinfectant. Advertising pitch: "Olinsol is a standard formulation prepared in accordance with the requirements of the Chinese Pharmacopoeia. It is a disinfectant with excellent bactericidal efficacy. Add a little to the bath; it can prevent all communicable infections—a necessary sanitary item for all households". *Credit* Shun Pao, Shanghai, 7 July 1935

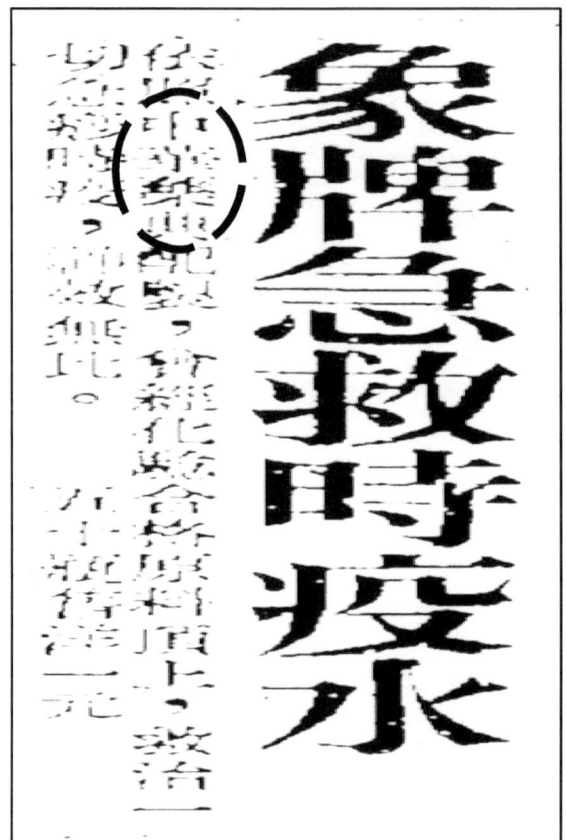

Fig. 8.10 Advertisement of the *Elephant* brand of first aid anti-epidemic solution. Advertising pitch: "The *Elephant* first aid solution possessing miraculous properties in epidemics". *Credit* Shun Pao, Shanghai, 15 August 1935

Notes and References

1. The "Self-Strengthening Movement" (自强运动) was inspired by Wei Yuan (魏源, 1794–1857), a philosopher and historian and headed by Prince Gong, a reformer of the Manchu Qing court.
2. Chang, Peng-Yuan, "Modernization and Revolution in China, 1860–1949", *Journal of Institute of Modern History, Academia Sinica,* June 1990, 19: 50–51. Accessed 22 April 2023. https://www.mh.sinica.edu.tw/MHDocument/PublicationDetail/PublicationDetail_879.pdf.
3. In 1885 the constitutional monarchy with the cabinet system of government was adopted in Japan. Ito Hirobumi (1841–1909) became Japan's first prime minister. The Constitution of the Empire of Japan was promulgated in 1889 when it established the political system with a national assembly and an electoral system of a modern state.
4. In 1900, China's 400 million population spread across a geographical area of 13.16 million square kilometres whereas Japan's 44 million lived in 0.38 million square kilometers.
5. Li Beibei 李桔桔Xu, Feng 徐峰, "Zhongguo jindai chengshi hua lu ji chengshi hua feeqi@, 中国近代城市化 率及城市化分期 [Urbanization Rate and Urbanization in Modern China],

Zhongguo chengshì yanjiu (dianzǐiqikan) 中国城市研究 (电子期刊), [E-Journal of China Urban Studies], 2, no. 2, 2007, 60–68 Accessed 29 September 2023. https://www.sinoss.net/uploadfile/2010/1130/7841.pdf.

6. Chang Yufa 张玉法, 1920 niandai zhongguo de zhengzhi sichao"1920年代中國的政治思潮 [Political Trends in China in the 1920s], *Zhongguo wenhua yanjiusuo xuebao* 中国文化研究所学报, [Journal of the Institute of Chinese Culture], no.7 (1998): 133–134. Accessed 29 September 2023. https://www.cuhk.edu.hk/ics/journal/articles/v38p133.pdf.

7. Dr. Heng J. Liu's rapid ascent from a surgeon at the PUMCH to that of the medical superintendent and director of PUMC was most likely due to a policy set by the the Nationalist government's Ministry of Education, requiring that all institutions including foreign-owned universities and colleges must have a Chinese director and an administration consisting of a majority of Chinese nationals.

8. Lei, Sean, *Neither Donkey Nor Horse*, (Chicago: The University of Chicago Press 2014): 65–66.

9. Dr. Heng J. Liu and the Conference participants lacked public consultations on the subject in the first place. Liu also seemed to underestimate the political reality that Chiang Kai-shek's rival within the Nationalist Party, Wang Jingwai 汪精卫(Wang Ching-wei) , supported the elitists' modernity drive.

10. Personal Interview of Madam Angela Chen-Lin 陈林颖曾女士, Chairperson, Lifu Medical Research, Cultural and Educational Foundation 财团法人立夫医药研究文教基金会, Taipei, 22 April 2019.

11. Chiang Kai-shek Is Baptized", *The Christian Century: A Journal of Religion*, XLVII, no. 45 (1930):1335–1337.

12. Chen Lifu 陈立夫, *Zhongguo Guomíndang Dangyuan Yu Xin Shenghuo Yundong* 中国国民党党员与新生活运动 [Chinese Nationliast (Kuomingtang) Party Members and New Life Movement], (Naning: Zhongzheng Books, 1934), 70–71. Accessed 29 September 2023. https://taiwanebook.ncl.edu.tw/en/book/NCL-002486642/reader.

13. Tseng, Husan-ching et al., 曾宣靜等 Min chu zhongyi yi yu fa quan zhi jiangou (1912–1949)—"yi zhongyi tiaolì" ji yishi fa" wei lunshu hexīn, 民初中医「医育法权」之建构 (1912–1949)—以《中医条例》及《医师法》为论述核心 [Creating Legal Rights for Chinese Medicine during the Early Years of the Republic of China (1912–1949): On the Chinese Medicine Ordinance of 1936 and the Physicians Act of 1943″], *Taiwan shida lishi xuebao* 台湾师大历史学报,[Bulletin of Historical Research], no.59, (2018): 57–60. Accessed 29 September 2023. https://wiww.his.ntnu.edu.tw/publish01/show_paper_list.php?issue_id=10.

14. Li Hanji 黎汉基 *Guangzhou yaowu gui guan zhengce bianqian (1921–1936)*, 广州药物规管政策变迁 (1921–1936) [Changes of Guangzhou Municipal Pharmaceutical Regulatory Policies During the Nationalist era, 1921–1936], *Chinese Social History Review*, no. 1 (2011): 243–246. Accessed 29 September 2023. https://www.sinoss.net/uploadfile/2013/0321/20130321114013297.pdf.

15. Social medicine was initiated by the Song emperors in the eleventh century, however, the system of public dispensaries offering affordable materia medica to the public gradually disappeared towards the end of the Ming dynasty in the late sixteenth century. By the seventeenth century, overseas monarchies and traders offered exotic materia medica, watches, wines and curios as tributary gifts to the Manchu Qing emperors and their senior imperial court officials. Hence, the market for expensive local or overseas products was almost non-existent in the eighteenth and nineteenth centuries except for opium as a leisure drug imported from India and Turkey.

16. Heuser, Robert, "The Chinese Trade Mark Law of 1904: A Preliminary Study of Exterritoriality, Competition, and Late Ch'ing Law Reform", *Oriens Extremus* 22, No. 2 (1975):192–194.

17. Motono, Eiichi, "Anglo-Japanese Trademark Conflict in China and the Birth of the Chinese Trademark Law (1923), 1906–26, *East Asian History*, no. 37, (2011): 10–11.

Accessed May 5, 2023. https://www.eastasianhistory.org/sites/default/files/article-content/2011-issue37/pdfs/EAH37-Motono.pdf.

18. Rendan (人丹)'s formulation was reportedly based on two ancient prescriptions listed in Li Shizhen's 李时珍 *Compendium of Materia Medica* 本草纲目 of 1596, with some unique ingredients.

19. Lee, Puitak 李培德, *Riben rendan zai hua de shìchang celue ji qí yu zhongguo ren dan de jìngzheng* 日本仁在华的市场策略及其与中国人丹的竞争 [The Marketing Strategy for Japanese Jintan in China and its Rivalry with Chinese Rendan], *Zhongyang yanjiuyuan jindaishi yanjiusuo jikan* 中央研究员近代史研究所集刊[Bulletin of the Institute of Modern History, Academia Sinica], 89, no. 9, (2015): 101.

20. Prior to the Communist take-over in October 1949, the National New Medicine Traders Association was a national wholesaler organization of western drugs formed by the provincial drug wholesaler associations of which the Shanghai New Medicine Traders Association was the largest one of all.

21. The core members of the Shanghai New Medicine Traders Association were the major retail pharmacy chains which also owned generic drug manufacturing houses. They distributed both the imported brands and local ones.

22. Chang Ning 张宁, "*A si pi ling zai zhongguo—minguo shiqi zhongguo xin yao ye yu deguo baier yao chang jian de shangbiao zhengsong*" 阿司匹灵在中国—民国时期中国新药业与德国拜耳药厂间的商标争讼 [Aspirin in China: Trade Mark Disputes between China's Pharmaceutical Industry and I.G. Faben], *Zhongyang yanjiuyuan jindaishi yanjiusuo jikan* 中央研究员近代史研究所集刊 [Bulletin of the Institute of Modern History, Academia Sinica] 59, no.3, 2008, 99–123, esp. 131–140.

23. He, Bian, *Know Your Remedies: Pharmacy and Culture in Early Modern China*, (Princeston: Princeston University Press, 2020), 44–47.

24. Li Hanji, "Minguo shiqi guangzhou yaowu", no. 18, 2011: 256–257.

25. Cameron, John, "Adulterations", *China Medical Journal,* Chinese Medical Journal Publishing Co. Ltd., April 1927: 345–347. Accessed 29 September 2023. https://mednexus.org/doi/epdf/10.3760/cma.j.issn.0366-6999.1927.04.108.

26. Cameron, John, "Pharmaceutical analysis in hospital pharmacies of China", *The Journal of the American Pharmaceutical Association* 16, no. 11 (1927): 1068–1071.

27. Cameron, John, "A Chinese Pharmacopoeia—When?" *The National Medical Journal* 13, no. 6 (1927):450–451.

28. Meng, M and Chen, P, "The Compilation of Chinese Pharmacopoeia I", *National Medical Journal of China* 16, no. 2 (1930): 190–209.

29. Zhao, Yuxin 赵宇新等 "Zhongguo yaodian de fazhan lishi ji qishi" 中国药典的发展历史及启示 [Development History and Enlightenment of the Chinese Pharmacopoeia], *Zhongguo yaopǐn biaozhun* 中国药 品标准 [Chinese Drug Standards] 21, no. 6 (2020). Accessed 29 September 2023. https://mp.weixin.qq.com/s?__biz=MzIzMzExNzEwNQ==&mid=2650167317&idx=1&sn=7a9e2382afd95373443e18d5ab8e9716&chksm=f0887ccbc7fff5dd7a882157268bc5559093bd6eece3eb22af3d271fa41ad520e0ddd8e952fe&scene=27.

30. Zhao, [Development History and Enlightenment], 27.

31. Lei, *Neither Donkey Nor Horse*: 65–66.

Chapter 9
Conclusion: Modern Pharmacy with Chinese Characteristics

Stretching across a span of over two millennia, this journey takes us from the Mausoleum of King Zhao Mo in Canton in 122 BCE to Tiananmen Square in Beijing when Chairman Mao Zedong announced the founding of the People's Republic on 1 October 1949. In the concluding chapter, a comprehensive summary will revisit the three fundamental questions raised at the outset of the book.

What events led diplomats, religious men, and traders to export exotic matera medica and modern medicines to China from faraway lands over the past two millennia, particularly in the nineteenth and twentieth centuries? What sparks occurred when chemists clashed with Chinese medicine dispensaries in the nineteenth century? What drove the shifting relationship between Chinese materia medica and biologicals, alkaloidal extracts, and chemical drugs during the late Manchu Qing dynasty to the early Republican period in China.

Firstly, many events led to the imports of exotic *matera medica* from faraway lands over the past two millennia and particularly in the nineteenth and twentieth centuries by China. Chapter 1 reveals the watershed moment that occurred with the opening of the ancient Silk Roads between the Western Han and its northern neighbors, spurred by Zhang Qian's groundbreaking expeditions to Central Asia, between 135 and 115 BCE. Following a period of turmoil after the decline of the Eastern Han dynasty (25–220), the reunification of China under the Sui dynasty (581–671) ushered in an era of heightened trade and religious interactions between China, Central Asia, and South Asia, encompassing both overland and maritime routes of the Silk Roads. The entry of Ayurvedic medicine and Buddhism enriched Chinese medicine with new medical philosophies such as Jivaka Pustaka and the introduction of Triphala. These foreign influences prompted Tao Hongjing and other Daoist medical philosophers to embark on experimental investigations with these non-Chinese materia medica imported from distant lands.

Emperor Taizong's reign (r. 626–649) of the Tang dynasty (618–907), ushered in an era of remarkable stability and prosperity, fueling a renaissance in both trade and religious practices. The capital city of Changan (now Xian) became a thriving hub,

© The Author(s), under exclusive license to Springer Nature Singapore Pte Ltd. 2023 193
P. Chiu, *A History of Western Pharmacy in China*,
https://doi.org/10.1007/978-981-99-8635-4_9

with Buddhist monasteries, Daoist temples, Nestorian churches, Jewish synagogues, and other religious institutions flourishing. During the tenth century, under the Song dynasty, the utilization of non-Chinese materia medica from overseas experienced an explosive growth. The Song emperors, who held a deep appreciation for medicine and healthy living, embraced new policies introduced by state chancellor Wang Anshi. These measures aimed to increase taxation and promote public health, ensuring the availability of affordable medicines. State-owned dispensaries offered prepackaged materia medica, Chinese and non-Chinese, for sale, resulting in approximately ten percent of the exotic materia medica originating from faraway lands.

During the Mongolian Yuan dynasty (1271–1368), attempts were made to introduce Islamic medicine and materia medica to China in the late fourteenth century, without success. Consequently, the presence of exotic elements of materia media from the overseas in Chinese medicine dispensaries remained relatively low. A few centuries later, the Governor General of Batavia in the Dutch East Indies, acting on behalf of the Kingdom of Netherlands, sent tributary gifts to Emperor Shunzhi (1638–1661) to establish trade with China in 1656. Among these gifts were cloves, cinnamon, and sandalwood. One notable contribution from the Roman Catholic Church was cinchona, a valuable exotic materia medica that Father Jean de Fontaney, was used to treat Emperor Kangxi's fever in July 1693. The Opium Wars, the 1st Sino-Japanese War, and the Boxer Movement in the late 19th and early twentieth centuries played a decisive role in China's eventual adoption of western medicine and pharmacy (See the next section on *Impacts of Western and Japanese Colonial Powers*).

Secondly, the sparks occurred, with some brighter than the others, and one or two burst into mighty flames when western chemists clashed with Chinese medicine dispensaries in the 100 years between the end of the First Opium War (1842) to the end of WWII (1945). The signing of the Treaty of Nanking in 1842, concluding the First Opium War and granting British entrepreneurs and missionaries settlement rights in five treaty ports. The cession of Hong Kong provided the U.K. with a strategic location for the opium trade. Following the end of the Second Opium War in 1860, Western chemists spread throughout the treaty ports in China. Advertisements for "opium cures" soon appeared in Shen Pao, Shanghai's first Chinese newspaper, in 1872. During the height of British imperialism in China in the 1870s, chemists in Hong Kong and Shanghai introduced branded proprietary medicines imported from Europe, the U.K., and the U.S. This retail pharmacy business inspired Chinese Medicine dispensary owners like Huang Chujiu to venture into western chemist trade, while Ningbo entrepreneurs, some worked as dispensing assistants at expatriate chemists, setup their own western chemists, and launched their locally produced brands of "opium cures." This localization movement eventually drove out the expatriate chemists or made them insignificant players by the 1930s (See the section on *Localization of Western Retail and Manufacturing Chemists* below).

Third and finally, the shifting relationship between the plant and animal based Chinese materia medica and biologicals, alkaloidal extracts, and chemical drugs emerged at the conclusion of World War I when the Allies and Germany finalized the terms of the Treaty of Versailles in 1919. Controversially, Germany's colony of

Qingdao (Tsingtao) in China was transferred to Japan, despite China being one of the Allies and expressing opposition. In response, young intellectuals spearheaded the May 4 Movement in 1919, advocating for a "New Culture" that embraced the values of "science" and "democracy." This movement led to a desire for "total westernization" in some circles with many individuals regarding proprietary medicines with foreign names, such as Dr. T.C. Yale Stimulant Remedy produced by western chemists, as far superior to remedies containing Chinese materia medica. The shift went into a higher gear when those western educated medical and pharmaceutical professionals became senior policy makers in the Nationalist government and led changes in building institutions and promulgating new laws and regulations in relation to medicine, pharmacy and healthcare. Dr. Heng J. Liu, as Minister of Health, setup the Republic's first Chinese Pharmacopoeia Commission, became its editor-in-chief and appointed a panel of five members with 4 pharmacists and a medical microbiologist in January 1929. Three out of four pharmacists and the medical microbiologist were educated and trained in Japan and one pharmacist, Moody Meng, was educated and qualified in the UK.

The First Public Health Conference was organized by the MoH in Shanghai from 23 to 26 February 1929. The main objective of the Conference was to "Abolish Chinese Medicine" and the eventual redundancy of Chinese medicine practitioners and Chinese materia medica. In defending their right, the Chinese medicine practitioners soon organized a parade, supported by the public and politicians, three weeks later in Nanjing, on 17 March 1929. With nationwide publicity and support, the decision to "Abolish Chinese Medicine" initiated by Dr. Heng J. Liu was stalled and a National Chinese Medicine Academy (中央国医馆, *Zhongayng Guoyi Guan*) was established to set standards and course curriculum and as a model to train qualified Chinese medicine practitioners in January 1930. In response, Dr. Heng J. Liu promptly completed the edition of the first edition of the Chinese Pharmacopoeia (CP) in May 1930. With only 8.5% or 60 Chinese materia medica listed in the modern Pharmacopoeia for use by the country's medical practitioners, a permanent tilt of the balance towards biologicals, alkaloidal extracts, and chemical drugs has become the Nationalist government's public health policy. The rest is history.

Impacts of Western and Japanese Colonial Powers

The arrival of Portuguese traders in Macau in 1557 turned a new leaf in world history. Macau became the primary gateway for trade with Canton, attracting British, European, and U.S. traders who used it as their home base during the winter and spring months when trade seasons were dormant. Another pivotal moment occurred when Hong Kong was ceded to the United Kingdom by China as a crown colony. This happened after China's defeat in the First Opium War (1839–1842), leading to the opening of five treaty ports in 1842. The Treaty of Nanking, signed in 1842, granted British traders and missionaries' permission to settle in these treaty ports. From 1843 onwards, Anglican and Protestant Churches, including the London Missionary

Society (LMS), began constructing hospitals in Hong Kong and the treaty ports. Retail chemists, operated by British, French, and German entrepreneurs, also emerged, and served as marine suppliers to the transiting freighters docking at Victoria Harbour in Hong Kong and the Huangpu River in Shanghai.

To manage their community affairs within the leased territory, the traders of Britain, France, and the U.S. established the Shanghai Municipal Council (1854–1941). In 1860, when the Convention of Peking was signed, Britain and the U.S. merged their concessions, leading to the formation of the enlarged Shanghai International Settlements in 1863. In the late nineteenth century, a fierce competition for influence over Korea unfolded between China and Japan, culminating in the First Sino-Japanese War (1894–1895). Following China's defeat, the Treaty of Shimonoseki was signed, wherein China acknowledged Korea's independence and relinquished Taiwan, the Penghu (Pescadores) Islands, and the Liaodong Peninsula. However, Russia maintained its occupation of the Liaodong Peninsula from 1895 to 1905 until the Russo-Japanese War (1904–1905) when both the Liaodong Peninsula and a substantial portion of the Chinese Eastern Railway in South Manchuria fell into Japan's control. The Boxer Rebellion (1900–1901) served as a catalyst for China to reform its millennium old Keju examination system, a move that mirrored Japan's Meiji Restoration in 1868, aimed at modernizing the state. China looked to Japan as a model, leading to an influx of thousands of students who sought higher education there. Some received government scholarships, while many self-financed their studies. Others received funding from the Boxers Indemnity Fund to pursue undergraduate studies in various fields in the United States, such as agriculture, mining, architecture, civil engineering, science, technology, law, and economics. Additionally, many Chinese students received financial support from British, French, and other European countries to pursue graduate studies abroad.

During this time, Western colonial powers solidified their presence in their respective colonies and occupied territories in China. Christian missionaries from Canada, the United States, and the United Kingdom played a significant role by establishing universities, medical colleges, and hospitals in Beijing, Canton, Shandong, Szechuan, and various inland provinces. Similarly, the Japanese South Manchurian Railway and the puppet state of Manchukuo established hospitals and university medical schools with pharmacy departments, educating and training pharmacy students from Korea, Manchuria, and Taiwan. Throughout the early twentieth century, Britain and Japan emerged as the main influencers shaping modern pharmacy in China, while France had a unique presence through institutions like St. Paul Hospitals in Hong Kong and the Aurora University, l'Université Franco-Chinoise, and Sainte-Marie Hospital in Shanghai. The Chinese Pharmacopoeia, published by the Republican government in 1930, represented a fusion of the British, Japanese, and U.S. Pharmacopeias, incorporating insights from four external pharmaceutical experts, including one from Japan and three from the United Kingdom.

Localization of Western Retail and Manufacturing Chemists

Today, class actions lodged against makers and distributors of habit-forming opiate drugs of fentanyl by consumers can result in bankruptcies which was not the case for opium or morphine in the nineteenth century. A few historians have extensively researched and written on narcotics and culture, however, the development of modern China's retail and manufacturing industries which evolved directly from this habit forming "opium cures" are worth mentioning here. The highly lucrative retail and wholesale "opium cures" in the treaty ports, particularly Shanghai, inspired local apprentices and dispensers working for western chemists to open their own retail chemists. The OTC market soon became "red hot" with Hong Kong or Shanghai based traders' increasing imports of laudanum and proprietary medicines and local chemists manufacturing their private label "opium cures" and proprietary medicines. A. S. Watson benefited from the "opium cures" directly for over three quarters of a century since 1870s until the arrival of Japanese Imperial Army in the mainland and the colony of Hong Kong in July 1937 and December 1941 respectively.

When Bayer of Germany discovered heroin in 1897, the global narcotic drug market entered a new phase. With Manchu Qing China's opium smokers' unabated appetite for "opium cures", the western retail chemist sector expanded into all corners of the eighty ports well in the 1910s. Sir Frederick Lugard, colonial Governor of Hong Kong from 1901 to 1928, reported before the Legislative Council meeting on 11 March 1909:

> Morphia (Latin for morphine) is not only imported in a liquid form for injection but also in the insidious form of so called "anti-opium pills", which are in vast quantities, as a cure for opium smoking. The Commissioner of Imperial Maritime Customs states that these morphia pills are obtainable in every medicine shop in Canton and their sale is increasing. Even in remote country villages morphia tabloids and hypodermic syringes are frequently seen, and a condition of things which allows a Chinaman I know to buy daily a dram bottle of Japanese morphia (60 grains) imperatively calls for restriction if not prohibition.[1]

In short, the cost attraction of morphine injection to opium smokers as articulated by Lugard was the key reason for the switch from opium smoking to morphine injection as the narcotic substitute (Table 9.1).

Hardly over a period of two decades, western chemists such as A.S. Watson grew from 30-odd dispensaries selling its brand of "opium cures" in 1890 to over a hundred in the mainland by 1910, all be benefiting from the high profit margins of narcotic drugs. By then, local chemists became serious competitors as they leveraged their retail, manufacturing, and wholesale business with the private label "opium cures"

Table 9.1 Cost comparison of narcotic drugs by weight and potency equivalence

Unit/use	Smoking	Eating opium	Eating morphia	Injected morphia
Quantity in grams	235.5 (4 mace)	12	2	1
Cost in cents	$ 1.32	11	14	7

Credit Hong Kong Government Gazette

and proprietary medicines. They were knowledgeable in producing the range of "opium cures" with its raw materials sourced from British, German and US agents in Shanghai. Their advantages were a lower cost base with salaries of local employees much lower than their expatriate counterparts. In addition, Shanghainese chemist and druggist owners could reach out to more provincial distributors. Gu Songquan (1857–1926), a former dispenser with the British Dispensary, opened the first locally owned Great China Dispensary in Shanghai's International Settlements in 1888. His move motivated other local dispensers of Chinese medicine dispensaries and western chemists to follow suit. As a result, they developed a thriving wholesale and manufacturing chemist business with leading brands of OTC products in the 1910s to 1940s period. A survey of the 1947 Shanghai Telephone Directory showed over 300 western pharmacies and a thousand drug stores had taken root in Shanghai—China's most cosmopolitan city.[2] Frank Dikotter et al. described the use of heroin replacing morphine:

> As an alternative to opium, heroin pills and powders only appeared on the market after the fall of the empire (in 1911). Although the main ingredient was heroin, those narcotic substances could include caffeine, quinine, and occasionally also cocaine to suit the predilections of different consumer groups.[3]

The same retail and manufacturing chemists in Hong Kong and Shanghai also produced and marketed their brands of proprietary medicines from the 1870s. For example, the use of hypodermic syringes in administering morphine subcutaneously to achieve euphoric effects for chronic users in the 1890s to the availability of Neo-Sypharsan in treating syphilis by intravenous injection gave rise to China's first sterile pharmaceutical manufacturers of Hypoule and Sine in Shanghai in the 1920s. By 1930, some of the original players, e.g., Koeffer Dispensary and new players such as New Asiatic and Sine, had moved into ethical pharmaceuticals giving rise to the modern pharmaceutical industry. In addition, Chinese chemists and pharmaceutical scientists gained experience and knowledge to extract high quality Chaulmoogra oil and ephedrine for domestic and export use in treating leprosy and paediatric asthma. "Opium cures", due to their high profitability as narcotic drugs, were the key driving force behind the entrenchment of western chemists in developing a modern supply chain from retail to wholesale and manufacturing all under one roof.

Apothecaries in the Anglophone world evolved in the mid-nineteenth century with the development of two professions: general practitioners, and chemists and druggists in the UK and colonies of the British empire, including India, Hong Kong, the Strait Colonies, and the treaty ports of China. Entrepreneurs associated with western chemists in the Shanghai International Settlements took the opportunity to import and sell "*opium cures*" in the late 1890s and then mass-produced the more lucrative "opium cures" and proprietary medicines in the 1900s. Chang Ning, a historian with expertise in the Shanghai retail drug market of the Republican era describes the rise of western pharmacy in modern China:

> We have observed the Chinese-owned chemists in Shanghai have continuously replicated what the western chemists have conducted in their retail pharmacy business since the late nineteenth century. Initially, they produced generic "opium cures", and other proprietary

medicines according to the same formulas (published in the British or the United States Pharmacopoeias). By then, the New Medicine industry in Shanghai and the major treaty ports had reached the stage as an established enterprise, and their members had also become assertive to fight back ....[4].

Education Reform and Bench Strength of Local Talents

The concept of "total westernization" was first mooted by Liang Qichao (梁启超, Liang Chichao, 1873–1929), a Confucian scholar turned liberal reformist, in the failed 1898 "Hundred Day Reform" (百日维新) movement led by his teacher, Kang Youwei (康有为, 1858–1927). One of the pressing items on the reform agenda was "education was for all and not for a privileged few". Liang's dream finally came true. After one thousand three hundred years, the new public education system consisting of primary, secondary, and tertiary levels was launched in 1905. The Manchu Qing imperial court held the last nationwide Keju examination in Kaifeng, Henan province in 1904, since installed in 605.

The Japanese model of a 7 + 4 primary and secondary school system was adopted by the Manchu Qing court in 1905 and was changed to a US model of 6 + 3 + 3 in 1922 by the Beiyang government as a direct result of the May 4 movement. After Chiang Kai-shek unified the young Republic in the successful Northern Expedition in 1928, the newly reorganized Ministry of Education further specified 4–6 years for university education; medicine and law at 5 years, normal universities or teaching training colleges at 4 years, and vocational schools with a minimum of 3 years. A university could have a minimum of three and up to eight academic colleges, including arts, science, law, education, agriculture, engineering, commerce, and medicine. For universities having only three academic colleges, they must include three of the four faculties of science, agriculture, engineering, and medicine. Pharmacy was not among the eight academic colleges but could be a department affiliated with a medical or science college in a university.

Since the mid-nineteenth century in Britain, retail chemists trained their dispensers in-house. As working hours were long, a few of those determined dispensers spent an average of five years as apprentices and, at the same time, attended part-time evening classes at one of the schools of pharmacy. When they passed the minor examination and qualified as a chemist and druggist, they registered as a member of the PSGB. Students who could afford a two-year full-time study at the PSGB-run School of Pharmacy became pharmaceutical chemists after passing the major examination. Those chemists who passed the minor examination could also upgrade their knowledge by attending a conversion course. Finally, after passing the major examination, they could register as a pharmaceutical chemist (PhC), a higher qualification deemed more prestigious.[5]

At the end of the nineteenth century, the British and American pharmaceutical education systems introduced more researched based subjects in their curriculum: pharmacology, microbiology, biochemistry, and pharmaceutics subjects. The purpose was to prepare pharmacy undergraduate students who had good degrees to pursue research and become scientists instead of being dispensing chemists in the retail market. In addition, pharmacy graduates could pursue their professional careers in the rapidly evolving sectors of the pharmaceutical industry, hospital pharmacy, and the academic world. This change in the curriculum of the pharmacy undergraduate course was a significant milestone for pharmacy in becoming a true profession independent from medicine. China's modern pharmacy education was half a century behind Europe or the US and thirty years behind that of Japan in the nineteenth century.

The Army Medical College in Canton provided the first modern pharmacy course in 1904 with Tomo Inokomori (猪森朋), a Japanese pharmacist, as the head of the pharmacy department, which became a public medical college in 1914 and eventually became the Sun Yat-sen University Medical College in 1926. In 1907.the renamed National Army Medical College in Tianjin also started to provide a pharmacy diploma course. The pharmacy curriculum followed the Imperial University of Tokyo, with an emphasis in pharmacognosy, studies of materia medica, and industrial pharmacy. They accepted high school graduates for a 3-year pharmacy course. Other pharmacy schools, except those missionary universities in Chengdu and Jinan, which opened before 1929, also followed the Japanese pharmaceutical education curriculum. Consequently, Japanese influence played a significant role in China's early adoption of western pharmacy and pharmaceutical practices, leaving a lasting impact on the field.

In July 1929, the Ministry of Education of the Nationalist government promulgated the "University Organization Law". A month later, the "University Regulations" were announced, with universities classified into state and privately funded academic institutions which could set up their own research institutes. The state-funded national, provincial, and municipal universities received funding from the respective levels of the governments. Private universities were mainly former Christian missionary universities such as the Shantung Christian University in Jinan, Southwest University in Chengdu, and St. John University in Shanghai. Moreover, the Nationalist central and provincial governments also commenced building public hospitals alongside the missionary hospitals, generating a demand for qualified pharmacists to work in both the public and private sectors. From 1929, the PUMC Hospital, in collaboration with the North China Pharmaceutical Association, in Beiping, offered a one-year dispensing evening class which later expanded to a 2-year evening dispensing class to train hospital pharmacy technicians. Other municipalities and major cities, such as Canton, Hangzhou, Shanghai, Shengyang (Mukden), and Suzhou, followed suit.

The five pharmacy schools of AMC, NCP, SMC, WCUU and Shenyang Medical College were better financed and staffed with qualified pharmacy academics. The Manchuria Medical University, founded by the South Manchuria Railway in 1911 as the Manchuria Medical College, started a pharmacy diploma programme which was approved as the 23rd school of pharmacy by the Ministry of Education of Japan in August 1937. Other schools of pharmacy were much thinner in their faculty members with many part-timers and the course contents were closer to the training of vocational pharmacy dispensers. Nevertheless, a handful to a dozen pharmacy students graduated from each school, and a couple hundred graduated as pharmacy technicians every year. With the increasing bench strength of pharmacy, graduates increased in the first three decades of the twentieth century. Some worked in hospitals, the enterprising ones joined the pharmaceutical industry or retail pharmacy and those academic ones stayed behind as lecturers or researchers with the five major pharmacy schools.

The bench strength for experienced and knowledgeable pharmacists and scientists also increased as those academics who received scholarships to study higher degrees abroad returned in the 1920s to the 1940s. The latter continued research in multiple disciplines at local universities and institutes and collaborated with overseas scholars and scientists. By 1949, the pharmacy profession had experienced notable growth, with over 3000 pharmacy graduates actively employed across various sectors. The majority of these graduates found employment in hospital and industrial pharmacy, while a significant number served in army medical supplies units. In contrast, the number of pharmacists working in western retail chemists, which mandated registration under the Pharmacist Registration Regulations, was less than 500. Additionally, nearly 1000 pharmacy technicians were employed in these chemists.

In summary, local talents and the returnees became another driving force to upgrade modern China's pharmaceutical research and manufacturing capability. With a period of two to three decades, local retail chemists and druggists in Shanghai evolved from a "cottage industry" making batch-size "opium cures" to that of an industrial pharmaceutical system for Chinese materia medica and western drugs. In the first three decades of the foundation of the People's Republic, most Western and Japanese educated health care policy makers continued to contribute and further developed the urban healthcare infrastructure in Mao Zedong's socialist state. One of the key drivers in the improvements of public health has been the investment in the human resources of healthcare professionals in China.

New Chinese Identity to Serve the Masses or a Privileged Few

After the 4 May Movement in 1919, many people were perplexed by the extreme views of the New Culture Movement. As a symbol for fostering a new Chinese identity, Dr. Sun Yat-sen officially advocated a new attire, the Zhongshan Suit, to replace the traditional robes and western suits for men in 1923. It was neither eastern nor western but a fusion of both (Table 9.1).[6],[7] However, the modernization of traditional medical practice in China faced significant challenges during its transition, as it involved multiple stakeholders such as politicians, Western-educated medical and pharmaceutical professionals, Chinese medicine practitioners, Chinese dispensaries owners and wholesalers, not to mention the medicinal herb growers. It became a highly controversial subject when changes to the 2000 years old Chinese medicine practice were imminent. To begin with, when the young Republic was transitioning from feudalism to modernity, nationalism was one of the key considerations, and controversy over the teaching medium soon arose when the UMC transited into the PUMC in 1915. The majority of the faculty of the PUMC had always in favour for Chinese to be the teaching medium for medicine.[8]

The Rockefeller Foundation had always supported an elitist approach to being a leader in medical education as a role model in modern China. Accordingly, the CMB insisted that English would be the sole teaching medium for the new PUMC and Hospital. However, school children living in the provinces would require a further three years to learn English, except for a few who had participated in missionary schools in the larger treaty ports. For example, the Chinese MoE's assessment of the PUMC in the mid-1930s urged that enrollment at the PUMC should be increased and that more classroom instruction should be in Chinese. Other recommendations soon followed: increase the courses in public health, parasitology, and bacteriology; teach Chinese medical terminology; and publish papers in both Chinese and English so that they would reach a larger audience except a few PUMC alumni. Suzanne Pepper summarizes the U-turn taken by CMB:

> The Rockefeller Foundation's response was especially interesting. In deference to the widespread demands in China for nationalistic forms of education with practical application, the Foundation directed its funding in the mid-1930s away from missionary schools and education aboard. The reports accompanying these decisions reflected the increasingly critical consensus that had hardened around these issues.
>
> The judgement on the Peking Union Medical College Hospital was equally harsh, which had received the bulk of Rockefeller's investment in China since 1913 (US $ 33 million out of a total of $37 million). Despite the high standards of modern medicine, it had introduced into China, a Foundation report concluded, the achievements were not commensurate with the investment. This was because its "stereotyped medical education" was not meeting China's medical and public health needs. The most scathing criticism, however, was reserved for education abroad and the returned students. As tickets to academic positions in China, degrees from foreign universities appeared to be the students' dominant ambition.[9]

When Chiang Kai-shek's Nationalist government re-established its governance in Nanjing in late 1928, the priorities of the MoE, and MoH were to build schools and universities and to provide health to the public. Commencing in 1929, public universities and provincial hospitals were built across the country to serve the masses and the role of missionary hospitals and universities have become diminished quickly. Although China's journey to modernity in the first half of the twentieth century was interrupted periodically with the War as the deadliest, however, the continuation of higher education during those War years remained as a top priority with Chen Lifu as the Minister of Education to preserve the strength for recovery after the War years.

One Country, Two Pharmacy Systems

Chinese people have relied on its indigenous materia medica for health needs through peaceful times and wars, pandemics, and natural disasters since time immemorial. In 1929, public health policymakers led by Dr. Heng J. Liu at the MoH intended to abandon Chinese medicine in the mainstream medical and health system. However, the historic First National Health Conference led by Dr. Heng J. Liu symbolizing the modernity of Chinese medicine began on 26 February 1929. In a swift and decisive response to Dr. Heng J. Liu's proposed elimination of the time-honored medical tradition, Ye Kaitai (叶开泰), a highly esteemed Chinese medicine practitioner hailing from Wuhan, took proactive measures. On March 17, 1929, he convened the National Congress of Chinese Medicine Alliance in Shanghai, where numerous Chinese medicine practitioners gathered. With a unanimous voice, they vehemently voiced their opposition to the encroachment of Western medical practitioners into the realm of Chinese medicine.

Chiang Kai-shek, and Chen Guofu and Lifu brothers were the only exceptions swimming against the tide as almost all Nationalist politicians and intellectuals. Led by Chiang's political opponent, Wang Jingwai, the Nationalists deemed Chinese medicine practitioners ignorant about enlightenment and modernity. As a compromise, the Central Committee of the Nationalist Party finally held its 26th political meeting on May 7, 1930, accepted the Chen brothers' recommendations, and formally established the legal status of Chinese medicine in deeds.

The publication of the first edition of The Chinese Pharmacopoeia (CP) in 1930 marked a significant milestone, indicating the future trajectory of China's modern healthcare system. Dr. Heng J. Liu and his appointed members of the editorial board of the CP decided only 60 Chinese materia medica out of 2608 listed in the Compendium of Materia Medica and its Supplement Edition, reflecting an astonishing decline of 98%. This drastic shift was evidently driven by the Western-educated elite, who actively embraced western medicine and pharmacy. The success of primarily European and Japanese medicine and pharmacy in the treaty ports of modern China could be a strategy taken concertedly by the Western powers; initially the Portuguese, Dutch, British, French in the 16th to the early nineteenth centuries and lately by Japan and the U.S. in the first half of the twentieth century to extend their influence beyond military might. Pratik Chakrabarti offered the following view:

> The Expansion of European commercial and cultural dominance led to the pre-eminence of European medical traditions and practices were part of colonial establishments. European (author's insertion "or equally applicable to American") hospitals, drugs such as quinine, vaccines, European medical colleges—which offered people Western medical degrees and recognized only western medicine—became dominant with the spread of colonial influence and power. As Europeans collected specimens in the tropics in the seventeenth century, they often extracted the materials used in the local drugs for their own medicines, but discouraged the adoption of those traditional medicines. They instead introduced and encouraged among the Europeans and the locals the use of their own medicines. Along with that, European (and American) colonial authorities controlled medical universities, degrees and licensing. These often linked to the marginalization of traditional forms of medicine.[10]

Although Chiang Kai-shek and the Chen brothers' interventions safeguarded the heritage of Chinese medicine and materia medica in 1929, Chinese medicine was not viewed as a scientific discipline by the western educated elite during their time on the mainland. As a result, Chinese medicine practitioners were struggling for survival until the newly founded communist state led by Mao Zedong's Chinese Communist Party who began to reverse the decision of *"Western Medicine First"* approach continued by those public health officials who stayed behind on the mainland after the Communist Revolution in 1949. However, the first edition of the Pharmacopoeia of the People's Republic of China was published 5 years after the Communists succeeded the Nationalists, in 1953. The form and structure were in line with the 1930 Pharmacopoeia with mostly western drugs except the number of drug monographs vastly reduced from 708 to 513, apparently due to many imported medicines were not available at the height of the Cold War in the 1950s. Substantial investments in the education and scientific development of Chinese medicine and pharmacy were made with dedicated universities, hospitals, generic drug houses and research institutes built since the mid-1950s.

A major shift occurred in 1963, again when the then Soviet Union fell apart with China which started to pursue an independent path in the research and development of chemical drugs without external help. Mao's dream for China to tap into its rich indigenous source of materia medica by incorporating clinically proven herbal remedies in its national pharmacopoeia came true after sixteen years when the second edition of the Pharmacopoeia of the PRC was published in 1965. The two volumes of Chinese, and modern drugs consisted of a total of 1113 drug monographs were documented with volume 1 consisted of 446 drug monographs of Chinese materia medica and 197 recipes and volume 2 consisted of 667 drug monographs of antibiotics, chemical drugs, vaccines and sera, and other inorganic substances. Consequently, many state-sponsored Chinese materia medica research projects came to fruition with one gained global attention when the active ingredients of Qinghaosu, an anti-malarial herbal drug, were synthesized. Its most active ingredient, artemisinin, was identified by Tu Youyou in 1972. Tu had received training under the guidance of Dr. Lou Zhichen, who himself pursued a Ph.D. in pharmacognosy at the University of London in the late 1940s through a British Boxer Indemnity scholarship. Tom Hayden, former Director of The Centers for Disease Control and Prevention (CDC), wrote of Tu Youyou's discovery of artemisinin:

> Tu Youyou is one of the few people who can say they have saved millions of lives. It is one thing to discover a folk remedy and quite another to find its medically active agent and turn it into a modern drug. The ancient recipe turned out to hold the key. Tu found that the active compound, now known as artemisinin, is destroyed by high heat. After she succeeded in extracting this chemical from the wormwood, her first test subject was herself. In 2015, Tu became the first woman in China to win a Nobel Prize. The World Health Organization has named artemisinin, now mankind's main line of defense against malaria, an essential drug. Although malaria has been eliminated in the U.S., it causes hundreds of thousands of deaths worldwide each year. Tu's discovery is a mainstay in the efforts to save those lives.[11]

Today, two compounds, artemether and artesunate, synthesized from Qinghaosu's research laboratories at the Chinese Academy of Chinese Medical Sciences remain as the active drugs in the Model Essential Drug List of the World Health Organization of 2023.[12] Madam Angela Chen-Lin, the chairperson of LiFu Medical Research, Cultural, and Educational Foundation summarized the integration of modern vaccine technologies and Chinese materia medica formulations in combating COVID-19 infections. She described it as a hybrid approach and a classic case study exemplifying the coexistence of *"One Country, Two Pharmacy Systems."*

With the foresight and wit of the Nationalist leaders, including the Chen Guofu and Lifu brothers, the co-existence of "One Country, Two Pharmacy Systems" of Chinese and western medicine in the Mainland and Taiwan has worked well in the past seventy-four years. It has become a unique fusion of medicine and pharmacy that contributes to the world's health and well-being. As shown in the recent COVID-19 pandemic, both Chinese materia medica formulations and COVID-19 vaccines employing modern technologies have helped tens of millions of Chinese people and those in the Global South recovered from their coronavirus illness without lingering symptoms.[13],[14]

The groundwork laid by ship surgeons, medical missionaries, expatriate chemists, Ningbo entrepreneurs, British and Japanese pharmacy educators, returnee pharmaceutical scientists, and healthcare policymakers have been pivotal since the early nineteenth century. They had collectively driven the dramatic transformation and modernization of China's pharmaceutical industry and the pharmacy profession until the fall of the Nationalist government in 1949. The policy makers who had received Western training remained in Communist China demonstrated adaptability by revising their public health strategies. They redirected their attention towards rural health programmes and embarked on widespread education initiatives for healthcare professionals. A remarkable transformation took place, evident in the significant increase in the number of pharmacists. From a modest figure of 3500 in 1949, the pharmacist workforce has soared to an astonishing 750,200 as of June 2023, representing a staggering 214-fold surge. This substantial pool of skilled professionals stands as one of China's invaluable assets in its pursuit of global leadership in the pharmaceutical and vaccine industries.

Notes and References

1. Lugard, Frederick Dealtry, *Memorandum Regarding the Restriction of Opium in Hong Kong and China,* Legislative Council Meeting, Hong Kong, 11 March 1909: 37–38. Accessed May 5, 2023.
2. Chemists and Druggists Section, Shanghai Telephone Directory and Buyer's Guide, 1947 Issue, Shanghai: Shanghai Telecommunication Administration, Ministry of Transportation, Republic of China, 1947: 31–33. Accessed 29 September 2023. https://books.google.co.uk/books?id=iSYMAQAAIAAJ&printsec=frontcover#v=onepage&q&f=false.
3. Dikkoter, D., Laamann, L., and Zhou, X. (2005). *Narcotic Culture: A History of Drugs in China* (London: C. Hurst & Co., London, 2004), 131.
4. Chang, [Aspirin in China], 151.
5. Both chemists and pharmaceutical chemists (PhC.) could open retail pharmacy shops. Those with a PhC qualification could advance their career in academia, hospital and industry sectors.
6. In Asia, the national dress for male students or adults was designed to foster a sense of national identity from the late nineteenth century to the mid-twentieth century. It is called *Gakuran* in Japan, *Zhongshan Suit* or now Mao *Suit* in modern China, and the *Nehru Jacket* in India. They look similar and yet have subtle differences such as with or without the front pockets or the sleeve buttons.
7. Dr. Sun Yat-sen's other names included *Zhongshan* (Chungshan). The "Zhongshan Suit" was named after him and symbolizes Confucian values with a modern spirit: The four pockets symbolize the four Confucian virtues of *li* (etiquette), *yi* (righteousness), *lian* (integrity*) and chi* (shame).

8. Medicine in China by the China Medical Board of the Rockefeller Foundation, New York, 1914: 83. https://centennial.chinamedicalboard.org.
9. Pepper, Suzanne, "Post-Mao Reforms in Chinese Education: Can the Ghosts of the Past be Laid to Rest", Ed. Epstein, Irving, *Chinese Education, Policies and Prospect* (New York: Garland Publishing, 1991), 1–41, esp. 4–12.
10. Chakarabarti, P., *Medicine and Empire, 1600–1960*, (Basingstoke: Palgrave Macmillian, 2014):182.
11. Hayden, Tom, "The 100 Most Influential People: Tu Youyou—Conqueror of Malady", *Time*, 21 April 2016. Accessed 29 September 2023. https://time.com/collection-post/4298237/tu-youyou-2016-time-100/.
12. Antimalarial medicines for curative treatment, *The selection and use of essential medicines*, Web Annex A, World Health Organization, Model List of Essential Medicines, 23rd list, 2023: 22–23. Accessed 29 September 2023. https://www.who.int/publications/i/item/WHO-MHP-HPS-EML-2023.02.
13. Personal Interview of Madam Angela Chen-Lin 陈林颖曾女士, Chairperson, Lifu Medical Research, Cultural and Educational Foundation 财团法人立夫医药研究文教基金会, Taipei, 12 November 2022.
14. The term "Global South" generally refers to those lower income countries with the majority located in or near the tropics. In 2023, the Global South represents 85% of the world's population and nearly 39% of global GDP. They include Brazil, India, Indonesia and China, which, along with Nigeria and Mexico, are the largest Southern states in terms of land area and population.

Author Index

© The Editor(s) (if applicable) and The Author(s), under exclusive license to Springer Nature Singapore Pte Ltd. 2023
P. Chiu, *A History of Western Pharmacy in China*,
https://doi.org/10.1007/978-981-99-8635-4

Index